Injection Procedures

Todd P. Stitik

Editor

Injection Procedures

Osteoarthritis and Related Conditions

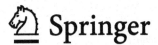 Springer

Editor
Todd P. Stitik
Professor, Physical Medicine and Rehabilitation
Co-Director, Musculoskeletal/Pain Management Fellowship
Director, Occupational/Musculoskeletal Medicine
Co-Director, Interventional Spine Injection Clinic
Department of Physical Medicine and Rehabilitation
New Jersey Medical School
Newark, NJ, USA
todd.stitik@gmail.com

ISBN 978-0-387-76594-5   e-ISBN 978-0-387-76595-2
DOI 10.1007/978-0-387-76595-2
Springer New York Dordrecht Heidelberg London

Library of Congress Control Number: PCN applied for

Springer is part of Springer Science+Business Media (www.springer.com)

I dedicate this book to my wife, Rossana, and children, Jeanette ("Jenna") and Luke, whose patience, understanding, sacrifice, and support were greatly appreciated and necessary for the project to be completed. Without them in my life, this book would not have been written.

Preface

It has been my belief, ever since I was a resident physician and performed my first musculoskeletal injection procedure (a carpal tunnel injection for a patient whom I had diagnosed by EMG testing with carpal tunnel syndrome), that better instructional material was needed for musculoskeletal medicine injection procedures. I recall in preparing for that injection that I had to refer to several different sources of information. Despite this, not one source adequately explained the entire procedure in a practical step-by-step fashion that also included helpful clinical pearls and pitfalls, and none of the sources provided me with a template that I could use to document the procedure in the medical record. The patient's gratitude when the injection subsequently greatly relieved his symptoms helped to convince me that I wanted to develop a musculoskeletal medicine practice with an emphasis on office-based injection procedures.

After struggling to learn and perform several other injection procedures while I was still a resident, I began to wonder why office-based musculoskeletal medicine injection procedures in general were not being performed at that time using some form of image guidance. It was my belief that image guidance could help with injection accuracy and that this would likely translate into better clinical results and help to minimize patient's discomfort and side effects. It is hard to prove with certainty for most procedures that the increased accuracy associated with image guidance compared to blind injection procedures results in better outcomes. However it is tough to deny that an image-guided injection procedure, that does *not* result in pain relief, more convincingly excludes the structure as a pain generator compared to lack of a beneficial response after a nonimage-guided injection.

When I began to teach musculoskeletal medicine, I quickly learned to enjoy the inevitable look of interest on the faces of the students, residents, and fellows when they witnessed a particular injection procedure for the first time. This interest is then usually replaced with a look of satisfaction and sometimes exhilaration when they eventually successfully perform a procedure themselves.

I also found that good and sometimes detailed procedural documentation is very important with respect to patient care (particularly for repeat procedures since a procedure note that documents any nuances encountered during a procedure will usually help guide future procedures on the same patient) and reimbursement and can be helpful in situations of alleged malpractice. However, any busy clinician can relate to the dilemma that is often posed by the desire to adequately document a procedure and the reality of significant time limitations.

Through these experiences with learning, performing, and then teaching musculoskeletal medicine injection procedures, I decided to someday attempt to write a comprehensive injection textbook with an emphasis on image guidance. When I finally and firmly committed to undertaking this project, it was clear to me that the field of musculoskeletal medicine was rapidly moving in the direction of image guidance as a tool for improving injection procedures. During the subsequent years during which this book has been written, the trend of image guidance has accelerated even more, particularly with the advent of musculoskeletal ultrasound into mainstream medicine in the USA. This trend further convinced me of the need for a text that emphasized image guidance.

In summary, this musculoskeletal medicine injection text has several purposes: to discuss as many of the different procedures as possible, reference the literature, instruct the physician in a step-by-step manner on how to perform the injection using images (not just drawings) from procedures performed on actual or simulated patients wherever possible, teach useful clinical pearls and warn of pitfalls, and provide ready-made documentation templates that could be adapted to a given clinical practice for the medical record. It was therefore my overall goal that this book would be much more than just an instructional manual on how to perform an injection. I hope that this has been achieved.

Newark, NJ   Todd P. Stitik

Acknowledgments

The following pharmaceuticals are often cited in the Procedure Instructions and the Injection Procedure Templates in Chaps. 6–12. As a space-saving device, the manufacturer, city, state/province, country are noted herewith instead of in the Instructions and Templates:

Betadine® (Purdue-Pharma LP, Stamford, CT, USA)
Depo-Medrol® (Pfizer, New York, NY, USA)
MyoJect™ (VIASYS Healthcare, San Diego, CA, USA)
Omnipaque™ (GE Healthcare, Waukesha, WI, USA)

Contents

Contributors

Eric L. Altschuler
Department of Physical Medicine and Rehabilitation, New Jersey Medical School, Newark, NJ, USA

Naimish Baxi
New Jersey Medical School, Newark, NJ, USA

Jose Santiago Campos
Department of Physical Medicine and Rehabilitation, New Jersey Medical School, Newark, NJ, USA

Christopher Castro
Northeastern Rehabilitation Associates, Bethlehem, PA, USA

Mohammad Hossein Dorri
Department of Physical Medicine and Rehabilitation,
New York College of Medicine, New York, NY, USA

Jeffrey J. Fossati
Department of Physical Medicine and Rehabilitation, New Jersey Medical School, Hackensack, NJ, USA

Patrick M. Foye
Department of Medicine and Rehabilitation, New Jersey Medical School, Newark, NJ, USA

Gregory Gazzillo
Department of Physical Medicine and Rehabilitation, Mayo Clinic, Rochester, MN, USA

Ladislav Habina, Jr.
Department of Pain and Rehabilitation Center, Seton Hall University, South Orange, NJ, USA

Jose Ibarbia
Department of Rehabilitation Medicine, New York – Presbyterian Hospital, Columbia University Medical Center and Weill Cornell Medical Center, New York, NY, USA

Debra S. Ibrahim
New Jersey Medical School, Newark, NJ, USA

Jong H. Kim
Department of Physical Medicine and Rehabilitation, New Jersey Medical
School, Newark, NJ, USA

Ajay Kumar
Physiatrist and Interventional Pain Specialist, Private Practice, East Stroundsburg,
PA, USA

Charles Lee
New York College of Podiatric Medicine, New York, NY, USA

Michael J. Mehnert
Department of Physical Medicine and Rehabilitation, Rothman Institute,
Thomas Jefferson Medical School, Philadelphia, PA, USA

Gregory J. Mulford
Department of Rehabilitation Medicine, Atlantic Health – Morristown Memorial
Hospital, Morristown, NJ, USA

Charles Sara
Department of Physical Medicine and Rehabilitation, Northern NJ Pain & Rehab,
Newark, Hackensack, USA

Lisa Schoenherr
Department of Physical Medicine and Rehabilitation, New Jersey Medical
School, Newark, NJ, USA

Todd P. Stitik
Department of Physical Medicine and Rehabilitation, New Jersey Medical
School, Newark, NJ, USA

Jiaxin J. Tran
New Jersey Medical School, Newark, NJ, USA

David J. Van Why
Department of Rehabilitation Medicine, Thomas Jefferson University Hospital,
Philadelphia, PA, USA

Brian F. White
Department of Surgery, Division of Physiatry, Bassett Medical Center,
Cooperstown, NY, USA

Peter P. Yonclas
Department of Physical Medicine and Rehabilitation, New Jersey Medical School,
Newark, NJ, USA

Part I
Introduction to Injection Procedures and Related Topics

Chapter 1
Basic Principles of Joint and Soft Tissue Injection Procedures

Todd P. Stitik, Jong H. Kim, and Gregory Gazzillo

Introduction

Joint and soft tissue injection procedures are commonly performed as part of a musculoskeletal medicine practice [1]. These procedures are very valuable diagnostic and therapeutic patient management tools. This chapter, along with Chap. 2, will review the basic principles behind these injection procedures and serve as the general framework from which these procedures are taught throughout this book.

The area of office-based musculoskeletal injection procedures is an evolving one. With the recognition that alarmingly poor accuracy has been documented with nonimage-guided injection procedures, particularly into the knee, shoulder regions, and hip regions [2–7], the use of image guidance for these procedures is becoming more commonplace. More recently, musculoskeletal ultrasound is now being used to help guide certain injection procedures. While indications for the use of musculoskeletal ultrasound as guidance for injection procedures are still being developed, this mode of image guidance provides an obvious advantage for some procedures. For other injection procedures, fluoroscopic guidance is more advantageous. Within the individual injection chapters, recommendations are made regarding the need for image guidance for a particular procedure.

The authors do not have a lot of experience with ultrasound guidance compared to fluoroscopic guidance for injection procedures due to the availability of fluoroscopy compared to ultrasound in their musculoskeletal practice at the time of this writing. At the time of this writing, the authors' practice is in the process of obtaining an ultrasound unit, and the authors expect their use of ultrasound guidance for many procedures to increase significantly; it may even replace fluoroscopic guidance as the image-guidance modality of choice for some of the injections.

T.P. Stitik (✉)
Department of Physical Medicine and Rehabilitation, New Jersey Medical School,
Newark, NJ, USA
e-mail: todd.stitik@gmail.com

T.P. Stitik (ed.), *Injection Procedures: Osteoarthritis and Related Conditions*,
DOI 10.1007/978-0-387-76595-2_1, © Springer Science+Business Media, LLC 2011

Indications

Indications for joint and soft tissue injection procedures can be grouped into diagnostic and therapeutic categories. While some injection and/or aspiration procedures are performed for purely diagnostic purposes, others are performed exclusively with therapeutic intent. Finally, some injection procedures serve the dual purpose of diagnosis and treatment.

Diagnostic Uses

The injection of a local anesthetic can be particularly helpful in determining if a given structure is a "pain generator." For example, despite a comprehensive patient history, review of imaging studies, and physical examination, it can be difficult to determine whether or not pain is emanating from the subacromial region within the shoulder and/or whether there is true rotator cuff weakness or simply pain-limited weakness. A properly placed subacromial lidocaine injection as part of an impingement test can help to readily determine if the subacromial region is a pain generator and can help to make the distinction between true weakness (such as can occur due to a rotator cuff tear) and pain-limited weakness. When utilizing a diagnostic local anesthetic injection, it is important to perform a targeted physical examination in order to identify specific maneuvers that reliably provoke the symptoms that the patient has been complaining of. These "provocative maneuvers" should then be repeated shortly after the injection in order to allow the physician and the patient to compare the signs and symptoms, respectively, before and after the injection. Use of a visual tool such as a simple visual analog scale (VAS) can help both patient and physician to distinguish the level of preprocedure and postprocedure pain (Fig. 1.1). When utilizing this tool, it is very important that the scale be explained in sufficient detail to the patient until the physician or other ancillary medical personnel is convinced that the patient understands how to use this. Many patients find the concept of a graphical representation of pain intensity difficult to grasp. In fact, if the patient is simply handed a diagram and asked to complete this on his/her own without sufficient explanation, it is quite likely that the wrong conclusion will be reached. If, despite detailed explanation, the patient simply does not appear to understand how to indicate pain level utilizing the VAS, it should be abandoned and the patient should simply be asked to report how much their pain level changed after the injection, and a decision regarding injection efficacy should be made based upon this verbal reporting.

If the patient appears to understand the concept, he or she should mark the VAS prior to diagnostic injection to indicate the amount of preinjection pain and then mark it again after the procedure to indicate the amount of postinjection pain. The physician then compares the two values, determines if this difference also correlates with what the patient is verbally reporting, and decides if this represents enough of a change, in order to conclude that the structure is a probable pain generator. While there are no validated absolute values for making this determination, certain general guidelines appear to be reasonable. For example, a greater than 50% improvement

Patient: _____ **Date:** ___ /___ /06

Provocative pain maneuver(s): _____

Diagnostic Injection Procedure: ☐-Right ☐-Left ☐-Bilateral_____

Patient instructions: Draw a vertical line through the scale to indicate the level of pain you are having now.

Example: This shows a patient with a _high_ amount of pain.

No Pain   *Unbearable Pain*

_____|_____

Example: This shows a patient with a _moderate_ amount of pain.

No Pain   *Unbearable Pain*

_____|_____

Example: This shows a patient with a _low_ amount of pain.

No Pain   *Unbearable Pain*

_____|_____

Pre-procedure pain: What is your pain RIGHT NOW? (Measure after the most painful provocative maneuver as follows:_____

No Pain   Unbearable Pain

_____

VAS mm: _____

Post-procedure pain: What is your pain RIGHT NOW? (Measure after repeating the most painful provocative maneuver listed above)

No Pain   Unbearable Pain

_____

VAS mm: _____

Change in VAS pain: [pre-procedure pain] – [post-procedure pain]= _____ mm

Fig. 1.1 Diagnostic pre- vs. post-procedure VAS pain

in the overall level of pain probably indicates that the structure is the major pain generator (i.e., causing at least half the amount of pain). Because the local anesthetic is being injected into a target structure and oftentimes inadvertently also into the overlying tissue, it is preferable that the provocative maneuver does not involve simple palpation of the structure. The fact that both the target structure and the overlying tissue have been injected with local anesthetic can make tissue palpation an unreliable indicator because discomfort associated with simple palpation may decrease simply as a result of the anesthetic deposited into the overlying tissue. For example, palpatory pain in the region of the antero-medial aspect of the proximal tibia/knee may occur secondary to either pes anserine bursitis or regional discomfort associated with knee osteoarthritis. The deposition of local anesthetic into this general region of palpatory tenderness would likely render subsequent palpation less painful. This still might not effectively determine whether or not the patient truly has pes anserine bursitis as a major pain generator. Rather than relying upon palpatory pain as the provocative maneuver, a more reliable maneuver would probably be pain with resisted knee flexion, as the pes anserine bursa presumably is compressed by the semitendinosus, sartorius, and gracilis tendons during resisted knee flexion. Subsequent pain relief during resisted knee flexion after a local anesthetic injection should prove to be more specific for pes anserine bursitis than for knee osteoarthritis. In this case, comparing pain associated with resisted knee flexion both before and after local anesthetic injection should be a more reliable provocative maneuver than simple palpation of tissue before and after local anesthetic injection. In a similar fashion, the physician should try to identify analogous pain provocative maneuvers for other diagnostic injection procedures. One would anticipate that pain relief should occur for a time period that is consistent with the duration of action of the local anesthetic (generally 1–4 h for usual doses of 1–2% lidocaine) and that duration is slightly prolonged when larger doses are used [8]. However, pain relief after diagnostic local anesthetic injections sometimes can occur for surprisingly long time periods as is discussed in greater detail in Chap. 2.

Bursal/Synovial Fluid Analysis

Aspiration of bursal or synovial fluid from a bursa or joint can yield important diagnostic information. Synovial fluid can in fact be classified into four groups based upon characteristics such as viscosity, appearance, white blood cell count (WBCC), and percentage of polymorphonucleocytes (% PMN) within the differential (Table 1.1). Although a specific classification system has not been developed for bursal fluid, the parameters used to classify synovial fluid have been used for bursal fluid as well [9].

In addition to actual laboratory analysis of bursal or synovial fluid, simple visual inspection can also provide rapid important diagnostic information. For example,

Table 1.1 Classification of synovial fluid

Synovial fluid type	Synovial fluid test parameter		
	Appearance	White blood cell count/mm^3	Percentage of polymorphonucleocytes
Normal	Clear	200	<25
Noninflammatory	Clear → Yellow	200–2 K	<25
Inflammatory	Yellow → Cloudy	2–50 K	>50
Septic	Purulent	>50 K	>80

Data from Holder L. Septic Arthritis. In EMedicine. Accessed 6/22/08

aspiration of a patient's knee after a traumatic injury can help with the diagnosis of osteochondral fracture or anterior cruciate ligament rupture, as these injuries are typically associated with grossly bloody effusions. In contrast, imaging modalities (including MRIs) used in clinical medicine are not capable of reliably distinguishing between bloody and nonbloody effusions. Inflammatory conditions are frequently associated with somewhat cloudy fluid whereas a septic structure usually yields a purulent-looking fluid. This immediate feedback gained from visual inspection of synovial fluid can be very helpful in guiding management while awaiting laboratory fluid analysis and/or imaging results.

Therapeutic Uses

Joint and soft tissue injection procedures – including bursal, tendon sheath, tendon insertion site, and intramuscular injections – have significant potential benefits. These benefits include those associated with fluid aspiration, corticosteroid administration, local anesthetic administration, viscosupplementation of osteoarthritic synovial joints, knee lavage, part of distention arthrography for shoulder adhesive capsulitis, and, more recently, autologous blood injections.

Simple fluid aspiration from a distended joint or bursa can provide prompt and significant pain relief. A typical example is a patient who presents with a large knee effusion and reports an impressive amount of pain relief immediately after aspiration of the knee. This degree of pain relief in fact can result in an immediate and very noticeable improvement in the patient's ability to extend the knee compared to the semi-flexed posture that the knee was held in prior to the aspiration, since the volume of a joint is maximal and therefore intra-articular pressure is least when it is in a position of relative flexion [10]. In addition, a very dramatic improvement in gait from an antalgic pattern to a nonantalgic pattern is often quite noticeable to the patient, physician, and any patients in the waiting room, who watched the patient hobble into the exam room and then walk out painfree!

Corticosteroid injections will be discussed in more detail in the Chap. 2. Briefly, however: Injectable corticosteroids have a long record of use particularly in conditions involving inflammation. Although there are varying degrees of evidence-based proof of efficacy for various conditions, it is generally felt that corticosteroid injections do offer some potential benefit.

In addition to their use in identifying pain generators as part of diagnostic injection procedures, local anesthetics are also of potential benefit when used as part of therapeutic injections [11]. In this setting, they are most typically combined with corticosteroids. Local anesthetics will also be discussed in more detail in Chap. 2.

Viscosupplementation is currently only FDA-approved within the United States for pain associated with knee osteoarthritis. In many countries outside of the United States, it is approved for use in any painful osteoarthritic joint. The efficacy of viscosupplements in providing pain relief in osteoarthritis patients has been reported in multiple controlled clinical trials and summarized in several meta-analyses [12–15].

Although conclusions from meta-analyses and individual clinical trials vary somewhat, the majority of the evidence, including that from the most comprehensive meta-analysis to date, is that it is both an effective and extremely safe intervention [12].

Contraindications

There are several contraindications for joint and soft tissue injection procedures in general. In addition, there are some specific contraindications for particular procedures. Injection procedures are generally contraindicated in patients with significant anticoagulation (i.e., a level of anticoagulation beyond the therapeutic range), bacteremia, cellulitis of the overlying skin and soft tissue, severe lymphedema of the target limb, and overlying skin lesions such as psoriatic skin plaques that can be extremely difficult to aseptically cleanse during preinjection skin preparation. Other contraindications pertain to the medications that are administered as part of the procedure. For example, a true allergy to a local anesthetic within the amide family of local anesthetics would contraindicate the use of lidocaine or any other amide local anesthetic. Although corticosteroid allergies are rare, they have been reported, and a true corticosteroid allergy would contraindicate injection of a corticosteroid [16]. While latex allergies do not contraindicate a given injection procedure, they do significantly affect the choice of materials used for the procedure beyond that of simply using latex-free gloves. Latex is also found within the rubber seal of the top of multiuse bottles. In circumstances of latex allergy, use of single-dose glass ampules is strongly preferred. In addition, the contrast agent Omnipaque™ (GE Healthcare, Waukesha, WI, USA) is typically stored in a bottle with a rubber stopper that is also latex containing. Nonlatex-containing Omnipaque™ bottles should instead be used in latex-allergic patients undergoing fluoroscopic-guided injection procedures.

Patients with avascular necrosis and those with joint arthroplasty are at an increased risk of infection from injection procedures [17]. It should also be noted that patients with joint replacements and synovitis at the site of previous joint replacement may have an infection at this site as the cause of the synovitis [18]. This is an important concept, because corticosteroid injections are often used as a treatment for noninfected synovitis. Synovitis after joint replacement can occur because residual synovial tissue is usually present even after the arthroplasty. Patients who are immunocompromised are also at obvious increased risk of infection [19]. Other relative contraindications to corticosteroid injections include an osteochondral fracture and severe osteoporosis in adjacent bone.

Step-by-Step Process

Office-based injection procedures can be conducted according to a step-by-step sequential process that is common to most, if not all, of these procedures. This step-by-step process is shown in Table 1.2 and will generally be used to describe the individual injection procedures discussed throughout this text.

Table 1.2 Step-by step process for office-based joint and soft tissue injection procedures

Step no.	Event
1	Informed consent
2	Patient positioning
3	Injection site marking and cleansing
4	Material preparation
5	Local anesthetic administration (optional)
6	Postprocedural care discussion
7	Aspiration (if applicable)
8	Injection
9	Immediate postprocedure phase and follow-up visit

Table 1.3 General informed consent topics relevant to most office-based injection procedures

General category	Details
Allergic reaction	Betadine® (Purdue-Pharma LP, Stamford, CT, USA) or other skin disinfectant
	Corticosteroid
	Latex
	Local anesthetic
	Omnipaque™ (GE Healthcare, Waukesha, WI, USA) or other contrast agent
	Viscosupplements
Hemarthrosis or Hemorrhagic bursitis	If patient is on anticoagulants or antiplatelet medication
Infection	Especially in diabetic or immunocompromised patients
Lipotrophy (aka lipoatrophy or fat atrophy)	Only pertains to corticosteroid injections
Postinjection pain flare	Usually pertains to corticosteroid injections, but postinjection arthralgias have also been described with viscosupplements
Severe acute inflammatory reaction (aka pseudoseptic reaction)	Hylan GF-20 Synvisc® (Genzyme Corporation, Cambridge, MA, USA)

Step 1: Informed Consent

Obtaining informed consent, either written or verbal, is an important consideration for physicians who perform procedures. Some rules governing the informed consent process are dictated by local hospital policies. For example, some hospitals may require that a particular consent form be used to document the informed consent process. While there are some differences in the actual informed consent process, there are certain informed-consent related issues that are particularly applicable to office-based joint and soft tissue injection procedures (Table 1.3).

The patient should be informed of the possibility of an allergic reaction to any substance that is injected during the procedure. The likelihood of allergic reaction to a local anesthetic is very dependent upon the class of local anesthetic that is used. Specifically, ester-type local anesthetics (e.g., Novocain®, Hospira, Lake Forest, IL, USA) carry a significantly higher likelihood of local anesthetic allergy compared to the amide class of local anesthetics (e.g., lidocaine). This higher likelihood of allergic reaction to the ester class of local anesthetics is a result of hydrolysis of the ester local anesthetic within the serum. This process creates an intermediary product that is much more likely to act as an allergen. Given the general public's familiarity with the term Novocain®, a useful screening question for the possibility of allergy to lidocaine is to ask the patient whether an allergic reaction resulted from administration of "novocaine" as part of a dental procedure. In reality, dentists actually administer lidocaine (rather than Novocain®) for procedures requiring local anesthetics. While the answer "yes" often requires further clarification as to what the "allergic reaction" really was, an answer of "no" is extremely likely to be predictive that the patient is not allergic to local anesthetics. Although an allergy to lidocaine is reportedly extremely rare (<1%), [20] the senior author (TS) did witness lidocaine-related allergic reactions on two occasions. Both occasions involved a lidocaine subacromial injection as part of impingement test. While one patient required treatment in the emergency room due to complaints of dyspnea, the other patient was managed in the office with the use of Benadryl® (McNeil-PCC, Inc., Fort Washington, PA, USA). Allergic reactions to corticosteroids have also been reported, but are extremely rare [16]. While the senior author (TS) has never personally witnessed this reaction despite having performed several thousand corticosteroid injections, there have been occasions during which a patient has reported a history of an allergy to corticosteroids. It was later determined after a referral to the Allergy and Immunology service and subsequent skin testing that a corticosteroid allergy in fact was not present. For both local anesthetics and corticosteroids, it should be kept in mind that multidose bottles of these injectates also contain a preservative. The probability in fact of allergy to the preservative is much more likely than allergy to the local anesthetic or corticosteroid [21, 22]. When fluoroscopic-guidance is used, a contrast agent, such as Omnipaque™, is also often injected. Allergic reactions to contrast dye used for fluoroscopic-guided injection procedures are actually relatively common compared to allergic reactions to local anesthetics and corticosteroid injections [16, 23]. A common screening question for a contrast dye allergic reaction is whether the patient is allergic to iodine. It has been previously taught that an allergy to shellfish is indicative of being allergic to the contrast dye, as both contain iodine. However, since the iodine found in shellfish is organic and is an essential element, individuals cannot have an allergic reaction to it [24]. Individuals with shellfish allergies do not have an allergy to iodine, but rather to other protein allergens, a major one being tropomyosin [25]. The contrast agents typically used nowadays for fluoroscopic-guided injection procedures are actually less likely to cause an IgE-mediated allergic reaction, as these contrast agents are nonionic [26]. The physician can screen for an allergic reaction to viscosupplements derived from rooster combs by asking whether patients are allergic to avian proteins. A useful screening question is whether a patient is allergic to eggs or feathers. A positive response to this question would contraindicate the administration of an avian-derived viscosupplement. Even though the purification process reportedly removes all avian proteins, avian proteins allergy is still considered to be a relative contraindication to viscosupplements. Under these circumstances, a bacterially derived viscosupplement (i.e., Euflexxa®, Ferring Pharmaceuticals, Inc., Saint-Prex, Switzerland) could instead be administered.

Other allergic reactions pertinent to office-based injection procedures include latex allergies and allergies to povidone–iodine skin antiseptics (e.g., Betadine®, Purdue-Pharma LP, Stamford, CT, USA). Positive responses to the screening questions would mandate modification of the procedure in such a manner so as to avoid contact with latex or Betadine®. In the latex-allergic patient, use of plastic gloves and single-dose medications stored in glass ampules (rather than in multiuse bottles with latex-containing rubber stoppers) are preferred. Of note, the bacterially derived viscosupplements (i.e., Euflexxa®) should be avoided in a latex allergic patient, as the rubber stopper on the prefilled syringe contains latex. At the time of this writing, efforts are being undertaken by the manufacturers of Euflexxa® to reformulate the prefilled syringe to exclude latex.

Certain patients should be specifically informed about the possibility of a hemarthrosis due to a joint injection procedure. Patients who are already relatively anticoagulated are at particular risk for this. This is especially true of patients on Coumadin® (Bristol-Myers Squibb, New York, NY, USA) and/or those who have an underlying coagulopathy such as sickle cell anemia, von Willebrand's disease, or other disorders involving the clotting mechanism. Depending upon the procedure, patients on oral antiplatelet agents may need to be informed of the risk of hemarthrosis.

Patients should be informed that infection due to joint and soft tissue injection procedures is always a possibility. Most of the literature regarding the incidence of such infections is derived from knee corticosteroid injections. The incidence of these is actually quite low (1:3,000–1:50,000) [27]. Infection due to these injection procedures, however, can have devastating consequences. For example, diabetic patients in particular have an increased risk of developing infections, especially of the skin [28]. Special precautions are warranted with diabetic patients.

Patients should be informed that they can develop subcutaneous fat atrophy (aka lipotrophy or lipoatrophy) as a result of a corticosteroid injection that has been inadvertently placed into subcutaneous tissues. This can occur in various body regions. The senior author (TS) has witnessed this in the gluteal region of a patient who had received corticosteroid trigger point injections while under the care of a previous practitioner (Fig. 1.2a, b).

Patients may experience a postinjection pain flare due to the corticosteroid. Although this is almost always self-limiting and symptomatically treated with rest, ice, NSAIDs, and/or simple analgesic, patients nonetheless should be advised of this possibility.

Patients can have acute postinjection arthralgias after viscosupplementation due to two possible mechanisms. These two reaction types will be briefly discussed here as they have been extensively reviewed elsewhere [29]. Severe acute inflammatory reactions (aka SAIRs or pseudoseptic reactions) can occur with the cross-liked viscosupplement, Synvisc® (Genzyme Corporation, Cambridge, MA, USA) (hylan GF-20). Clinically, it presents similar to a septic knee; however, cultures are negative. The development of antibodies to chicken proteins and hylan and the general requirement for a prior exposure suggests an immunologic basis for the severe acute

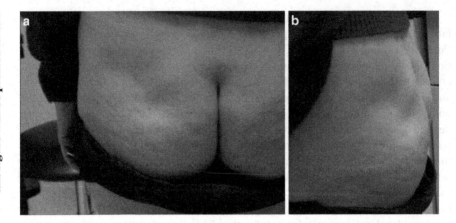

Fig. 1.2 (**a, b**) Patient with subcutaneous fat atrophy (aka lipotrophy or lipoatrophy) as a result of a corticosteroid injection that has been inadvertently placed into subcutaneous tissues

inflammatory reaction [30, 31]. The frequency of pseudoseptic reactions have been estimated in the literature to occur with a range from 1.8 to 27% of treated patients and with higher rates associated with repeat Synvisc® treatment courses [32]. The occurrence of the potential side effect is frequent enough that patient should be specifically consented about the possibility. In contrast, pseudoseptic reactions are not known to occur with noncross-linked viscosupplements such as Hyalgan® (sodium hyaluronate) (Sanofi-Aventis, Bridgewater, NJ, USA). Patients with a known history of pseudogout should probably be informed that an acute exacerbation of this can occur after administration of a viscosupplement [30]. This side effect is generally transient and often managed successfully with NSAIDs.

Step 2: Patient Positioning

There are several principles regarding positioning of patients for injection procedures. Specifically, patients should be positioned in such a manner that they are physically comfortable during the procedure. In addition to patient comfort, physician comfort during the procedure is also quite important, particularly for those procedures in which some difficulty in completion of the procedure is encountered. Since difficulty with a procedure can be an unpredictable event, the physician should assume that he/she may need to be in a particular position for an extended time period and should therefore positions him-/herself in as comfortable a position as possible. Another principle governing patient positioning for procedures involves taking into account the likelihood of a vasovagal reaction due to the procedure. Since it can be difficult to predict which patients are likely to develop a vasovagal reaction during the procedure, they should be positioned whenever possible in a prone or supine position so that they can be put into the Trendelenburg position in a prompt manner. Other factors involved with patient positioning include the desirability of not allowing patients to see the medication preparation step of the procedure, as this often involves the use of large gauge needles used to draw up medications. It is also preferable to not allow the patients to see the procedure itself, particularly at the time of needle insertion. Strategic positioning of the patient relative to an exam room curtain during a procedure can help to block their view. For example, for injection procedures performed into the wrist or hand, positioning the patient seated with the affected limb on a table in an exam room with a curtain pulled cross the upper forearm can be quite helpful. In the senior author's (TS) experience, most patients welcome the fact that the view of the procedure is blocked by the curtain.

Step 3: Injection Site Marking and Cleansing

The site of injection should be marked in such a manner that it can be readily identified by visual inspection after the site has been sterilized. Although different methods are available for marking the injection site, the most commonly used methods include depressing the overlying skin with a plastic needle cap, depressing the overlying skin with a retracted ballpoint pen, or marking the overlying skin with either a pen or a skin marker. After the injection site has been marked, the skin should then be sterilely prepped. Physicians may have their own preference for the type of skin disinfectant to use. Commonly used ones include Betadine® (povidone-iodine 10%), ChloraPrep One-Step® (CareFusion Corporation, San Diego, CA, USA) (2% chlorhexidine and 70% isopropyl alcohol), Techni-Care® (Care-Tech Laboratories, Inc., St. Louis, MO, USA) (parachlorometaxylenol), or some combination of these. Each disinfectant has its own profile of organism-spectrum, rapidity of onset, and potential toxicity (Table 1.4) [33].

The method used in the senior author's (TS) practice for cleansing the skin involves swabbing the skin with Betadine®-soaked gauze pads in a circular direction, starting from the injection site, and moving outward. Three such applications should be sufficient. After this, the Betadine® ideally should be allowed to dry. While the literature contains some differences regarding the general recommendation for drying time, it is likely that a 2-min drying time should sufficiently allow the Betadine® to significantly reduce the skin flora load. In order to help with the drying process, a timing device containing an audible alarm can be kept in the exam room or on an injection cart and set for 2 min and then allowed to count down. As 2 min can seem like an inordinate amount of time in the exam room, this time should be put to efficient use. At this point in time, the physician can move on to the next step: material preparation [33]. Of note, the senior author (TS) is considering changing his cleansing preparation to chlorhexidine/alcohol.

Step 4: Material Preparation

Preparation of materials used for injection procedures can be a rather time-consuming process. However, this can be performed more efficiently by having all necessary materials in the room already, so that time is not wasted by leaving the

Table 1.4 Properties of antiseptic agents

Class (example)	Onset	Antimicrobial activity				Side effects and toxicity
		Gram positive bacteria	Gram negative bacteria	Virus	Fungi	
Iodine/iodophors (Betadine®, Purdue-Pharma LP, Stamford, CT, USA)	Intermediate	Excellent	Good	Good	Good	Skin irritation
Chlorhexidine	Intermediate	Excellent	Good	Good	Fair	Ototoxicity, keratitis
Isopropyl Alcohol	Rapid	Excellent	Excellent	Good	Good	Skin drying, volatile
Parachlorometaxylenol (meta-xylenol 1 3% phospholipid PTC) (Techni-Care®, Care-Tech Laboratories, Inc., St. Louis, MO, USA)	Intermediate	Good	Fair	Fair	Fair	None reported

Data from Larson EL. Guideline for use of topical antimicrobial agents. *Am J Infect Control* 1988; 16:253–266

Table 1.5 Materials for inclusion on an injection cart

Category	Material
Skin preparation	Betadine® (Purdue-Pharma LP, Stamford, CT, USA) bottles or swabs
	Chlorhexidine
	Alcohol prep pads
	Sterile gauze pads
Gloves	Nonsterile
	Sterile
Needles	18 gauge–30 gauge size range
Syringes	1 cm³–20 cm³ size range
Medications	Lidocaine (without epinephrine): 1% and 2%; single-use ampules preferred
	Marcaine® (Hospira, Lake Forest, IL, USA): 0.05%; single-use bottle
	Corticosteroid: single-use bottles preferred
Other	Normal saline
	Clamp (hemostat)
Emergency	EpiPen® (Dey Pharma LP, Napa, CA, USA)
Optional	Vapocoolant spray
	Laboratory materials
	Timing device for skin drying

room in order to gather supplies. The senior author (TS) has found that an injection cart, which can be wheeled into an examination room, can be extremely helpful. Prior to the use of an injection cart, the author's practice attempted to stock each of the individual exam rooms. This, however, invariably led to numerous occurrences of a particular exam room running out of a given supply. In contrast, the injection cart was a much more effective way of stocking the needed materials. Since only this location needs to be restocked, the incidence of not having a particular injection procedure-related supply significantly decreased. A list of materials for inclusion into an injection cart is shown in Table 1.5.

The choice of nonsterile vs. sterile gloves is dependent upon whether or not the needle injection site needs to be palpated again after it has been cleansed. As a general rule, the majority of office-based peripheral injection procedures can be accomplished with the use of nonsterile gloves. The so-called "no-touch technique" essentially involves wearing nonsterile gloves but applying sterile technique at the procedure site. In contrast, spinal injection procedures should be performed with the use of sterile gloves as portions of spinal needle that subsequently enter into the patient sometimes need to be touched by the physician during the procedure.

Choice of needle gauge and length for a given procedure is dependent upon factors including the target structure (e.g., small or large joint), body habitus, the need to aspirate joint or bursal fluid (larger gauge needles preferred), a patient's level of anxiety about a procedure (smaller gauges for "needle phobic" patients), a physician's level of comfort with a given needle, etc. The general guiding principle for needle selection is to use the smallest gauge needle that is capable of successfully performing the procedure. Smaller gauge needles offer many advantages. One obvious advantage is that smaller gauge needles tend to be less painful and cause less tissue damage. If the patient requests to see the needle, it can also be a psychological advantage to display a small gauge needle, particularly if it is attached to a small syringe to a patient prior to an injection procedure. Another, perhaps, less obvious advantage of a small gauge needle is that there is less of a chance that skin will be taken along with the needle after the needle penetrates the skin surface into the target structure. This skin fragment may in fact be a means of causing a joint or soft tissue infection. Therefore, the risk of infection is perhaps less with smaller gauge needles.

In addition to choosing needle gauge and length, the physician has a choice of a straight needle or a spinal-type needle. When image guidance is used for an injection procedure, the physician can take advantage of a spinal needle, as this type of needle is beveled at the end. The beveling will cause the needle to travel in a direction opposite to that of the opening due to a force vector that it encounters as it traverses tissue (Fig. 1.3). The physician can therefore precisely direct the needle in circumstances when this degree of needle control is needed. In contrast, if image guidance is not being used, a straight needle might be more appropriate in order to prevent the needle from inadvertently steering off course. Choice of syringe is also dependent upon several technical factors. One apparent misconception is that a large volume syringe should be chosen in situations where the physician believes that additional "aspirating power" is needed to aspirate out a small effusion. It has been suggested that "if the ratio of the syringe diameter to the needle diameter is too large, a large negative pressure develops quickly without fine control of the degree of vacuum. In this situation, an instantaneously high flow rate is more likely to entrain the debris or a synovial frond, which can be sucked down onto the bevel and block flow."[34].

Whenever possible, single-dose ampules of preservative-free lidocaine as well as single dose Marcaine® (Hospira, Lake Forest, IL, USA) and corticosteroid bottles should be used. If multidose bottles are used, the tops of multidose bottles

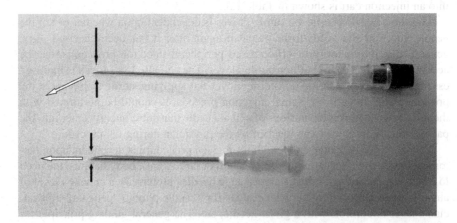

Fig. 1.3 Spinal needles with vector forces acting on them while the needle penetrates tissue. These forces push the needle in a direction away from the opening. In contrast, a typical hypodermic needle is not similarly beveled and will therefore tend to continue along a straight path when entering the tissue

(aka vials) should be cleansed off before drawing up medication from them in order to help ensure sterility. These bottles have a rubber cap that is designed to be penetrated by the needle and then to self-seal. If a multidose bottle is used for local anesthetics and corticosteroids, the local anesthetic should be drawn up first. Ideally, this should be followed by changing the needle, so as to decrease the probability that local anesthetic will subsequently get into the corticosteroid bottle when drawing up the corticosteroid. If instead the corticosteroid is drawn up first, some of the corticosteroid can inadvertently get into the local anesthetic bottle. This will give a partly cloudy appearance. It would then be unclear as to whether or not this cloudiness represented bacterial growth or steroid contamination. When faced with this scenario, it is most prudent to assume bacterial contamination and discard the bottle. Therefore, when using multidose bottles from which solutions are drawn up into one syringe, the local anesthetic should be drawn up first followed by the corticosteroid. This situation can be avoided, of course, by changing the needle between drawing up the local anesthetic and corticosteroid or, best yet, by restricting use to medications contained in single-use glass ampules. Once the injectate is drawn into the syringe, it is probably best to keep the syringe tip covered with the needle rather than removing the needle at that point and exposing the syringe opening to the ambient air. For viscosupplements, prefilled syringes are more efficient than bottles that require viscosupplements be drawn up.

In terms of medication selection, some general corticosteroid dosing guidelines have been developed based upon given joint/bursa sizes. Chapter 2 reviews this information, and each of the individual injection chapters gives recommended dosages. The choice of recommended dosages and the concentrations for concomitant local anesthetics are dependent upon the purpose of the procedure and the size of the structure. For example, a diagnostic injection into a medium- to large-sized joint or bursa might necessitate a relatively large volume of lidocaine in order to coat most, if not all, of the nociceptive structures lining of the target structure. Under these circumstances, 1% lidocaine would be preferred because local anesthetics are relatively more toxic in more concentrated solutions. Therefore, even though a relatively large volume of local anesthetic is being injected, the total amount of local anesthetic is half the amount for 1% lidocaine compared to 2% lidocaine. In contrast, for situations in which a diagnostic injection is being performed into a small target structure, the use of 2% lidocaine is probably an advantage in order to deliver a greater total amount of local anesthetic to a given structure without encountering potential local anesthetic toxicity, as the total dosage of the local anesthetic is still relatively small. Guidelines have been developed for the maximum allowable dose of certain local anesthetics. For example, the maximum dose of lidocaine is 300 mg (4–5 mg/kg) and of Marcaine® it is 175 mg (2.5 mg/kg) [35]. These dosages translate into maximum volumes for a 1% lidocaine solution of 30 mL (0.4–0.5 mL/kg), a 2% lidocaine solution of 15 mL (0.2–0.25 mL/kg), a 0.25% Marcaine® solution of 70 mL (1 mL/kg), and a 0.5% Marcaine® solution of 35 mL (0.5 mL/kg). When a therapeutic injection procedure is being performed, the addition of local anesthetic to the corticosteroid solution does offer some advantages. The immediate pain relief associated with the local anesthetic can offer the patient significant psychological comfort, particularly if the procedure was otherwise poorly tolerated. If rapid pain relief is achieved, the patient may leave the office thinking that, despite the pain from the procedure, "Even though it hurt, it was still well worth it." Of course, the patient will need to be counseled that the effect from the local anesthetic is usually transient so that they are not instead ultimately left with the impression of, "It hurt and the benefit did not even last." The response to the local anesthetic component of the injection can also provide the physician with important immediate feedback from the procedure. For example, pain relief from the injection can help confirm the suspected diagnoses, whereas a lack of response to the local anesthetic could make the physician reconsider the diagnosis. The choice between the lidocaine and a longer acting local anesthetic such as Marcaine® is also dependent upon whether or not the intent of the procedure is for diagnosis or treatment. For example, lidocaine is often used for most diagnostic joint and soft tissue injection procedures, because its relatively quick onset should allow the physician to observe the effects of the injection within a reasonable amount of time. For therapeutic procedures, however, Marcaine® can be used instead of or in addition to the lidocaine. Marcaine® offers the advantage of more prolonged analgesia. This can help to better bridge the gap between pain recurrence when the local anesthetic wears off and pain relief when the corticosteroid begins to take effect. By using both lidocaine and Marcaine®, the advantages of quick onset pain relief from the lidocaine and more prolonged pain relief from the Marcaine® can be realized. Of note however, very serious toxicity can result from either the administration of a dose that exceeds the maximum allowable for Marcaine® or inadvertent intravascular injection of Marcaine®. The physician should take this into consideration when deciding whether or not to use Marcaine®.

Step 5: Local Anesthetic Administration (Optional)

Local anesthetic injections into the overlying skin and soft tissue provide cutaneous and subcutaneous anesthesia for some injection procedures. The advantages of local anesthetic injections include increased patient physical comfort as well as the provision of significant psychological comfort to patients who are undergoing these injection procedures. The administration of local anesthetic is a way of "locating the injection target" by assisting with determination of the desirable needle entrance angle and depth required to reach the target. When the aspiration and/or injection needle is subsequently placed, the physician simply has to follow the path used for the local anesthetic needle that was successful in reaching the target. For some procedures, this can be a major advantage. For example, when performing an intra-articular knee injection, the injection of local anesthetic can significantly help with injection accuracy, particularly for physicians-in-training and those physicians who are less familiar with the procedure. For some non ultrasound-guided procedures, the injection of a local anesthetic into subcutaneous tissue can obscure landmarks used for the injection and therefore be a disadvantage. For example, during a non ultrasound-guided peritendinous injection in patients with deQuer to pray vain's tenosynovitis, the senior author (TS) believes that the injection of local anesthetic somewhat impedes the ability to perform the injection, because the tendons become less apparent on visual inspection.

An unpleasant burning sensation due to local anesthetics can and often does occur as a result of its relatively low pH: acid pH helps to prolong the shelf life. This burning can be minimized by buffering the local anesthetic with sodium bicarbonate. Buffering the local anesthetic also speeds its onset of local anesthesia [6]. Although buffering the anesthetic adds yet another step to the procedure, this extra step can be minimized by making a supply of buffered lidocaine at the beginning of the workday and then discarding it at the end of the day. The senior author (TS) often uses this approach for local skin anesthesia as part of spinal injection procedures. Although multidose bottles of local anesthetic containing a preservative are used for creating the buffered lidocaine supply, it is unclear if the buffering process neutralizes the preservative and therefore renders the solution susceptible to bacterial growth if it is stored beyond the end of the day. Therefore, it is probably wisest to make fresh buffered lidocaine every day. Sodium bicarbonate bottles are fortunately quite economical. Of note, the sodium bicarbonate bottle itself does not contain a preservative. Therefore, the used bottle of bicarbonate should also be discarded at the end of the day. Buffered lidocaine can be made by mixing lidocaine and sodium bicarbonate in a 5:1 ratio. This is often most easily performed by aspirating out at least 10 cm³ of air from a 50 cm³ multidose lidocaine bottle and then injecting 10 cm³ of sodium bicarbonate into the bottle. Aspiration of air is necessary in order to provide enough room within the bottle for the injection of the sodium bicarbonate. The physician, in fact, can emphasize that the local anesthetic is going to be used to "numb" the area prior to the procedure. In the senior author's (TS) experience, a statement such as this can make the difference between a patient who is very anxious about the procedure and one who is not. Since patient anxiety can sometimes cause physician anxiety, it is the senior author's (TS) opinion that physician performance improves in the setting of a nonanxious patient.

When injecting a local anesthetic, a very small gauge needle (e.g., 25 gauge or 30 gauge) should be used. Skin traction can also be applied to facilitate this initial needle entry. After needle entry, a wheel of local anesthetic can be raised. The needle can then be advanced towards the target structure as local anesthetic is given after aspirating back to check for inadvertent vascular entry. Additional local anesthetic can be administered while withdrawing the needle out of the subcutaneous tissue and skin.

Another disadvantage of local anesthetic administration is the potential for local anesthetic toxicity. Unless the injection has been inadvertently administered intravascularly, in which case local anesthetic toxicity can occur abruptly, local anesthetic toxicity is quite unlikely unless recommended doses are exceeded. Local anesthetic toxicity can be recognized by its central nervous system (CNS) and cardiovascular (CV) manifestations [35]. Local anesthetic toxicity can initially present as perioral numbness, ringing in the ears, a metallic taste, anxiety, or tremulousness [36]. Physicians should be aware of these early symptoms of local anesthetic toxicity in order to quickly recognize this so as to provide supportive treatment in a monitored setting.

At low doses, local anesthetics also have a sedative effect causing light-headedness, dizziness, and drowsiness. As plasma levels increase, CNS excitation occurs, which can lead into a tonic-clonic seizure. Other CNS manifestations include neuronal apoptosis, cauda equina syndrome, and anterior spinal artery syndrome. CV system toxicity of local anesthetics involves relaxation of arteriolar smooth muscle and cardiac depression, causing hypotension and a decreased cardiac output. Slowed conduction may occur as well, showing prolongation of the P-R and QRS intervals on an electrocardiogram.

An alternative to a local anesthetic injection is the use of vapocoolant spray applied to the skin surface. When applying this topical refrigerant, the skin surface should be sprayed until it just begins to turn white, thus indicating that it has anesthetized cutaneous nerve endings. While this is a relatively convenient option, the potential disadvantage is that there is no guarantee of the sterility of the vapocoolant liquid. The coolant is optimally applied by quickly inserting the injection needle after the spray has been applied. Given the absence of a guarantee of the sterility, this could potentially contaminate the previously sterilized skin injection site. While additional Betadine® or chlorhexidine/alcohol could be quickly applied after the spray, the absence of time to allow the Betadine® or chlorhexidine/alcohol to dry might therefore not sterilize the skin surface again. The vapocoolant spray is not guaranteed for sterility, and this substance is technically classified as a medical device rather than a medication. Medical devices are not held to the standard of sterility as are medications. While there are no known published cases of infection due to vapocoolant spray, the senior author (TS) is aware of one lawsuit involving an infection whereby it was alleged that the vapocoolant spray may have been responsible.

In order to anesthetize the skin and underlying subcutaneous tissue, it is important to allow enough time for the medication to take effect before commencing with the procedure. Lidocaine's onset of action for infiltration anesthesia ranges from ½ to 1 min and is related to the total volume administered (the higher the volume administered, the faster the onset) and the percent of lidocaine used (the higher the percentage, the faster the onset) [37]. During the slight lag time between administration of the lidocaine and the onset of skin/subcutaneous anesthesia, postprocedural care discussion can take place.

Step 6: Postprocedural Care Discussion

While allowing time for the local anesthetic to take effect, important information can be conveyed to the patient. For example, a frequent source of confusion for patients who have undergone a diagnostic injection of local anesthetic is the fact that they might not understand that pain will return after the local anesthetic wears off. If patients are not specifically told this, it has been the senior author's (TS) experience that patients will misinterpret this to indicate that either the procedure was unsuccessful or that the procedure itself caused the pain. Not infrequently, this will result in a call to the office either later that day/night or over the next several days. In order to avoid this, the patient should be specifically educated that the local anesthetic will wear off ("like at the dentist's office when the novocaine wears off") and therefore pain will return. In fact, the initial level of postprocedural pain might be slightly worse given the fact that a needle was used to deliver the injectate and local discomfort from needle trauma to tissue can also add to the pain.

An important additional topic of discussion involves the procedure for communication between the patient and physician. It is the senior author's (TS) strong belief that any problems related to a procedure should be communicated by the patient or patient's caregiver directly to the attending physician who performed the procedure. If this is not possible, a physician who is covering for the attending physician should assume that role. This is preferable to the patient communicating this information to his/her primary care physician or to an emergency room. Inadvertent miscommunication is unfortunately likely to occur, if the patient or caregiver communicates with a physician who is different from the physician who performed the procedure. It is also extremely important to the ongoing education of the physician to become aware of potential procedure-related side effects. The likelihood of prompt treatment of a side effect is also presumably improved if it is being directed by the physician performing the injection, who is most familiar with potential procedure-related side effects. From a practical point of view, communication directly to the physician performing the injection procedure also allows for "damage control" after a procedure in the case of a true complication.

A very common question on the part of patients is their allowable activity level after the procedure. This is a topic of some controversy as it pertains to advisable activity levels after a corticosteroid injection into a joint. Recommendations range from complete rest of the injected joint to no significant change in activities. Complete joint rest theoretically allows the corticosteroid to take effect on the joint by remaining in contact with the joint surface and therefore binding to receptors. Resting of the joint as well as the application of ice likely decreases the rate of clearance of the corticosteroid from the joint [38]. Relative rest is also believed by some to decrease the likelihood of a postinjection corticosteroid flare [39]. While the senior author (TS) does not generally prescribe complete best rest after a corticosteroid injection, he does ask that patients modify their activity for a few days to exclude strenuous activities and will often prescribe an orthotic device to further help rest the structure.

Postprocedural modality use can also be discussed with the patient. This includes the use of ice after procedure. General guidelines for icing a body region include doing this often for 20–30 min time intervals and no more frequently than every 2 h. These guidelines have been developed based upon 20–30 min application times being the optimal time frame for the effect of ice. The general guideline that ice should not be used more frequently than every 2 h is based upon the chance of cutaneous nerve injury with more frequent application. Recommendations in review articles range from 10 to 20 min 2–4 times per day, up to 20–30 min, or 30–45 min every 2 h [40, 41]. If the physician believes that ice application at home is important, the use of this modality can be demonstrated to the patient by applying ice to the affected body region in the physician's office immediately after the procedure. This will not only demonstrate to the patient how to actually apply the modality but should also set an example to the patient of the importance of applying the modality. The patient may very well think to himself/herself, "If the doctor took the time to apply the ice, it must be important!"

Wound care issues such as instructions for cleansing the injection site and bandage removal/changing can also be reviewed at this point. If instruction in application of a bandage is needed, then this can instead occur in the immediate postprocedure phase, at which time the patient can be shown how to apply a bandage.

If additional time is still available at this point while waiting for the local anesthetic to take effect, relevant paperwork can be completed. This paperwork can involve prescriptions, physician notes to allow activity modification at work or home and completion of a portion of an office note.

Step 7: Aspiration (If Applicable)

If it is applicable to a given procedure (e.g., knee arthrocentesis), an attempt can be made to aspirate from the target structure by inserting a needle of appropriate size attached to an aspirating syringe. In performing the aspiration, the same needle trajectory should be followed as was used for administration of the local anesthetic. Once the needle enters the target structure, aspiration can then be conducted. If it is difficult to aspirate the structure, several possibilities exist. First, the target structure may not have been actually entered. Adjustment of needle position, followed by a repeat attempt at aspiration, can clarify this. Secondly, even if the target structure is entered, it might not contain enough of an effusion for aspiration. Alternatively, the needle may be positioned within the target structure in such a way that aspiration is not possible. For example, the needle bevel might be situated against synovial tissue, which is blocking the needle opening. In contrast, the aspirate might be so thick that it cannot fit through the needle. Under these circumstances, thinning out the aspirate via injecting normal saline or local anesthetic through the aspirating needle could be helpful. Alternatively, if some effusion has already been aspirated, tissue could have subsequently occluded the needle opening. Some of the aspirate can then be gently injected through the needle back into the target structure in order to clear the debris from the needle tip. Gravity can also assist with aspiration. For example, when aspirating a patient's knee, the knee can be turned gently toward the aspirating needle while the physician holds the aspirating syringe/needle and guides it down into a gravity-dependent position in order to assist with flow through the needle. Another strategy is for a smaller syringe to be connected to the aspirating needle: see Material Preparation section in this chapter for rationale for using a smaller syringe. If an effusion persists despite needle reposition, dilution of the effusion, the use of gravity, and the use of a smaller aspirating syringe, final additional measures such as needle reentry into the structure using a larger needle and/or different approach can be considered.

If it is extremely important to obtain any synovial fluid sample (e.g., rule out infected joint) but attempted aspiration was negative, a technique known as the "wash and retrieve" can be used [34]. Specifically, an appropriate quantity (e.g., 20 ml for a knee joint) of sterile saline can be injected into the target structure and then aspirated out; then the resulting wash is sent for culture. When using this technique, it is important to realize that increased resistance to injection of the normal saline suggests that the needle tip is not within the target structure. Under those circumstances, no more normal saline should be injected.

Depending upon the appearance of the aspirate, the fluid may need to be sent to the laboratory for analysis. If this is the case, the initial portion of the aspirate should be used for culture and gram staining, if this is applicable. By utilizing the first portion of the aspirate for these analyses, this should minimize the chance that the aspirate has become contaminated through the needle that is being used to transfer the aspirate into the specimen containers. If an effusion is still present despite filling up the syringe, this syringe can simply be reattached to the needle after the syringe has been emptied as long as sterility has been maintained throughout the process. Alternatively, a new syringe can be attached. Aspiration can then proceed until the full extent of the aspirate is removed. If an initially nonbloody effusion becomes blood-tinged during removal, this often indicates that the needle opening is now lodged against synovium. Another clue to this is the frequent occurrence of complaints of some discomfort as the synovium makes contact with the needle tip. This traumatic-type effusion can sometimes be confused with a truly bloody effusion. This can be an important distinction to make as it does affect the differential diagnosis of the effusion.

Step 8: Injection

If aspiration has been performed and completed, the aspirating syringe should be unclamped from the needle and a syringe containing the injectate should be clamped onto the needle. Figure 1.4 shows components of needle and syringe. This unclamping and clamping process should be performed, such that the clamp is applied to that portion of the needle hilt where needle and plastic come together (Fig. 1.5). In contrast, the clamp should not be applied to the needle itself (Fig. 1.6), as this would contaminate a portion of the needle, unless the clamp had been previously sterilized. In addition, a clamp should not be applied to the portion of the needle hilt where only plastic is present (Fig. 1.7), as this might crack the plastic. The senior author (TS) in fact witnessed this on one occasion during a knee viscosupplementation procedure, when his resident physician clamped the needle hilt in this region and cracked the plastic. The needle then had to be withdrawn, and another needle had to be inserted.

The technique for the injection depends upon the type of structure being injected. For example, a joint injection procedure is generally straightforward, particularly if synovial fluid is first aspirated from the joint, as this would clearly indicate that the needle is in joint. Under these circumstances, the injectate can simply be deposited into the joint. Even if the injection is actually delivered outside of the joint, it is generally believed that corticosteroids can nonetheless diffuse into the joint and be

Fig. 1.4 Components of a needle and syringe

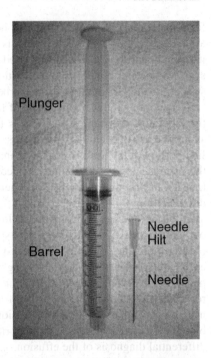

Plunger

Needle
Hilt

Barrel

Needle

Fig. 1.5 Correct location to
apply clamp: needle covered
by plastic portion of hilt

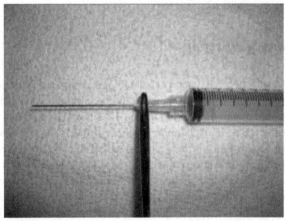

of benefit. In contrast, viscosupplements are unable to diffuse into the joint through the capsule and synovium, and therefore they require precise injection into the joint.

A peritendinous injection is more difficult. If ultrasound guidance is not being used, this procedure is performed by attempting to first place the needle opening gently against the tendon. This placement is confirmed by the inability to readily inject the medication due to a significant amount of pressure associated with an attempted injection. Next, while maintaining pressure against the hub of the syringe, the needle is then withdrawn in as small increments as possible until there is a sudden loss of resistance.

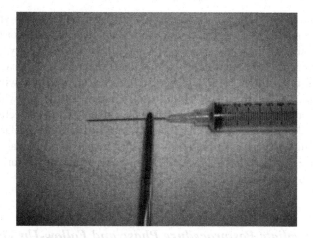

Fig. 1.6 Incorrect location to apply clamp: exposed needle

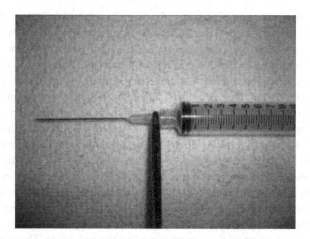

Fig. 1.7 Incorrect location to apply clamp: plastic portion of needle hilt

At this point, the injectate is delivered, and the needle tip ideally lies between the tendon and the surrounding tendon sheath. This placement can sometimes be confirmed by noticing a retrograde filling of the tendon sheath. In contrast, a localized accumulation of fluid suggests that the needle tip is located outside of the tendon sheath. Regardless of the fact that the needle tip may have been placed outside of the tendon sheath, corticosteroids are believed to be soluble enough that a beneficial effect can still occur via diffusion through the tendon sheath as long as they are deposited in the close vicinity of the tendon sheath. Ultrasound guidance can help to avoid these inaccuracies.

When injecting into a bursa, aspiration prior to the injection may reveal the presence of bursal fluid, thus confirming accurate needle placement. Unfortunately, however, bursal fluid often cannot be aspirated from a bursal structure, unless it is extremely distended. Alternatively, ultrasound guidance can help with aspiration of small amounts of bursal fluid.

For all soft tissue injection procedures, including joint, tendon sheath, and bursae, aspiration prior to final injection should be conducted in order to rule out inadvertent intravascular entry. In cases of inadvertent vascular entry, the needle should be repositioned. Fluoroscopic-guided injection procedures have the added advantage of recognition of an inadvertent intravascular pattern with contrast administration. The senior author (TS) has seen a number of cases in which aspiration failed to reveal blood return but subsequent Omnipaque™ injection readily revealed that the injection would have been performed into a vascular structure. Ultrasound guidance can also help to avoid inadvertent intravascular injections. This fact argues for the increased use of fluoroscopic guidance for various office-based injection procedures.

Step 9: Immediate Postprocedure Phase and Follow-Up Visit

Immediately after the procedure, the skin can be cleansed free of Betadine®. Betadine® can most efficiently be removed by using a hospital towel: wet part of it, wash off the Betadine®, and then dry off the structure with the dry portion of the towel. The wound site can then be covered with bandage. After this has been done, the patient should be observed for any adverse reactions, as these can occur due to inadvertent intravascular local anesthetic injection. Because the maximum arterial plasma concentrations of anesthetics develop within 10–25 min, consideration should be given for monitoring a patient for toxic effects for 30 min after the procedure [42]. For several reasons, a follow-up visit should be considered for any patient who has undergone an injection procedure. First, the physician can sometimes learn a great deal from the postinjection follow-up visit regarding tolerability, efficacy, and other issues. In this way, the physician should begin to develop a better understanding of where the injection procedures fit into the physician's therapeutic armamentarium. In addition, this is an opportunity for the physician to learn about any misconceptions that may exist on the part of the patient regarding the procedure. These can then be cleared up at the follow-up visit. Finally, it is the senior author's (TS) belief that patients appreciate being given a follow-up visit after having undergone an injection procedure. Perhaps this adds a degree of psychological comfort to the patient.

Final Words of Advice About Injection Procedures

The following advice comes from having performed several thousand office-based injection procedures over more than a decade and a half. While some of this information has been derived from successful injection procedures, the old adage, "You learn most from your mistakes" is definitely applicable to office-based injection procedures. It is hoped that the information imparted in this section will serve particularly to help prevent physicians from making errors.

The first topic pertains to adverse events. Any actual or perceived adverse event on the part of the patient should be fully documented within the medical record. This can prove to be extremely valuable in cases of threatened or actual medical malpractice suits. Fully documenting what actually occurred and what the physician's responses were to the situation is invaluable and should be encouraged. Gaps within the medical record leave a lot of room for possible negative interpretation on the part of an attorney or peer reviewer. In contrast, a detailed accounting of what the physician was considering, his/her actions based upon these considerations, and the patient's compliance or noncompliance with these instructions can remove much of this possible negative interpretation.

Documentation is also facilitated by the use of a procedure flow sheet. This can be very helpful in order to quickly review the number and type of injection procedures performed on any given patient. Ideally, the flow sheet is kept within the patient's chart in a readily accessible location for rapid retrieval, review, and updating at the time that a procedure is being considered or actually performed. Patients with chronic conditions that often require injection procedures (e.g., osteoarthritis) can undergo a surprisingly large number of injections over time. For example, a patient with lumbar spinal stenosis might undergo a series of corticosteroid spinal injection procedures, undergo intermittent corticosteroid knee injections, and undergo corticosteroid injections to treat associated pes anserine bursitis and trochanteric bursitis. Use of a flow sheet can help the physician to realize how many corticosteroid injections have already been performed and what the time course for these procedures has been. This is a clinically relevant question given the traditional teachings that no more than three corticosteroid injections per year [43] and no more than 20 corticosteroid injections in a lifetime [44] should be performed into any given osteoarthritic joint due to the possibility of accelerated osteoarthritis as is discussed in more detail in Chap. 2. However, a more recent study concluded that long-term, repetitive corticosteroid injection use has no significant harmful effects and is therefore safe [45]. Without use of a flow sheet, the physician must rely upon memory or individual office notes in order to count and track these procedures. This method of accounting can make this task much more difficult than it needs to be. A simple injection flow sheet that lists procedure date, body region injected, type of injection performed (i.e., diagnostic and/or therapeutic), corticosteroid dose for therapeutic injections, and response to the injection is very easy to construct and can pay significant long-term dividends. As noted previously, such charting can be performed while Betadine® is drying or while waiting for local anesthetic to take effect.

Patient anxiety about injection procedures can play a significant role with respect to how patients perceive and possibly respond to injection procedures. By placing some priority on minimizing patient anxiety, the physician can increase the likelihood that such a patient will perceive the entire experience as having been helpful and is more likely to allow future injection procedures. Unfortunately, the literature is limited on techniques that might be helpful with preprocedural psychological care, and most of the research has been conducted in the setting of elective surgery, both in the inpatient and outpatient settings [46]. It has been correctly explained that the medical aspects of care usually take precedence over the "psychoeducational" aspects of care, particularly in light of the increasingly severe time restrictions involved with patient care [47]. Preprocedural anxiety, however, is an important issue in the opinion of the senior author (TS). It has been his clinical experience that patients who have had a more negative experience with a procedure due to excessive anxiety and/or pain from the procedure tend to view the entire experience as relatively unfavorable and do not generally report a dramatic improvement from the injection procedure. In addition, those patients are very unlikely to allow another injection procedure, either to that body region or into other body regions for a different musculoskeletal problem. The physician can do several things to alleviate this anxiety.

If there is an office visit prior to the injection procedure, the physician has the opportunity to identify those patients with an "anxious predisposition" [48]. At this time, the physician can prescribe a short-acting anxiolytic medication to any patient who is exhibiting signs of excessive anxiety about the upcoming procedure. On the day of the procedure, if the patient has brought a friend or relative to the office, this person should be allowed to accompany the patient to the procedure as long as it is likely that they will be of help in alleviating the anxiety. This situation is somewhat complicated for fluoroscopic-guided injection procedures due to the exposure to radiation during the procedure. However, even under these circumstances, if the friend and/or family member is not at risk of being pregnant at the time of the procedure and if the physician judges that this would be of significant benefit to the patient, the friend or relative can be allowed to enter the procedure room and given appropriate radiation protection including a radiation vest and thyroid collar.

Anatomic models can be extremely useful in alleviating patient anxiety if they are used in such a way as to demonstrate the procedure that will be performed. By speaking to the patient in simple terms and showing the patient a model of the relevant anatomy, the physician can often explain the procedure in such a way that the patient will get the sense that it is relatively straightforward. In the senior author's (TS) experience, use of these models is also an extremely important teaching tool for medical students, residents, and fellows who might also be present for the procedure. Quite frankly, use of an anatomic teaching model can also help the attending physician to quickly refresh his/her memory of the relevant anatomy for procedures that he/she might not commonly perform. This review can easily be concealed under the guise of explaining the procedure to the patient and/or teaching the other medical personnel in the room.

During the actual procedure, it can be quite helpful to distract the patient with light conversation involving the patient. In contrast, the physician should resist the temptation to engage in nonmedical conversation amongst medical personnel that would exclude the patient. When the medical team is discussing nonmedical issues during the performance of the procedure, patients will likely perceive this as the medical team being distracted from the actual procedure. The patient may in fact blame a less than optimal outcome as well as any adverse events from the procedure as having been caused by this "distraction."

As was noted previously, blocking the patient's view from needles both during the medication preparation step and during the actual procedure can be of significant benefit. For those patients who specifically request to see the needle, it is wisest to show them the small gauge (i.e., 25 gauge or 30 gauge) needle/syringe combination that will be used for anesthetic administration, rather than showing them the larger gauge needle/syringe combination that will be used for the subsequent aspiration and/or injection. In the senior author's (TS) experience, patients have often shown a look of great relief when they have been shown a 30 gauge needle attached to a 1-cm^3 syringe and have been told that this is the needle that they will actually feel very briefly as the "numbing medicine" is being given to numb the area. If they still wish to see the actual procedure needle, they should be shown that.

As was also noted previously, strategic use of exam room curtains can help to physically block the view that the patient has of a procedure. This is particularly applicable to injection procedures performed on the hand and wrist regions, as it is quite natural for a patient to be sitting in an exam room chair placed at one end of the exam room table, while they place the affected extremity onto the surface of the table. The exam room curtain can then be pulled across the upper forearm region.

The body position that the patient is placed into during the injection procedure can also be put to one's advantage. Specifically, a supine or prone position is preferable whenever feasible, as patients tend to relax more when they are recumbent; in case of a vasovagal reaction, they do not run the risk of falling to the floor, and they can be relatively easily placed into the Trendelenburg position to help treat the reaction. The patient should then be monitored by someone until they can safely ambulate on his/her own. The occurrence of the vasovagal reaction, the steps used to assess the patient and treat the reaction, as well as the patient's condition upon leaving the office then should all be documented. Although the incidence of vasovagal reactions during peripheral joint and soft tissue injections is not currently known, phlebotomy (0.87%) and epidural spinal injection (caudal 0.8%, transforaminal lumbar 0.3%, interlaminar cervical 1.7%) related causes have been documented [49–52]. While these rates are actually quite low, the physician who performs a large number of these procedures will inevitably encounter vasovagal reactions.

Finally, if, despite all of the above measures, a patient remains extremely anxious, serious consideration should be given for canceling the procedure on that day. The procedure can then be rescheduled to allow for the prescription of anxiolytic medication, if that had not been prescribed prior to the procedure, or a prescription of a higher dose of anxiolytic medication if one had already been prescribed and was not successful at alleviating patient anxiety. Alternatively, some physicians have access to surgical centers and hospital-based procedure rooms where patients can be given intravenous sedation as well. For example, a small dose of intravenous Versed® (Roche, Nutley, NJ, USA) with or without fentanyl can be very effective in alleviating anxiety. However, an interesting trade-off is that the procedure is then conducted in a setting which implies a greater level of intervention compared to when it is to be performed in a simple examination room. The pros and cons of this selection should be weighed and a decision made based upon the individual patient.

References

1. Liddell WC, Carmichael CR, McHugh NJ. Joint and soft tissue injections: a survey of general practitioners. Rheumatology 2005; 44:1043–1046.
2. Bliddal H. Placement of intra-articular injections verified by mini-air arthrography. Ann Rheum Dis 1999; 58:641–643.
3. Jackson DW, Evans NA, Thomas BM. Accuracy of needle placement of intra-articular steroid injections. J Bone Joint Surgery Am 2002; 84:1522–1527.
4. Jones A, Regan M, Ledingham J, Pattrick M, Manhire A, Doherty M. Importance of placement of intra-articular steroid injections. BMJ 1993; 307:1329–1330.
5. Partington PF, Broome GH, Diagnostic injection around the shoulder: hit and miss? A cadaveric study of injection accuracy. J Shoulder Elbow Surg 1998; 7(2):147–150.
6. Williams MJ. Local Anesthetics. In Raj PP, ed. Pain Medicine: A Comprehensive Review. St. Louis: Mosby; 1996:162–175.
7. Cohen SP, Narvaez JC, Lebovits AH, Stojanovic MP. Corticosteroid injections for trochanteric bursitis: is fluoroscopy necessary? A pilot study. Br J Anaesth 2005; 94(1):100–106.
8. Brandt, KD. Synovial fluid analysis. An Atlas of Osteoarthritis. New York: The Parthenon Publishing Group Inc.; 2001:60.
9. Canoso JJ, D, Yood RA Acute gouty bursitis: report of 15 cases. Ann Rheum Dis 1979; 38:326–328.
10. Vegter J. The influence of joint posture on intra-articular pressure. J Bone Joint Surg 1987; 69-B(1):71–74.
11. Carbonell AM, Harold KL, Mahmutovic AJ, Hassan R, Matthews BD, Kercher KW et al. Local injection for the treatment of suture site pain after laparoscopic ventral hernia repair. Am Surg 2003; 69(8):688–691.
12. Bellamy N, Campbell J, Robinson V, Gee T, Bourne R, Wells G. Viscosupplementation for the treatment of osteoarthritis of the knee. Cochrane Database Syst Rev 2006; (2):CD005321.
13. Lo GH, LaValley M, McAlindon T, Felson DT. Intra-articular hyaluronic acid in treatment of knee osteoarthritis. JAMA 2003; 290:3115–3121.
14. Wang CT, Lin J, Chang CJ, Lin YT, Hou SM. Therapeutic effects of hyaluronic acid on osteoarthritis of the knee: a meta-analysis of randomized controlled trials. J Bone Joint Surg 2004; 86A:538–545.
15. Arrich J, Piribauer F, Mad P, Schmid D, Klaushofer K, Mullner M. Intra-articular hyaluronic acid for the treatment of osteoarthritis of the knee: systematic review and meta-analysis. CMAJ 2005; 172:1039–1041.
16. Matura M, Goossens A. Contact allergy to corticosteroids. Allergy 2000; 55:698–704.
17. Hernigou P, Bachir D, Galacteros F. Avascular necrosis of the femoral head in sickle-cell disease. Treatment of collapse by the injection of acrylic cement. J Bone Joint Surg Br 1993; 75(6):875–880.
18. Vanderwilde RS, Morrey BF, Melberg MW, Vinh TN. Inflammatory arthritis after failure of silicone rubber replacement of the radial head. J Bone Joint Surg Br 1994; 76(1):78–81.
19. Neth OW, Bajaj-Elliott M, Turner MW, Klein NJ. Susceptibility to infection in patients with neutropenia: the role of the innate immune system. Br J Haematol 2005; 129(6):713.
20. Finucane BT. Allergies to local anesthetics – the real truth/Les allergies aux anesthésiques locaux – la vraie vérité. Can J Anesth 2003; 50:869–874.
21. Dance D, Basti S, Koch DD. Use of preservative-free lidocaine for cataract surgery in a patient allergic to "caines." J Cataract Refract Surg 2005; 31(4):848–850.
22. Achar S, Kundu S. Principles of office anesthesia: Part I. Infiltrative anesthesia. Am Fam Physician 2002; 66(1):91–94.
23. Rydberg J, Charles J, Aspelin P. Frequency of late allergy-like adverse reactions following injection of intravascular non-ionic contrast media: a retrospective study comparing a non-ionic monomeric contrast medium with a non-ionic dimeric contrast medium. Acta Radio 1998; 39(3):219–222.

24. Bettmann MA. Frequently asked questions: iodinated contrast agents. RadioGraphics 2004; 24:S3–S10.

25. Lehrer SB, Ayuso R, Reese G. Seafood allergy and allergens: a review. Mar Biotechnol 2003; 5(4):339–348.

26. Mortele KJ, Oliva MR, Ondategui S, Ros PR, Silverman SG. Universal use of nonionic iodinated contrast medium for CT: evaluation of safety in a large urban teaching hospital. AJR 2005; 184:31–34.

27. Charalambous CP, Tryfonidis M, Sadiq S, Hirst P, Paul A. Septic arthritis following intra-articular steroid injection of the knee – a survey of current practice regarding antiseptic technique used during intra-articular steroid injection of the knee. Clin Rheumatol 2003; 22(6):386–390.

28. Muller LM, Gorter KJ, Hak E, Goudzwaard WL, Schellevis FG, Hoepelman AI Increased risk of common infections in patients with type 1 and type 2 diabetes mellitus. Clin Infect Dis 2005; 41:281–288.

29. Hammesfahr R, Knopf AB, Stitik TP. Safety of Intra-articular Hyaluronates for Pain Associated with Osteoarthritis of the Knee. Am J Orthop 2003; 32(6):277–283.

30. Hamburger M, Settles M, Teutsch J. Identification of an immunogenic candidate for the elicitation of severe acute inflammatory reactions (SAIRs) to hylan G-F 20. Osteoarthr Cartil 2005; 13(3):266–268.

31. Hamburger MI, Lakhanpal S, Mooar PA, Oster D. Intra-articular hyaluronans: a review of product-specific safety profiles. Semin Arthritis Rheum 2003; 32(5):296–309.

32. Goldberg VM, Coutts, RD. Pseudoseptic reactions to Hylan viscosupplementation: diagnosis and management. Clin Orthop 2004; 419:130–137.

33. Hsieh HF, Chiu HH, Lee FP. Surgical hand scrubs in relation to microbial counts: systematic literature review. J Adv Nurs 2006; 55(1):68–78.

34. Roberts WN. Primer: pitfalls of aspiration and injection. Nat Clin Pract Rheumatol 2007; 3(8):464–472.

35. Cox B, Durieux ME, Marcus MAE. Toxicity of local anaesthetics. Best Pract Res Clin Anaesth 2003; 17(1):111–136.

36. Klein SM, Greengrass RA, Gleason DH, Nunley JA, Steele SM. Major ambulatory surgery with continuous regional anesthesia and a disposable infusion pump. Anesthesiology 1999; 91:563–565.

37. Stitik TP, Klecz R, Greenwald B. Pharmacotherapy of Disability. In DeLisa JA, ed. Rehabilitation Medicine: Principles and Practices. Fourth edition. Philadelphia, PA: JB Lippincott Co; 2005:1205–1252.

38. Schumacher HR, Chen LX. Injectable corticosteroids in treatment of arthritis of the knee. Am J Med 2005; 118(11):1208–1214.

39. Chakravarty K, Scott DGI. A randomized controlled study of post-injection rest following intra-articular steroid therapy for knee synovitis. Br J Rheumatol 1994; 33:464–468.

40. Bleakley C, McDonough S, MacAuley D. The use of ice in the treatment of acute soft-tissue injury. Am J Sports Med 2004; 32:251–261.

41. Stitik TP, Nadler SF. Sports injuries: when-and how-to use cold most effectively. Consult Consult Prim Care 1999; 39(1):2881–2890.

42. Kesson M, Atkins E, Davies I, eds. Essential Equipment, Safety Cautions and Emergency Situations. In Musculoskeletal Injection Skills. Section I: Principles of Musculoskeletal Injections. Philadelphia, PA: Elsevier Science; 2003:10–17.

43. Katz JN, Simmons BP. Carpal tunnel syndrome. N Eng J Med 2002; 346(23):1807–1812.

44. Beary JP. Osteoarthritis. In Beary JP, Christian CL, Johanson NA, eds. Manual of Rheumatology and Outpatient Orthopedic Disorders: Diagnosis and Therapy. Boston, MA: Little, Brown and Company; 1987:187–198.

45. Raynauld JP, Buckland-Wright C, Ward R, Choquette D, Haraoui B, Martel-Pelletier Jet al Safety and efficacy of long-term intraarticular steroid injections in osteoarthritis of the knee: a randomized, double-blind, placebo-controlled trial. Arthritis Rheum 2003; 48(2):370–377.

46. Mitchell M. Patient anxiety and modern elective surgery: a literature review. J Clin Nurs 2003; 12:806–815.

47. Fung D, Cohen M. What do out-patients value most in their anesthesia care? Can J Anesth 2001; 48(1):12–19.
48. Voulgari A, Papanikolaou MN, Lykouras L, Alevizos B, Alexiou E, Christodoulou GN. Prevention of postoperative anxiety and depression. Bibl Psychiatr 1994; 165:49–55.
49. Zervou E, Ziciadis K, Karabini F, Xanthi E, Chrisostomou E, Tzolou A. Vasovagal reactions in blood donors during or immediately after blood donation. Transfus Med 2005; 15(5):389–394.
50. Botwin KP, Gruber RD, Bouchlas CG, Torres-Ramos FM, Hanna A, Rittenberg J et al. Complications of fluoroscopically guided caudal epidural injections. Am J Phys Med Rehabil 2001; 80(6):416–424.
51. Botwin K P, Castellanos R, Rao S, Hanna AF, Torres-Ramos FM, Gruber RD et al. Complications of Fluoroscopically Guided Interlaminar Cervical Epidural Injections. Arch Phys Med Rehabil 2003; 84:627–633.
52. Botwin KP, Gruber RD, Bouchlas CG, Torres-Ramos FM, Freeman TL, Slaten WK. Complications of Fluoroscopically Guided Transforaminal Lumbar Epidural Injections Arch Phys Med Rehabil 2000; 81:1045–1050.

Chapter 2
Pharmacotherapy of Joint and Soft Tissue Injections

Todd P. Stitik, Ajay Kumar, Jong H. Kim, Jiaxin J. Tran, and Charles Lee

Introduction

The most common medications used for office-based joint and soft tissue injection procedures include injectable corticosteroids and local anesthetics. In particular, the intra-articular administration of corticosteroids has been used for more than 50 years to help diagnose and/or treat various joint disorders [1]. Corticosteroids are also often injected into bursae, into tendon sheaths, at tendon insertion sites, and into muscular trigger points. Although corticosteroid injections (CSIs) may not cure the underlying disease process and can potentially worsen it, they can act rapidly and be extremely effective in relieving pain and inflammation [2]

To be most effective, CSIs should be used in conjunction with other therapeutic modalities. They especially represent a suitable alternative for those patients in whom NSAIDs and COX-2 inhibitors are felt to be contraindicated. This has recently become especially important due to the documented problems and concerns with COX-2 inhibitors. Amongst practitioners of musculoskeletal medicine, the use of CSIs in patients with osteoarthritis (OA), in particular, has increased given the increased frequency with which physiatrists and other musculoskeletal medicine practitioners now perform injection procedures as well as the increasing prevalence of OA.

Despite their use for many years in the management of OA and other musculoskeletal conditions, several aspects of CSIs remain controversial, including the exact mechanism of action, relative efficacy and duration, and some of the potential deleterious effects. One purpose of this chapter is to provide a good blend of basic science and clinical information on their mechanism of action, relevant pharmacokinetics, dosing, potential side effects, and common uses.

T.P. Stitik (✉)
Department of Physical Medicine and Rehabilitation, New Jersey Medical School,
Newark, NJ, USA
e-mail: todd.stitik@gmail.com

T.P. Stitik (ed.), *Injection Procedures: Osteoarthritis and Related Conditions*,
DOI 10.1007/978-0-387-76595-2_2, © Springer Science+Business Media, LLC 2011

Local anesthetics are also commonly used for office-based injection procedures. As was mentioned in Chap. 1, they are used both for diagnostic and therapeutic reasons. When used for therapeutic injections, they are often administered in conjunction with corticosteroids. Another major purpose of this chapter is to review basic science and clinical information on their mechanism of action, relevant pharmacokinetics, dosing, potential side effects, and common uses. Finally, contrast agents such as Omnipaque™ (GE Healthcare, Waukesha, WI, USA) are often administered as part of fluoroscopic-guided injections procedures in order to enhance visualization of the procedure.

Other less commonly used injectates include the viscosupplements, botulinum toxin, solutions used for prolotherapy (e.g., dextrose, phenol, glycerine, or cod liver oil extract) autologous blood products such as platelet rich plasma (PRP), platelet poor plasma (PPP), and thrombin, mesenchymal stem cells, and substances used for mesotherapy including plant extracts, vitamins, and medications such as NSAIDs. These substances will not be discussed in any detail as they are outside of the scope of this text.

Corticosteroids

Mechanism of Action and Pharmacokinetics of Injectable Corticosteroids

CSIs generally relieve pain and inflammation within the target structure. They are usually mixed with a local anesthetic for injection into a joint or bursa. An arthrocentesis or a bursal aspiration may sometimes precede the injection as well. This aspiration, along with the local anesthetic, may account for part of the analgesic effect. Specifically, arthrocentesis and bursal aspirations can decrease mechanical pressure associated with a joint or bursal effusions and likely help to remove inflammatory mediators [3]. However, the exact mechanism of action from the steroid itself is still unclear and could be due to local and/or systemic effects. Possible mechanism(s) of corticosteroids are summarized in Table 2.1 [7, 12, 13].

Some insight into the reason for the relatively short duration of clinical benefit from CSIs can be inferred from a study by Klint and colleagues [14]. Specifically, marked reductions in acute inflammatory mediators such as synovial T lymphocytes, tumor necrosis factor, and interluekin-1 beta were observed in association with beneficial clinical effects in RA patients who received one intra-articular CSI [14]. In contrast, less acute markers such as macrophage infiltration and proinflammatory endothelial cytokine expression remained unchanged.

Corticosteroids can be classified into short-acting, intermediate-acting, and long-acting preparations based on their duration of action (Table 2.2). In general, the less water soluble a corticosteroid is, the slower its onset of action and the longer its duration. Duration is particularly brief in joint inflammation, as the inflamed synovium is highly vascular and it rapidly clears the corticosteroid. Thus, short

Table 2.1 Intra-articular corticosteroid injection mechanism of action theories

Category	Individual mechanism
Effect on WBCs	Decreased synovial membrane permeability [4]
	Synovial WBC cell count reduction due to interference with leukocyte chemotaxis and direct effect on leukocyte motility [5]
Effect on other inflammatory mediators	Complement level reduction [6]
	Lysosomal membrane stabilization and reduction in acid phosphatase [7]
	Suppression of delayed hypersensitivity [8–10]
	Impairment of macrophage recruitment to inflammatory sites [8–10]
	Suppression of cytokine release [8–10]
	Reduction in antibody production [8–10]
	Reduction in interleukin-1 alpha and interlukin-1 beta synthesis [11]

duration corticosteroid preparations are rarely used for intra-articular procedures, as their half-life in the joint is less than 2 h [15].

Corticosteroids appropriate for intra-articular injections are modified chemically to decrease their water solubility and therefore increase their duration of action. Although precise information on the rate of systemic absorption of intra-articular steroids is not well known, long-acting corticosteroids are believed to be initially absorbed systemically within 48 h and then continue to be absorbed slowly over 2–3 weeks [16]. This estimate is based on the symptomatic improvement in joints remote from the injected one.

A corticosteroid preparation with a slow onset and long duration would be the ideal choice in chronic diseases such as OA. In situations such as an exacerbation of a disease in a physically active patient, a combination preparation of a short- and long-acting corticosteroid such as betamethasone phosphate and betamethasone acetate (celestone soluspan) may be a good choice.

Specific Corticosteroid Agents

Commonly used corticosteroid preparations include hydrocortisone, dexamethasone, methylprednisolone, and triamcinolone. Of these, dexamethasone has the strongest glucocorticoid (anti-inflammatory) properties, whereas hydrocortisone has the strongest mineralocorticoid properties. However, intra-articular potencies of corticosteroid preparations relative to one another are not entirely accurate and are based on the degree of hypothalamic–pituitary–adrenal axis (HPA) suppression following systemic steroid administration [16] (Table 2.2).

These potency estimates are not based upon their intrasynovial anti-inflammatory properties, and their relative values are not known. In a survey conducted among

Table 2.2 Corticosteroid equivalencies, solubilities, potencies, and durations of action, listed in order of increasing antiinflammatory potency

Corticosteroid preparation	Hydrocortisone equivalent	Solubility (% wt/vol)	Duration of action	Equivalent oral dose (mg)	Mineralocorticoid potency	Antiinflammatory potency
Hydrocortisone acetate	1	0.002	Intermediate	20	2	1
Methylprednisolone acetate	5	0.001	Intermediate	4	0	5
Triamcinolone acetonide susp	5	0.004	Intermediate	4	0	5
Triamcinolone hexacetonide	5	0.0002	Long	4	0	5
Betamethasone sodium phosphate and acetate suspension	25	NA	Long	0.6	0	20–30
Dexamethasone sodium phosphate suspension	25	0.01	Short	0.75	0	20–30
Dexamethasone acetate suspension	25	NA	Long	0.75	0	20–30

rheumatologists [17], methylprednisolone acetate was the preferred steroid by rheumatologist trained in the eastern US; triamcinolone acetonide was preferred by those trained in the West; and triamcinolone hexacetonide was preferred by those trained in the Midwest and Southwest.

Dexamethasone

Dexamethasone sodium phosphate is a rapid onset and short acting preparation of dexamethsaone. It is a logical choice for the treatment acute disorders, such as acute shoulder pain secondary to subacromial bursitis, but not for chronic conditions such as OA. Decadron® (Merck & Co., Whitehouse Station, NJ, USA) (dexamethasone acetate), which is relatively insoluble, may be a better alternative in OA given its high potency and long duration of action.

Of note, dexamethasone sodium phosphate contains sodium bisulfite, a preservative that may cause allergic-type reactions including life-threatening anaphylactic symptoms or less severe asthmatic episodes in certain susceptible patients. Dexamethasone is approved for the treatment of OA, rheumatoid arthritis (RA), tendonitis, tenosynovitis, and bursitis [18].

Triamcinolone

Triamcinolone hexaacetonide (Aristospan®, Sandoz, Princeton, NJ, USA) and triamcinolone acetonide (Kenalog® Britol-Myers Squibb, Princeton, NJ, USA) are commonly used triamcinolone salts for intra-articular injections. Triamcinolone has essentially no mineralocorticoid activity. It is approved for the treatment of OA, RA, bursitis, tendonitis, epicondylitis, gouty arthritis, as well as for use in epidural injections. However, it has a high incidence of dermatological complications including facial/neck flushing, subcutaneous atrophy, and depigmentation.

Methylprednisolone

This corticosteroid has an intermediate duration of action and therefore represents a good balance in terms of onset of action and duration. It is therefore the corticosteroid that is referenced in terms of recommended doses throughout the individual chapters of this book. It is available as a methylprednisolone acetate salt. Its glucocorticoid potency is about 1/5–1/7 of dexamethasone. In a study on the efficacy of triamcinolone hexacetonide (THA) and methylprednisolone acetate (MPA) in patients with symptomatic knee OA with effusion, both were found to be temporarily effective.

THA had a slight advantage for pain relief at 3 weeks, but its effect was lost by week 8. MPA, however, still had an effect at week 8 [19]. Methylprednisolone is approved for the same indications as triamcinolone for bursitis, tendonitis, or arthritis but not for the use as an epidural injection.

Efficacy in Osteoarthritis

CSIs have been used most commonly in knee OA. While previous evidence for CSI efficacy was weak and largely anecdotal [11, 20, 21], a large Cochrane meta-analysis found short-term efficacy of intra-articular corticosteroids for knee OA treatment with few side effects [22]. This review concluded that intra-articular corticosteroids were superior to placebo and intra-articular hyaluronans (aka viscosupplements) between 1 and 3 weeks postinjection, but not from 4 to 24 weeks.

However, hyaluronans were more efficacious as compared to corticosteroids for several other parameters (WOMAC OA index, Lequesne Index, pain, range of motion, and number of responders). These findings suggest a similar onset of action for intra-articular corticosteroids and hyaluronans, but hyaluronans provide a longer lasting benefit. There is some evidence that high doses of corticosteroids (i.e., doses of 50 mg equivalent of prednisone) may achieve a longer response [23].

Although there is now relatively good evidence for the short-term efficacy of corticosteroids, [23–28] longer duration of benefit has still not been confirmed [27, 29]. As discussed previously, CSIs have been found to be beneficial only for short duration with varying lengths of benefit. This variation could be due partly to inaccurate injections. In fact, one study documented a 29% rate of inadvertent extra-articular injection [24].

Moreover, if a patient with OA has underlying calcium pyrophosphate deposition disease, a disease that generally responds well to IA steroids, he/she may respond very well to a CSI. In contrast, an exacerbation of OA itself may not respond as well to this. This could lead to a misinterpretation of the response to CSI, as it is difficult to distinguish these entities without synovial fluid analysis.

It is not clear whether CSIs can lead to improved quadriceps muscle strength in knee OA. Jones and Doherty reported no improvement in isometric quadriceps strength of knee OA patients who received a CSI [24]. This is an important issue to settle, as muscle weakness is an important determinant of disability in OA [30].

CSI efficacy data are more limited for hip OA than for knee OA. Pain relief with CSIs for hip OA has been supported by controlled studies. However, only a short-lived effect varying from 4 to 8 weeks has been demonstrated [31–35]. Pain at rest [34] and at night [35] improved most substantially. In another study, pain relief and 10° of improved hip internal rotation, both lasting for 8 weeks, were seen in 50–90% of patients with mild to moderate OA (according to American College of Rheumatology Classification) after intra-articular CSIs [36].

A very small number of patients with severe hip OA demonstrated pain relief lasting for 8 weeks. None of the patients with severe hip OA showed any improvement in internal rotation after CSIs [30]. Greater symptomatic improvement has also been noted with steroids and local anesthetic injections compared to local anesthetics alone [34, 37]. Similar to knee OA, there is some evidence that higher doses of corticosteroid injections may result in a longer response [31].

There is some anecdotal evidence that CSIs into small joints, such as the first carpometacarpal (CMC) joint, the first metatarsophalangeal (MTP) joint, and the first acromioclavicular (AC) joint, may give a lasting benefit [38, 39]. However, a randomized controlled trial of intra-articular CSIs into the first CMC joint in moderate to severe OA showed no clinical benefit as compared to placebo [40]. In another study, pain relief lasting for 1 month was observed with CSIs to the first CMC joint [41]. CSIs have also been used effectively for the treatment of synovial cysts of the fingers that are causing pain and/or disfigurement. CSIs can shrink synovial cysts when they are administered into an underlying joint or directly into the cysts, which normally overlie the distal or proximal interphalangeal joints [42, 43].

There have been several studies involving intra-articular corticosteroid injections for shoulder pain with mixed diagnoses (e.g., adhesive capsulitis, rotator cuff tendonitis). It is difficult to draw conclusions from these studies because of the non-uniformity of the diagnosis and combined injection procedures that were performed. Two such studies, a Cochrane systematic review in 2003 and another meta-analysis in 1998, concluded that there is little evidence to support the efficacy of subacromial and glenohumeral joint corticosteroid injections for rotator cuff tendonitis and adhesive capsulitis [44, 45].

Although subacromial and intra-articular CSI may be beneficial for pain relief only for a short period of time compared to placebo [45], subacromial injections have been found to be helpful in improving the range of abduction in rotator cuff tendonitis [44]. In another meta-analysis, the authors concluded that subacromial corticosteroid injections may be effective in rotator cuff tendonitis up to a 9-month period. They were found to be more effective than NSAIDs for this disorder [46].

As the natural history of adhesive capsulitis is generally good, there are no long-term differences among treatment approaches for this condition, including no treatment at all. CSIs are increasingly performed by physiatrists into osteoarthritic cervical, thoracic, and lumbar zygapophyseal (facet) joints. The literature is limited to several uncontrolled studies on the use of these in patients with degenerative changes in the facets [47, 48].

These studies did suggest sustained pain relief after the injections. However, there is a general inability to determine whether OA changes seen on radiographic studies are the actual pain generators, since radiographic changes of OA have been found to be equally common in symptomatic and asymptomatic patients [38–40]. Second, diagnostic fluoroscopically confirmed intra-articular anesthetic injections have been shown to relieve low back pain whether or not arthritic changes are radiographically evident in the lumbar facet joints [49, 50].

A critical review on the therapeutic benefit of these injections for facet-mediated pain found only level III (moderate) to level IV (limited) evidence in favor of this intervention [51]. For example, a small ($n = 97$) randomized, placebo-controlled trial of lumbar facet fluoroscopic-guided CSIs concluded that this intervention was of limited value in chronic low back pain [52]. Conversely, a larger controlled study of 449 fluoroscopic-guided lumbar facet joint injections concluded that this could have a useful palliative effect for chronic low back pain [53].

Lumbar zygapophyseal joint cysts are potential pain generators in patients with axial pain and/or lower-limb radicular pain. The traditional treatment of symptomatic cysts that do not respond to conservative measures is surgical decompression. Preliminary studies suggest that facet joint aspiration and injection under fluoroscopic guidance have a role in the treatment of axial radicular pain due to synovial zygapophyseal joint cysts. Two studies have reported a success rate of 29–50% with synovial cyst aspiration and injection for synovial cyst induced radicular pain [54, 55].

Literature is not available on the efficacy of CSI for ankle and subtalar joint arthritis. CSI and local anesthetics under fluoroscopic guidance have been found to be useful to localize the source of pain in foot/ankle disorders, especially before planning for surgery (i.e., arthrodesis) [56, 57].

Response Indicators in OA Patients

Two studies have identified subgroups of OA patients who were most likely to benefit maximally from a CSI. Specifically, the best responses were in patients with signs of inflammation, such as warmth and effusion, that could be detected clinically or aspirated [20, 21]. However, in another study, no definite correlation could be found between response to the injection and markers of local inflammation, although local tenderness did have some predictive power in unadjusted analysis [19].

In contrast, laboratory markers of inflammation, including synovial fluid cell counts, do not seem to predict pain relief from a CSI [21]. Response to CSI has not been found to correlate with other markers of disease severity including range of movement, anxiety score, synovial thickening, depression score, Stanford health assessment questionnaire (HAQ) score, lower limb HAQ score, quadriceps strength [19], and radiographic severity [21, 29].

Poorer response to CSIs has been seen in patients who had severe hip pain, hip arthritis of more than 5-years duration, or radiographic evidence of concentric arthritis on hip X-rays [26]. However, in one study, image findings were not found to predict response to corticosteroid injections [58].

Efficacy in Other Selected Musculoskeletal Conditions

Local CSIs often provide beneficial results, particularly short term, in various musculoskeletal disorders that do not otherwise respond to the conventional conservative treatments. Although corticosteroid injections are a commonly used treatment modality specifically for chronic tendon disorders, there is a lack of solid trials regarding the need and effectiveness of such injections. Caution should be exercised with all tendon sheath injections as inadvertent intratendinous injections have been associated with tendon rupture. In fact, CSIs into the immediate vicinity of weight-bearing tendons (i.e., Achilles tendon, patellar tendon, and posterior tibial tendon) are believed by many to be relatively contraindicated [59].

The following is a brief review of the literature regarding the efficacy of CSIs for selected musculoskeletal disorders. These conditions were chosen based upon the likelihood that the musculoskeletal clinician would encounter them in a typical clinical practice.

Bicipital Tendonitis

There are no published studies on the efficacy, accuracy, or side effects associated with bicipital tendon sheath injections. The authors believe that these injections are often not necessarily indicated, as bicipital tendonitis is usually associated with subacromial bursitis/rotator cuff tendinopathy as a secondary pathologic process. As such, most cases of bicipital tendonitis can be treated effectively by performing an injection into the subacromial space and directing other treatment at the subacromial pathology. This approach directly treats the primary pathology (i.e., subacromial bursitis/rotator cuff tendinopathy) and indirectly treats the secondary pathologic processes (i.e., bicipital tendonitis). Alternatively, the bicipital "tendinitis" might actually represent a glenohumeral joint effusion as an indicator of underlying pathology within the glenohumeral joint.

Lateral Epicondylitis (Epicondylosis)

There are several published studies on the efficacy of CSIs for lateral epicondylitis. Although firm conclusions on its effectiveness cannot necessarily be drawn mainly because of study heterogeneity [60–63], corticosteroid injections appear to be relatively safe and superior compared to physiotherapy and the "wait-and-see" approach in the short term (2–6 weeks) treatment of lateral epicondylitis. However, intermediate (>6 weeks to 6 months) and long-term (≥6 months) patient follow-up found that there was no lasting beneficial effect from CSIs. Interestingly, a systematic review found that, at the 12-month follow-up, physiotherapy (91%) and the wait-and-see policy (83%) were slightly superior to CSI (69%) [64]. With the increased use of diagnostic ultrasound, it is becoming more evident that these cases often do not involve acute inflammation, but instead are due to chronic tendonopathy. As such, other injection procedures such as percutaneous needle tenotomy (PNT) and PRP are probably more beneficial.

Medial Epicondylitis (Epicondylosis)

Medial epicondylitis is rather uncommon compared to lateral epicondylitis. This perhaps at least in part explains why there is a paucity of literature and very limited evidence on the efficacy of CSIs for medial epicondylitis. The literature that is available suggests that CSIs seem to provide only short-term benefits in its treatment [65]. Caution should be observed with CSIs for medial epicondylitis as the needle can injure the ulnar nerve, which lies just behind the medial epicondyle and/ or the medial antebrachial cutaneous nerve [66, 67]. Ultrasound-guided injections can minimize if not eliminate this risk. Similar to the situation for lateral "epicondylitis", the usual underlying pathologic process is more likely a chronic tendonopathy, then it is an acute inflammatory process.

Carpal Tunnel Syndrome

Local corticosteroid injection has been used in an attempt to relieve the pain, numbness, and tingling often associated with carpal tunnel syndrome (CTS). However, its efficacy in this setting is still not well established. Evidence in the form of a Cochrane review suggests that CSIs may be helpful in CTS only for up to 1 month after injection as compared to placebo but also provided significantly greater clinical improvement compared to oral steroid up to 3 months after treatment [68]. This review looked at patients with all grades (i.e., mild, moderate, and severe) of CTS.

In contrast, an individual study that specifically looked at patients with mild CTS found a longer duration of benefit. Specifically, CSIs were found to be effective up to 16 months (79% of patients) for relief of symptoms in mild CTS [69] and were associated with normalization of electrophysiological parameters in half of the cases. Compared to other usual treatment (specifically oral anti-inflammatory medications and splinting), no significant difference in clinical outcome with CSIs was found by 8 weeks from the time of the injection or initiation of splinting and oral anti-inflammatory medications [68, 70].

Low injection doses of steroids (25-mg hydrocortisone) are probably as effective as high doses for the relief of symptoms [71]. This information suggests that a low dose corticosteroid injection into a patient with mild CTS can be helpful for the short-term management of symptoms and can provide a treatment alternative to those patients who are not amenable to splinting and/or oral anti-inflammatory medication. Ultrasound guidance for these injections permits use of a higher volume of injectate in an attempt to "hydrodissect" the median nerve free from potential fibrous adhesions.

de Quervain's Tenosynovitis

Corticosteroid injection in the tendon sheath is considered by some to be first line treatment for deQuervain's tenosynovitis [72, 73], as a success rate of 80–90% has been reported [74, 75]. The presence of a separate compartment for the extensor pollicis brevis is cited as the most common reason for failure of the CSI [76]. Ultrasound guidance offers the advantage of being able to recognize the situation and adjust the injection accordingly so as to target both compartments. There is controversy regarding the need for placing the CSI into the tendon sheath.

Two studies have shown that true intra-sheath injection offers no apparent advantage over subcutaneous injection in the treatment of deQuervain's tenosynovitis [77, 78]. A case was reported of subdermal atrophy following local hydrocortisone injection, which was believed to predispose to the development of cheiralgia paresthetica after wearing a watch [79].

Trigger Finger

A corticosteroid injection into a tendon sheath is a safe and potentially effective treatment for trigger finger (flexor tenosynovitis of the hand) [80–82]. A success rate of nearly 90% with single or multiple CSIs was found in 58 patients with 77 total episodes of trigger finger that were resistant to rest, therapy with nonsteroidal anti-inflammatory drugs, and/or splinting [83]. No adverse effects were encountered. CSIs, however, are not as effective in diabetic patients with trigger fingers, and a relatively high rate of recurrence has been documented [84, 85]. One study reported a 33% rate of recurrence with CSI in the treatment of trigger finger during the first year of follow-up [86]. Ultrasound guidance allows for more accurate targeting of the injection into the tendon sheath or into the actual A-1 pulley mechanism.

Trochanteric Bursitis (Tendonopathy)

There is a paucity of studies on the efficacy of CSI for trochanteric bursitis. The limited available evidence suggests that corticosteroid and lidocaine injections for trochanteric bursitis appear to be an effective and safe therapy with prolonged benefit [87, 88]. One case, however, of necrotizing fasciitis after a trochanteric bursa CSI has been reported [89]. The concept of a chronic tendonopathy of the hip external rotators rather than a true bursitis is an emerging concept.

Achilles Tendonopathy

Although it has been traditionally believed that CSIs are potentially contraindicated in Achilles tendonopathy, this issue remains controversial [90, 91]. The rationale behind the belief that CSIs are contraindicated is that the Achilles tendon is a weight-bearing tendon and CSIs may therefore result in tendon rupture. However, in a retrospective cohort study, 43 patients with Achilles tendinopathy were given low volume peritendinous injections under fluoroscopic guidance and were followed up for 2 years [92]. Neither tendon rupture nor any other major complications was reported, and 40% of the patients continued to report improvement in pain after a 2-year follow-up. This study suggests that, when placed accurately using fluoroscopic guidance, low volume peritendinous CSIs may be safe for patients with Achilles tendinopathy. Ultrasound visualization makes possible other procedures such as PNT and PRP in cases of chronic tendonopathy.

Plantar Fasciitis

There is limited evidence for the effectiveness of local corticosteroid therapy for plantar fasciitis. CSIs seem to be helpful in the short term to a small degree [93, 94]. Moreover, the effectiveness of other frequently employed treatments in altering the clinical course of plantar heel pain has not been established in randomized controlled trials [93, 94].

However, CSIs for plantar fasciitis are associated with a risk of plantar fat pad atrophy and a relatively high risk of plantar fascia rupture [95]. Interestingly, in two studies, ultrasound-guided CSI and palpation-guided CSI of the plantar fascia were found to give significant pain relief on long-term follow up (12 months). Of note, the heel pad was less disturbed, and there was a decrease in recurrence of heel pain for the ultrasound-guided injection as compared to palpation guidance [58, 96, 97].

Side Effects

A summary of side effects associated with CSIs and suggestions to minimize their occurrence are listed in Table 2.3 [98].

Allergic reactions to steroids could be due to preservatives or due to the steroid itself. For example, dexamethasone sodium phosphate contains metabisulphite, a preservative that can cause allergic reactions ranging from anaphylaxis to less severe asthmatic episodes in susceptible individuals. Preservative-free steroids are preferable for use in patients who have multiple allergies.

The literature is much more extensive with respect to allergic reactions from corticosteroids administered orally and parenterally. Allergic reactions due to intra-articular and soft tissue CSIs have been rarely reported [99, 100]. The allergic reactions can vary in range from drug-fixed eruption to severe anaphylaxis [101–103]. Usually, an allergy to one corticosteroid precludes injections with other corticosteroids [101, 102].

It is not clear whether aspirin-sensitive asthmatic patients are as predisposed to corticosteroid-induced allergic reactions from the intra-articular route as they are

Table 2.3 Side effects, complications, and suggestions to minimize complications from intra-articular corticosteroid injections

System	Side effect	Suggestions to minimize chance of complication
Dermatologic	Facial flushing ("steroid flush")	Flush needle tip with local anesthetic or normal saline prior to needle withdrawal from skin
	Skin depigmentation	Check for negative aspirate before the intra-articular injection
	Subcutaneous atrophy	
	Nicolau's syndrome	
Immunologic	Hypersensitivity reactions	Use preservative-free corticosteroid/preservative-free local anesthetic in patients with a history of allergic reactions in general
		Consider prophylaxis prior to the procedure with:
		Prednisone 50 mg po q 6 h × 3, start 18 h before the procedure
		Benadryl® (McNeil-PCC Inc., Fort Washington, PA, USA) 50 mg po 1 h before the procedure
		Epipen® (Mylan, Inc., Pittsburgh, PA, USA) 0.3 mg IM to thigh if having severe allergic reaction (anaphylaxis)
		Consider allergy and immunology consult for possible skin testing in order to determine if patient has corticosteroid or other injectate allergy
Musculoskeletal	Steroid arthropathy	Stay within recommended dosing and duration guidelines
	Avascular necrosis	Consider appropriate imaging (e.g., hip MRI) to rule out early onset avascular necrosis, especially in patients with preexisting risk factors for this condition
	Delayed healing	Always perform injections using sterile technique
	Joint capsule calcification	Only perform if strongly indicated in patients who are predisposed to hematogenous seeding of joints
	Joint infection	
	Direct or Indirect from hemato-genous seeding	
	Osteoporosis	Use judiciously in patients with documented significant osteoporosis
	Tendon/ligament rupture	Do not inject in regions of weight-bearing tendons (e.g., patellar tendon, Achilles' tendon, posterior tibial tendon). Stay within recommended dosing and duration guidelines
	Tachon's syndrome	Check for negative aspirate before the injection
	Post injection steroid flare	Consider some degree of postinjection relative rest and use a preservative-free corticosteroid/local anesthetic particularly in patients with history of worsens pain after previous corticosteroid injections

(continued)

Table 2.3 (continued)

System	Side effect	Suggestions to minimize chance of complication
Endocrine	Adrenal insufficiency	Appropriate laboratory monitoring
	Electrolyte imbalance, especially in patients with diabetes	Stay within recommended dosage and duration guidelines
	Glucose intolerance exacerbation	
	Hypercorticism	
	Disturbance in menstruation	

with systemic administration [104]. This question is of potential clinical importance in aspirin-sensitive asthmatic OA patients because both traditional NSAIDs and COX-2 inhibitors would be contraindicated in these patients. Therefore, they depend more upon CSIs as a treatment for OA flares.

Cutaneous complications include skin depigmentation, subcutaneous atrophy, and facial/neck flushing. They usually occur in less than 1% of patients, and, as mentioned previously, are most common with triamcinolone preparations, particularly triamcinolone acetonide (Kenalog®) [39, 105]. Facial/neck flushing is believed to be due to the systemic absorption of the corticosteroid [106]. It usually occurs rapidly within minutes to hours of the injection and can last for as long as 1–2 days [106]. CSIs into osteoarthritic first CMC joint can cause depigmentation of the overlying skin. Depigmentation can be cosmetically unacceptable in dark-skinned individuals, as it is more recognizable. However, it usually resolves over a period of time [107, 108].

Skin depigmentation is more common in body regions containing a relatively small amount of subcutaneous tissue. For example, cutaneous linear atrophy along the abductor pollicis tendon after a local CSI for de Quervain's tenosynovitis has been reported and personally observed by the senior author (TS) [109]. In comparison, subcutaneous fat atrophy (fat necrosis) usually occurs in regions with a large amount of subcutaneous tissue overlying the given structure (Chap. 1, Figs. 1.2 and 1.3). Unlike skin depigmentation, which is usually temporary, subcutaneous fat atrophy can be permanent [39].

Three cases of Nicolau's syndrome [110] (livedo-like dermatitis due to acute arterial thrombosis occurring immediately after intravascular injection of an insoluble drug substance) induced by intra-articular glucocorticoid injections have been reported [111]. The original cases described by Nicolau were initially referred to as "livedoid dermatitis" and occurred after intramuscular injections of bismuth suspensions to treat syphilis in 1925. Similar manifestations were reported with delayed-action penicillin suspensions and NSAID injections [110].

These cases of Nicolau's syndrome manifested as severe, excruciating pain in the buttock immediately after the injection and rapid development of cyanotic patches. A livedoid pattern followed. The syndrome terminated with a rapid resolution of the pain and a slow clearing of the skin changes in most patients. Three typical cases were also reported after intra-articular CSIs [111]. Symptoms of both severe pain and skin changes were found, along with two other patients who had incomplete variants without skin abnormalities [111]. Each of these five patients had received an injection of a glucocorticoid in a crystalline suspension in or about a joint.

In terms of mechanism of this disorder, the earlier cases seen after bismuth injections were thought to occur due to mechanical blockade of the arteries by the oil-based suspension. In contrast, glucocorticoids, NSAIDs, and penicillins are aqueous suspensions and probably cause acute vascular spasm due to penetration of microcrystals into the vessel. It is, therefore, believed that confirming a negative blood aspirate before injecting the medication may decrease the risk of this disorder.

Endocrine side effects of intra-articular corticosteroids can vary from adrenal crisis due to HPA axis suppression of adrenal function to iatrogenic Cushing's syndrome [112]. Endocrine side effects are due to systemic absorption of the medication and usually occur more commonly with water-soluble corticosteroids and when the corticosteroid is injected into multiple joints. Systemic absorption appears to be related to the absorptive area of the total amount of synovium exposed to the injectate [39].

Orally administered corticosteroids have a higher rate of systemic HPA axis suppression compared to locally administered corticosteroids. HPA axis suppression has been reported to occur within 24 h of a CSI and is maximal at 2–4 days status postinjection [113, 114]. There are no studies available about the maximum safe dose of corticosteroid that can be injected intra-articularly. However, general guidelines based on the size of a given joint have been developed and are shown in Table 2.4.

A typical intra-articular injection suppresses the HPA axis for 2–7 days [39]. As discussed previously, the degree of systemic absorption is enhanced when the same amount of steroid is injected into multiple joints as compared to a single joint. Ideally, only one large joint should be injected at a time, and a gap of at least several weeks between injections should be considered. Repeat injections can cause HPA suppression for up to 3 months and can lead to adrenal insufficiency [115]. Thus, patients who receive a CSI should be covered with appropriate oral replacement corticosteroids if they are to undergo a major surgical procedure, such as total joint replacement.

Hypercorticism has also been reported after CSIs, but not as commonly as has adrenal insufficiency. The literature contains reports of patients who developed signs and symptoms of hypercortisolism that appeared 4–6 weeks after intra-articular administration of triamcinolone acetonide and lasted for 4–6 months [2–116,

Table 2.4 General dosage guidelines for intra-articular corticosteroid injection in osteoarthritis

Joint size	Dosage of methyl prednisolone acetate (mg)	Triamcinolone acetonide (mg)	Dosage of dexamethasone (mg)	Example
Small	5–10	2.5–5	2–4	Interphalangeal
Medium	10–40	5–10	1–2	Elbow, wrist, ankle, AC joint
Large	40–80	10–20	0.8–1	Hip, knee, shoulder

116–119, 119–196]. Manifestations of hypercorticism, such as hypertension and glucose intolerance, have also been noted [39].

Corticosteroids used for intra-articular injections have very little or no mineralocorticoid activity. Though the risk is very small, they may cause fluid and electrolyte disturbances. This is especially true of hydrocortisone acetate, which has definite mineralocorticoid activity (Table 2.2). CSIs can cause sodium retention, fluid retention, and lead to congestive heart failure in susceptible patients. In such patients, CSIs should be used with caution, and corticosteroids with no mineralocorticoid activity (Table 2.2) are preferable; electrolyte blood work can be considered before the procedure. Adrenal insufficiency leading to electrolyte imbalance has also been documented in diabetic patients after intra-articular CSIs [120].

Patients with peripheral polyneuropathy (e.g., diabetic neuropathy) and vascular insufficiency are at high risk to develop Charcot joints. CSIs should be used with caution in this subgroup because of their potential adverse effect on articular cartilage. It can enhance the development of Charcot-like joints, though it is controversial; this will be discussed in detail later in this chapter.

Serum glucose level elevations can occur in diabetic patients undergoing CSIs, particularly when water-soluble preparations are used [119, 196]. The general belief is that intra-articular CSIs cause glucose elevations only in diabetic patients. The only major literature review on this topic concluded that even small intra-articular doses can trigger hyperglycemia and glycosuria [119]. However, this may not be the case for intra-articular CSIs in all diabetic patients [196]. For example, a study of fasting blood glucose levels for 2 weeks in eight diabetic patients after a single injection of 40 mg of methylprednisolone into either the trochanteric bursa or subacromial space did not find any significant increases in glucose levels [121].

Disturbance of menstrual pattern after intramuscular CSIs is well documented [122–124]. In contrast, there have been very few reports in the literature of disturbance of menstruation after intra-articular and periarticular CSIs [117, 118, 125, 126]. In one study, menstrual disturbance was noticed by 39 of the 77 (51%) women who received their first local injection of triamcinolone acetonide [46 intra-articular, 24 in soft tissue (bursa, tendon, tendon sheath), 7 epidural] [125]. In this study, both increased and decreased menstruations were reported. Although the exact mechanism of interference with menstruation is unclear, it likely involves progesterone receptor interaction as has been shown with triamcinolone acetonide [127, 128].

Much has been written about musculoskeletal complications of intra-articular CSIs. The most common is postinjection flare ("steroid flare"), that is, acute postprocedural joint pain and swelling. Postinjection steroid flare is estimated to occur in up to 10% of injections in RA patients, and it is much less common in OA patients [10, 119]. This phenomenon is due to the rapid intracellular ingestion of crystalline steroid ester by PMN cells, and therefore it has been also referred to as "crystalline gout-like arthropathy." [129, 130]

Steroid crystals have been detected in synovial fluid more than 1 month after the injection [131]. Steroid crystals can be confused with other crystals, such as monosodium urate or calcium pyrophosphate, and thus can mistakenly lead to the diagnosis of gout or pseudogout, respectively. Since crystal ingestion by macrophages is believed to be involved, it seems reasonable that it is more common with microcrystalline steroid preparations such as triamcinolone hexacetonide. However, one source has reported that it possibly occurs at a lower frequency with triamcinolone preparations [132]. Likewise, Friedman and Moore found a similar frequency with triamcinolone hexacetonide compared to an equal volume of the vehicle alone [27]. Regardless of mechanism or etiology, a postinjection flare usually begins 6–12 h after the injection and may cause a high degree of inflammation so that it can be easily confused with an iatrogenic joint infection. Synovial fluid pleocytosis with WBC counts exceeding 100,000 cells/mm³ and fever can occur. It usually resolves spontaneously within 1–3 days.

Concomitant lidocaine administration is thought to diminish the chance of this side effect [133, 134]. This issue is not clear-cut, as steroid crystals are thought to precipitate at an increased rate in the presence of the preservative methylparaben. Since single-dose lidocaine does not contain this preservative, the likelihood of steroid flare should be diminished with the use of single-dose (i.e., preservative-free) lidocaine compared with multidose lidocaine [135]. A common recommendation to decrease the chance of a postinjection flare is for patients to limit activity involving the injected joint for 2–3 days after the injection. However, support for this recommendation is lacking.

There is also no absolute consensus on the need for or the duration of activity modification after a corticosteroid injection in order to maximize therapeutic benefit. In knee OA patients, a randomized controlled study suggested benefit with 24-h postinjection bed rest following an intra-articular CSI [136]. Postinjection rest, whether relative or absolute, is believed to increase the retention of corticosteroid in the joint, thereby allowing a longer contact period with the joint surface and delaying the systemic absorption of the corticosteroid [137]. Some physicians also recommend to patients that they ice the affected site every 2 h as needed after the injection. However, this probably has more of an effect upon local postinjection soft tissue pain as compared to a true postinjection flare. A prior postinjection flare is not believed to predict subsequent flares [197].

Perhaps the issue most relevant to OA patients is the potential for "steroid arthropathy" (synovial joint destruction due to intra-articular steroid injections). This is a very controversial topic with conflicting evidence. Reports of steroid arthropathy have appeared in the literature over the years [138–142]. Although the exact incidence of this is still not known, Hollander and colleagues estimated it to be <1% based upon his routine follow-up of 100 patients' records over a 7-year time period [143].

The mechanism of steroid arthropathy is unclear, but there is laboratory evidence from studies in nonprimate OA animal models, especially in rabbits, of a deleterious effect on proteoglycan synthesis [144]. This altered cartilage structural protein biosynthesis is believed to make cartilage more susceptible to injury [144–147]. Another proposed mechanism for steroid arthropathy includes analgesia leading to a Charcot-like joint [148]. However, additional evidence suggests a protective effect of intra-articular CSIs on articular cartilage in guinea pig and dog models of OA [149]. Specifically, there was a marked reduction in size and extent of osteophyte formation in joints that received intra-articular CSIs. Moreover, electron microscopic examination of these joints did not show any evidence of chondrocyte degeneration or death. Hence, whether steroid arthropathy actually occurs is still not settled, but some guidelines have been developed in an attempt to help reduce its potential until the issue is resolved. These guidelines include limiting injections of any one joint to a maximum of 3 times per year and 20 times in a lifetime [150]. However, in a double blind randomized placebo-controlled study, 68 patients with knee OA received a triamnicolone acetonide (34 patients) injection every 3 months for 2 years. The study demonstrated no decrease in joint space narrowing, but a decrease in stiffness and improvement in function as compared to patients who received intra-articular saline (34 patients) [151]. Another recommendation is to limit the frequency of injection into any single joint to at least 3 months intervals [152]. But as discussed earlier, there is a lack of rigorous scientific evidence for these guidelines [153]. In addition to these restrictions, postinjection activity limitations may be useful as the early cases of steroid arthropathy may have actually been due to relative joint overuse because of the pain relief from the injections. Thus, avoiding unduly strenuous postprocedural activity is logical [154].

It is probably prudent to follow dosing and activity restrictions, unless it is ultimately proven that steroid arthropathy does not occur. Some physicians take an even more conservative approach and believe that intra-articular CSIs may be unnecessary since pericapsular or periligamentous injections in areas of tenderness around joints will also provide some benefit [155]. Whether depositing steroid outside the joint per se protects against steroid arthropathy is unknown.

Avascular necrosis (AVN) is another potential CSI-related side effect. In contrast to steroid arthropathy, where the primary pathology is within the cartilage of a synovial joint, the primary pathologic process in AVN involves the subchondral bone, with a secondary effect on the cartilage. This is a rare complication that can occur after administering multiple intra-articular CSIs into a given joint, but this generally does not occur after a single injection [156]. Proposed mechanisms for AVN include steroid-induced articular blood vessel hypercoagulability [157, 158] and/or steroid-induced vasculitis [157]. It is unclear as to whether AVN can occur in a joint remote from the site of the actual CSI. In contrast, AVN of the femoral head is a well-documented potential side effect of oral corticosteroids, especially if used chronically.

Calcification of an overlying joint capsule has been reported with repeated CSI injections. It is most common in the hand, where it is often punctate, asymptomatic, and resorbs spontaneously [159, 160]. It can also be more extensive and become a source of pain and cause a loss of motion [161, 162].

Steroid "chalk" (steroid "paste") on the surface of synovium and cartilage has been reported during surgery involving previously injected OA joints [163]. Although its clinical significance is not clear, analysis of steroid chalk has shown it to be an admixture of preservative-containing steroid and local anesthetic.

Tendon rupture is very rarely attributable to intra-articular CSIs without inadvertent intratendinous injection. There have been case reports in the literature of tendon rupture after soft tissue CSIs, but none have been reported after intra-articular injections [163]. The risk of tendon rupture seems to be the highest in the area of the Achilles tendon [164]. Plantar fascia ruptures have also been reported and have been estimated to be as high as 10% after a steroid injection [165].

There have been rare reports of Tachon's syndrome (highly acute back and thoracic pain after local CSI). In a French study, 318 cases of Tachon's syndrome were reported by 92 rheumatologists (one event per 8,000 injections) following injections into lumbar epidural space, the upper limb, the lower limb, and other locations [166]. Symptoms typically occurred within 1–5 min in more than 75% of the cases and in less than 1 min in the remainder of the cases.

Patients reported highly acute axial pain, which usually lasted for less than 5–15 min in 50% of the cases and less than 5 min in about one third of the cases. Apart from pain in lumbar (84%) and/or dorsal regions (25%), other manifestations were: anxiety (87%), shortness of breath (64%), facial flushing (64%), diffuse sweating (41%), agitation (29%), transient cough (23%), abdominal pain (20%), transient hypertension (15%), paleness (10%), hypotension (8%), diarrhea (3%), and headache (3%). These patients were not known to have any allergy to corticosteroids.

The outcome was favorable in all cases, and only four patients were transiently hospitalized. 146/318 (46%) of cases were given another injection, and Tachon's syndrome recurred in only 20 (14%) patients. The exact mechanism of Tachon's syndrome is not very clear, but it is believed to be the venous equivalent of Nicolau's syndrome with some differences [166].

The authors hypothesized that, in Tachon's syndrome, the usual delay of 5–15 min between injection and the appearance of first clinical signs points toward corticosteroid suspension entering the blood stream through a large vein rather than via direct intra-arterial injection [166]. They theorized that this is due to the fact that these areas have a rich venous plexus (e.g., heel, epidural space) or are under pressure (e.g., epicondyle where tissue is compressed by tendinous insertions). This is controversial since one would expect to see a high incidence of Tachon's syndrome after intravenous corticosteroid administration.

Osteoporosis is a well-known risk of systemic steroids. However, steroid-induced osteoporosis from CSIs is a controversial issue. There are no published studies in the literature comparing pre- and postinjection bone mineral density testing values in OA patients. A study on RA patients revealed a transient 2-week decrease in osteocalcin levels [167]. As osteocalcin is a marker of osteoblast activity, this suggests that repeat intra-articular CSIs may adversely affect bone mass.

Joint infection due to an intra-articular CSI is a potentially serious, but rare, complication. Infection can occur by two main mechanisms (1) direct infection of the joint during the procedure and (2) indirect hematogenous seeding of the joint. Direct infection of the joint can come from endogenous skin flora, in which case it is generally caused by *Staphylococcus aureus* [168, 169]. A study suggested that inserting a needle into a joint can carry a small fragment of skin tissue into the joint space [170]. Bacterial nucleic acid detected by polymerase chain reaction was found in about a third of these cases.

Considering the rarity of joint infection, these findings suggest that bacterium introduced at the time of arthrocentesis is either not viable or quickly cleared in almost all cases. Direct infection can also occur from a contaminated multi-dose corticosteroid vial [171], which can lead to atypical joint infections. Given this possibility, some clinicians emphasize using only single-dose corticosteroid ampules. Indirect infection due to joint seeding is more common in a patient with a systemic infection. Therefore, elective arthrocentesis and/or CSI are relatively contraindicated in a patient with a systemic infection.

Infection rates for injections performed using sterile skin preparation and without masks or gloves have been reported in the range of 1/14,000–50,000 injections [172–174]. In a retrospective study in France, the rate of infection was seven times lower when the corticosteroid was prepackaged in a sterile syringe (1/162,000) as compared to when it was not (1/21,000) [174]. Other issues involving skin preparation and the use of sterile gloves were studied, but no relationship was found between these factors and the incidence of infection [174]. The authors of this chapter agree with the recommendation that drapes and sterile gloves are unnecessary. (Protective gloves are advisable for any invasive procedure.)

Neurological side effects are rare after CSIs as compared to orally administered corticosteroids. In fact, the only CNS side effect that has been reported was a case of frank psychosis after an intra-articular steroid injection [118]. A number of reports of median nerve injury due to direct needle trauma during a CSI for CTS have been described [175–177]. However, peripheral nerve injury due to direct needle trauma following an intra-articular injection is extremely rare. Only one case of saphenous nerve injury following intra-articular viscosupplementation injection for knee OA has been reported in the literature [178].

Although there have been no such reports during CSIs, the authors of that report felt that direct needle trauma during the injection was the cause of the injury and not the particular injectate. Thus, the injury could have just as likely occurred during a CSI. It has been speculated that fluoroscopic guidance may decrease the risk of such injuries by facilitating a more direct entry into the joint and minimize the need to maneuver the needle through soft tissue on the way into the joint [179].

There have been anecdotal reports of ophthalmologic side effects from intra-articular CSIs [39]. Specifically, posterior subcapsular cataracts have been reported in a number of middle-aged patients who have received multiple intra-articular CSIs (Table 2.3).

Contraindications

Joint or soft tissue injections may be contraindicated in certain group of patients who otherwise might benefit from the procedure. As discussed earlier, contraindications could be due to corticosteroids and local anesthetics as well as to the injection itself (Table 2.5).

In summary, CSIs are thought to be beneficial for limited time periods in most patients with OA and for patients with some other musculoskeletal conditions. They

Table 2.5 Contraindications to local anesthetic/corticosteroid injection procedures

Allergy to injectate
Unstable or inaccessible joints
Primary severe coagulopathy
Uncontrolled diabetes
Charcot joint
Generalized infection
Septic arthritis
Lack of response to two or three prior injections
Weight-bearing tendons (e.g., Achilles tendon, patellar tendon)
Osteomyelitis of an adjacent bone
Need for a high degree of anticoagulant therapy
Osteochondral fracture of adjacent bone

are especially used for knee OA flares, particularly if associated with symptomatic effusion or with underlying calcium pyrophosphate deposition disease. This should ideally be used in conjunction with a comprehensive rehabilitation program.

Local Anesthetics

Local anesthetics are generally added to corticosteroids for intra-articular injections so that the synovial membrane lining of the joint can be more fully bathed by the injectate solution. Moreover, they can provide immediate pain relief to the patient and afford treatment feedback information to the physician. The ability of local anesthetics to relieve pain can also be used diagnostically to confirm the source of pain, that is, they can help to identify a pain generator. The short acting local anesthetic, lidocaine, is the most commonly used agent for percutaneous infiltration anesthesia as well as diagnostic blocks and injections.

Mechanism of Action and Pharmacokinetics of Local Anesthetics

Local anesthetics are subdivided into amides (e.g., lidocaine [Xylocaine®, APP Pharamaceuticals, Schaumburg, IL, USA] and bupivacaine [Marcaine®, Hospira, Lake Forest, IL, USA]) and esters (procaine [novocaine]) based upon their chemical structure. Both classes act by increasing electrical excitation threshold and thereby slowing of nerve conduction. Although the exact mechanism for this is not completely clear, sodium channel blockade is believed to be involved. They usually affect small unmyelinated fibers before large myelinated fibers.

After neural blockade, the sense of pain is first lost, followed by temperature, touch, proprioception, and skeletal muscle tone, in that order. Commonly used amino amides include lidocaine [Xylocaine®], mepivacaine [Carbocaine®, Hospira, Lake Forest, IL, USA], prilocaine [Citanest®, AstraZeneca AB, Wilmington, DE, USA], bupivacaine [Marcaine®], etidocaine [Duranest®, AstraZenaca AB, Wilmington, DE, USA], and dibucaine [Nupercainal®, Novartis, Basel, Switzerland]. Commonly used amino esters include tetracaine, procaine (novocaine), chloroprocaine (Nesacaine® APP Pharmaceuticals, Schaumburg, IL, USA), cocaine, and benzocain (Cetacaine® Cetylite Industries, Pennsauken, NJ, USA). Of all the local anesthetics, Marcaine® and lidocaine are the most commonly used agents in clinical practice (Table 2.6).

One easy way to remember which drug belongs in which category is that all of the amino amides contain the letter "i" twice, as does the term "amino amides." Local anesthetics exist in ionized and nonionized forms. Onset of action of local anesthetics is directly proportional to the lipid solubility and inversely proportional to the pKa of the anesthetic; the pH at which ionized and nonionized form exist in equal amounts. It is the nonionized portion that is capable of diffusing across nerve membranes and blocks sodium channels, producing analgesia.

Anesthetics with nonionized portions have a faster onset of action. Local anesthetics differ with respect to the pH at which the ionized and nonionized forms are present at equilibrium. The more closely the pKa for a given anesthetic approaches the physiologic pH of tissues, the more rapid the onset of action.

A decrease in pH shifts equilibrium toward the ionized form, delaying the onset of action. This explains why local anesthetics are slower in onset of action and less effective in the presence of inflammation, which creates a more acidic environment with lower pH. The amides are less allergenic than the ester local anesthetics. Therefore, amides are more frequently used in local and intra-articular as well as spinal injection procedures.

Amides local anesthetics are hepatically metabolized. Hence, patients with hepatic failure or decreased hepatic flow (patients on beta blocker or congestive heart failure) are more sensitive to these agents, and a lower dose should be used in such patients. Ester anesthetics are quickly hydrolyzed by plasma pseudocholineesterase enzymes into para-amino benzoic acid (PABA) and other compounds that are excreted unchanged in the urine. Esters anesthetics are more allergenic, and PABA is a known allergen in susceptible individuals. However, its rapid metabolism lowers the potential for toxicity.

Allergic reactions to amide local anesthetics are usually related to the preservative methylparaben, not to the anesthetic itself. The use of a single-dose preservative-free local anesthetic minimizes the risk of an allergic reaction. Toxicity of local anesthetics usually involves the CNS and the cardiovascular system; it is generally not an issue with joint and soft tissue injection procedures, since the amount of local anesthetic used is relatively small.

Anesthetic potency is directly related to lipid solubility, for example, bupivacaine (Marcaine®) is more lipid-soluble produce analgesia at relatively lower concentration (e.g., 0.25% or 0.5%) as compared with less lipid-soluble local anesthetics, such as lidocaine, which require higher concentration.

The potential cardiovascular side effects associated with epinephrine can be avoided by using local anesthetic solutions without epinephrine. The addition of a vasoconstrictor hastens the onset and improves the quality and duration of action but is not necessary for joint and soft tissue infections [180].

Table 2.6 Common injectable local anesthetics used in clinical practice

Drug (trade name)	Class	Onset	Duration (with epinephrine)	Usual dosage joint injection small (large)	Maximum dose (with epinephrine)
Lidocaine (Xylocaine®, APP Pharamaceuticals, Schaumburg, IL, USA)	Amide	Rapid (½–1 min)	½–1 h (2 h)	1/2–2 (2–9 ml)	4.5 mg/kg (7 mg)
Bupivacaine (Marcaine®, Hospira, Lake Forest, IL, USA; Sensorcaine®, APP Pharmaceuticals, Schaumburg, IL, USA)	Amide	Slow (5 min)	2–4 h (8 h)	1–2 (2–4 ml)	2.5 mg/kg (3 mg)

Contrast Agents: Omnipaque™ (GE Healthcare, Waukesha, WI, USA)

Background Information

Omnipaque™ (iohexol) is a colorless to pale-yellow radiographic contrast agent used to enhance visualization during radiographic procedures. Omnipaque™ may be used for intrathecal, intravascular, and oral/body cavity injection procedures. It is a nonionic, water-soluble solution that contains iodine. Compared to conventional ionic contrast agents, which are hypertonic (high osmolality), nonionic contrast agents are considered to be safer agents mainly due to their reduced tonicity. The reason for the increased osmolality in ionic contrast agents is due to the fact that they dissociate and yield two solute particles per molecule of the original substance when dissolved with water, blood, or cerebral spinal fluid [181].

Comparison Among Contrast Agents

Omnipaque™ was compared with two ionic contrast agents: Hexabrix® 320 (Mallinckrodt, St. Louis, MO, USA) (ioxaglate sodium meglumine) and isopaque (metrizoate) in knee arthrography [182]. Postprocedural pain was noted by 10/39 (25.6%) patients in the Omnipaque™ group, 20/39 (51.3%) patients in the Hexabrix® group, and 24/38 (63.2%) patients of the isopaque group. The study suggested that the substantially lower postprocedural pain with Omnipaque™ was due to its non-ionicity [183] and the absence of sodium salts [184].

Omnipaque™ was compared with another nonionic contrast agent, Amipaque® (Sanofi Pharmaceuticals, Bridgewater, NJ, USA) (metrizamide), in a study involving lumbar myelography[1]. The results indicated that Omnipaque™ displayed generally the same capabilities as Amipaque®, but with a notably lesser rate of morbidity than Amipaque®. Headaches, nausea, and vomiting were common, but there was a greater incidence of these in the Amipaque® group than the Omnipaque™ group. Headaches were reported in 36/175 (21%) patients using Omnipaque™ as opposed to 67/175 (38%) patients using Amipaque®. Nausea was reported in 17/175 (10%) Omnipaque™ patients and 29/175 (17%) Amipaque® patients. Vomiting was noted in 5/175 (3%) Omnipaque™ patients but in 14/175 (8%) Amipaque® patients.

A study compared the morbidity between the use of Omnipaque™ and Hypaque® (GE Healthcare, Princeton, NJ, USA) (meglumine diatrizoate) in temporomandibular joint (TMJ) arthrography [185]. The study indicated that, although one contrast agent was nonionic and the other was ionic, there was no major statistical discrepancy in pain during or after the injection procedure.

None of the patients from either of the Omnipaque™ or Hypaque® groups complained of pain during injection. Pain 30 min postinjection was reported in 7/20 patients from the Omnipaque™ group and in 5/20 patients from the Hypaque®

group. At the 24-h postinjection mark, seven Omnipaque™ patients experienced pain while 11 patients experienced pain in the Hypaque® group. Thus, the conclusion from this study was that, in the TMJ, the ionicity of the contrast agent did not make any substantial statistical difference in procedural-related pain.

Pharmacokinetics

The pharmacokinetics of Omnipaque™ has been extensively reviewed elsewhere [186]. Summarized herewith is information that is most relevant to the musculoskeletal medicine physician. Distribution and elimination of Omnipaque™ is dependent upon its route of administration. Specifically, for most body cavities, the injection of Omnipaque™ is taken up by the neighboring tissue and excreted by the kidneys and bowel. For intravascular injections, Omnipaque™ is dispersed in the extracellular fluid compartment and is eliminated by glomerular filtration.

Urine concentrations are at their height 1-h postinjection, and roughly 90% of the injected dose is eliminated from the system within the first 24 h. When administered by the intrathecal route, Omnipaque™ is absorbed by the cerebral spinal fluid into the blood stream and eliminated via renal excretion. After administration into the lumbar subarachnoid space and tracked using computerized tomography, contrast medium was found in the thoracic region in about 1 h, in the cervical region in approximately 2 h, and in the basal cisterns in 3–3 h.

Side Effects

Compared to conventional ionic contrast agents such as Hypaque® and Conray® (Mallinckrodt, St. Louis, MO, USA) (meglumine iothalamate), Omnipaque™ and other nonionic contrast agents have been shown to have less systemic toxicity and neurotoxicity [187]. In addition, preliminary data indicate that nonionic contrast agents cause less patient discomfort, if they are inadvertently injected intra-arterially during a musculoskeletal injection procedure [188]. The hyperosmolality of the ionic contrast agents significantly increases their toxic effects, whereas the low osmolality of the nonionic contrast agents such as Omnipaque™ at 300 mg/mL iodine is equal to the osmolality of blood, thus being safer contrast agents.

Side effects of Omnipaque™ have been extensively reviewed elsewhere [186, 189–195]. Although the occurrence of such incidences are relatively low, the most common side effects due to the use of Omnipaque™ are headaches, nausea, vomiting, mild to moderate pain, stiffness, backaches, and neckaches. Reactions typically present themselves within the first 10-h postinjection and almost all take place within 24-h postinjection. The side effects will persist for only a few hours and should cease within 24 h.

For body cavity injections, the most frequent complaint was pain and swelling, which was mainly due to the procedure itself rather than the use of Omnipaque™. The use of iodine-containing contrast agents (including Omnipaque™) has been linked to serious and life-threatening side effects, with the main source being cardiovascular in origin. Although a feeling of warmth and pain can occur due to the injection of contrast agents in general, these are not as common or as serious with Omnipaque™ compared to several other contrast agents.

Summary and Conclusion

Office-based musculoskeletal injection procedures most often involve a local anesthetic, as part of preprocedural skin and soft tissue anesthesia and/or as part of the injection itself, and a corticosteroid preparation. Fluoroscopic-guided procedures also generally include a contrast agent such as Omnipaque.™ Contrast agents are available in both ionic and nonionic forms. The nonionic ones such as Omnipaque™ seem to be preferable with respect to potential side effects including postprocedural pain. While several different choices of local anesthetics are available, perhaps the most commonly injected ones include two amides, the short-acting agent lidocaine and the long-acting agent Marcaine®. Serious toxicity can result from doses exceeding the recommended ones and from inadvertent intravascular injection. Several different injectable corticosteroid preparations are available, with durations ranging from short-acting to long-acting depending upon their degree of lipid solubility. Although their potential side effects vary somewhat depending upon the exact preparation, most of them are common to all corticosteroid preparations. Controversy still exists regarding the existence of steroid arthropathy and issues such as the optimal amount of postprocedural rest, if any, to help limit postinjection flares and to maximize therapeutic benefit. Other injectable agents such as viscosupplements are discussed elsewhere in this book.

References

1. Hollander JL. Prednisone and prednisolone: newest corticosteroids. Merck Rep 1955; 64(4):3–7.
2. Siegmeth W, Krepelka M, Supper A. Intra-articular injections in arthrosis of the small and medium size joints. Wiener Medizinische Wochenschrift 1995;145(5):117–9.
3. Stefanich RJ. Intra-articular corticosteroids in treatment of osteoarthritis. Orthop Rev 1986; 15:65–71.
4. Eymontt MJ, Gordon GV, Schumacher HR, Hansell JR. The effects on synovial permeability and synovial fluid leukocyte counts in symptomatic osteoarthritis after intraarticular corticosteroid administration. J Rheumatol 1982;9(2):198–203.
5. Goetzl EJ, Bianco NE, Alpert JS, Sledge, CB, Schur PH. Effects of intra-articular corticosteroids in vivo on synovial fluid variables in rheumatoid arthritis. Ann Rheum Dis 1974;33:62–6.
6. Hunder GC, McDuffie FC. Effect of intra-articular hydrocortisone on complement in synovial fluid. J Lab Clin Med 1972;79:62–74.

7. Mazanec DJ. Pharmacology of corticosteroids in synovial joints. Phys Med Rehabil Clin North Am 1995;6:815–21.
8. Butler WT, Rossen RD. Effects of corticosteroids on immunity in man. J Clin Invest 1973;52:2629–40.
9. Fauci AS, Dale DC, Balow JE. Glucocorticoid therapy: mechanisms of action and clinical considerations. Ann Intern Med 1976;84:304–15.
10. Saxon A, Stevens RH, Ramer SJ. Glucocorticoids administered in vivo inhibit human suppressor T lymphocyte function and diminish B lymphocyte responsiveness in vitro immunoglobulin synthesis. J Clin Invest 1977;60:922–30.
11. Pelletier JP, McCollum R, DiBattista J, Loose LD, Cloutier JM, Martel-Pelletier J. Regulation of human normal and osteoarthritic chondrocyte interleukin-1 receptor by antirheumatic drugs. Arthritis Rheum 1993;36:1517–27.
12. Ito K, Lim S, Caramori G, Cosio B, Chung KF, Adcock IM, Barnes PJ. A molecular mechanism of action of theophylline: induction of histone deacetylase activity to decrease inflammatory gene expression. Proc Natl Acad Sci USA 2002;99(13):8921–6. Epub 2002 Jun 17.
13. Creamer P. Intra-articular corticosteroid injections in osteoarthritis: do they work and if so, how? Ann Rheum Dis 1997;56:634–6.
14. Klint E, Grundtman C, Engstrom M, Catrina AI, Makrygiannakis D, Klareskog L et al. Intraarticular glucocorticoid treatment reduces inflammation in synovial cell infiltrations more efficiently than in synovial blood vessels. Arthritis Rheum 2005;52(12):3880–9.
15. Gray RG, Tenenbaum J, Gotlieb NL. Local corticosteroid treatment in rheumatic disorders. Semin Arthritis Rheum 1981;10:231–54.
16. Meikle AW, Tyler FH. Potency and duration of action of glucocorticoids: effects of hydrocortisone, prednisone and dexamethasone on human pituitary-adrenal function. Am J Med 1978;63:200.
17. Centeno LM, Moore ME. Preferred intraarticular corticosteroids and associated practice: a survey of members of the American College of Rheumatology. Arthritis Care Res 1994;7(3):151–5.
18. Olin BR. Hormones. Adrenal corticosteroids. In Olin BR, ed. Facts and Comparisons. St. Louis: Wolters Kluwer; 1993:465–86.
19. Pyne D, Ioannou Y, Mootoo R, Bhanji A. Intra-articular steroid in knee osteoarthritis: a comparative study of triamcinolone hexacetonide and methylprednisolone acetate. Clin Rheumatol 2004;23(2):116–20.
20. Bird HA, Ring EFJ. Therapeutic value of arthroscopy. Ann Rheum Dis 1978;37:78–9.
21. Lane NE, Thompson JM. Management of osteoarthritis in the primary-care setting: an evidence-based approach to treatment. Am J Med 1997;103(6A):25S–30S.
22. Bellamy N, Campbell J, Welch V, Gee TL, Bourne R, Wells GA. Intraarticular corticosteroid for treatment of osteoarthritis and the knee (Review). Cochrane Database Syst Rev 2005; 2:CD005328.
23. Arroll B, Goodyear-Smith F. Corticosteroid injections for osteoarthritis of the knee: meta-analysis. BMJ 2004;328:86.
24. Jones A, Doherty M. Intra-articular corticosteroids are effective in osteoarthritis but there are no clinical predictors of response. Ann Rheum Dis 1996;55:829–32.
25. Gaffney K, Ledingham J, Perry JD. Intra-articular hexacetonide in knee osteoarthritis: factors influencing the clinical response. Ann Rheum Dis 1995;54:379–81.
26. Dieppe PA, Sathapatayavavongs B, Jones HE, Bacon PA, Ring EFJ. Intra-articular steroids in osteoarthritis. Rheumatol Rehabil 1980;19:212–17.
27. Friedman DM, Moore ME. The efficacy of intra-articular steroids in OA; a double blind study. J Rheumatol 1980;7:850–6.
28. Ravaud P, Moulinier L, Giraudeau B. Effects of joint lavage and steroid injection in patients with osteoarthritis of the knee: results of a multicenter, randomized controlled trial. Arthritis Rheum 1999;42(3):475–82.
29. Godwin M, Dawes M. Intra-articular steroid injections for painful knees. Can Fam Physician 2004;50:241–8.

30. McAlindon TE, Cooper C, Kirwan JR, Dieppe PA. Determinants of disability in osteoarthritis of the knee. Ann Rheum Dis 1993;52:258–62.
31. Robinson P, Keenan AM, Conaghan PG. Clinical effectiveness and dose response of image-guided intra-articular corticosteroid injection for hip osteoarthritis. J Rheumatol 2005; 32(7):1305–6.
32. Flanagan J, Casale FF, Thomas TL, Desai KB. Intraarticular injection for pain relief in patients awaiting hip replacement. Ann R Coll Surg Engl 1988;70:156–7.
33. Qvistgaard E, Christensen R, Torp-Pedersen S, Bliddal H. Intraarticular treatment of hip osteoarthritis: a randomized trial of hyaluronic acid, corticosteroid and isotonic saline. Osteoarthr Cartil 2006;14(2):163–7.
34. Kullenberg B, Runesson R, Tuvhag R, Olsson C, Resch S. Intraarticular corticosteroid injection: pain relief in osteoarthritis of the hip. J Rheumatol 2004;31(11):2265–8.
35. Plant MJ, Borg AA, Dziedzic K, Saklatvala J, Dawes PT. Radiographic patterns and response to corticosteroid hip injection. Ann Rheum Dis 1997;56:476–80.
36. Margules KR. Fluoroscopically directed steroid instillation in the treatment of hip osteoarthritis: safety and efficacy in 510 cases. Arthritis Rheum 2001;44:2449–50.
37. Leveaux VM, Quin CE. Local injections of hydrocortisone and procaine in osteoarthritis of the hip. Ann Rheum Dis 1956;15:330.
38. Dieppe PA. Are intra-articular steroid injections useful for the treatment of the osteoarthritis joint? Br J Rheum 1991;30:199.
39. Gray RG, Gottlieb NL. Intra-articular corticosteroids: an updated assessment. Clin Orthop Relat Res 1983;177:235–62.
40. Meenagh GK, Patton J, Kynes C, Wright GD A randomized controlled trial of intra-articular corticosteroid injection of the carpometacarpal joint of the thumb in osteoarthritis. Ann Rheum Dis 2004;63:1260–63.
41. Joshi R. Intra-articular corticosteroid injection for first carpometacarpal osteoarthritis. J Rheumatol 2005;32(7):1305–6.
42. Dodge LR, Brown RL, Niebauer JJ, McCaroll HR. The treatment of mucous cysts: long term follow up in sixty two cases. J Hand Surg 1984;9A:901–4.
43. Breidahl WH, Adler RS. Ultrasound guided injection of ganglia with corticosteroids. Skeletal Radiol 1996;25(7):635–8.
44. Arrol B, Goodyear- Smith F. Corticosteroid injections for painful shoulder; a metaanalysis. Br J Gen Pract 2005;55(512):224–8.
45. Slipman CW, Lipetz JS, Wakeshima Y, Jackson HB. Nonsurgical treatment of zygapophyseal joint cyst-induced radicular pain. Arch Phys Med Rehabil 2000;81(7):973–7.
46. Buchbinder R, Green S, Youd JM. Corticosteroid injections for shoulder pain. Cochrane Database Syst Rev 2003;(1):CD004016.
47. Carrera GF, Williams AL. Current concepts in evaluation of the lumbar facet joints. Crit Rev Diagn Imaging 1984;21(2):85–104.
48. Helbig T, Lee CK. The lumbar facet syndrome. Spine 1988;13(1):61–4.
49. Revel ME, Listrat VM, Chevalier XJ, Dougados M, N'guyen MP, Vallee C et al. Facet joint block for low back pain: identifying predictors of a good response. Arch Phys Med Rehabil 1992;73(9):824–8.
50. Murtagh FR. Computed tomography and fluoroscopically guided anesthesia and steroid injection and facet syndrome. Spine 1992;13:686–9.
51. Slipman CW, Bhat AL, Gilchrist RV, Issac Z, Chou L, Lenrow DA. A critical review of the evidence for the use of zygapophysial injections and radiofrequency denervation in the treatment of low back pain. Spine J 2003;3(4):310–6.
52. Carette S, Marcoux S, Truchon R, Grondin C, Gagnon J, Allard Y. Controlled trial of corticosteroid injections into facet joints for chronic low back pain. [Randomized controlled trial]. N Eng J Med 1991;325(14):1002–7.
53. Shih C, Lin GY, Yueh KC, Lin JJ. Lumbar zygapophyseal joint injections in patients with chronic lower back pain. J Chin Med Assoc 2005;68(2):59–64.

54. Sabers SR, Ross SR, Grogg BE, Lauder TD. Procedure-based nonsurgical management of lumbar zygapophyseal joint cyst-induced radicular pain. Arch Phys Med Rehabil 2005; 86(9):1767–71.
55. Lutz GE, Shen TC. Fluoroscopically guided aspiration of a symptomatic lumbar zygapophyseal joint cyst: a case report. Arch Phys Med Rehabil 2004;85(12):2071–2.
56. Khoury NJ, el-Khoury GY, Saltzman CL, Brandser EA. Intraarticular foot and ankle injections to identify source of pain before arthrodesis. AJR Am J Roentgenol 1996;167(3):669–73.
57. Tallia AF, Cardone DA. Diagnostic and therapeutic injection of the ankle and foot. Am Fam Physician 2003;68(7):1356–62.
58. Robinson P, Keenan AM, Conaghan PG. Clinical effectiveness and dose response of image-guided intra-articular corticosteroid injection for hip osteoarthritis. Rheumatology (Oxford) 2006 Jul 26 online.
59. Rifat SF, Moeller JL. Basics of joint injection: general techniques and tips for safe, effective use. Postgrad Med 2001;109(1):157–160, 165–166.
60. Korthals-de Bos IB, Smidt N, van Tulder MW, Rutten-van Mölken MPMH, Adèr HJ, van der Windt DAWM et al. Cost effectiveness of interventions for lateral epicondylitis: results from a randomised controlled trial in primary care. Pharmocoeconomics 2004;22(3): 185–95.
61. Smidt N, Smidt N, Assendelft WJ, van der Windt DA, Hay EM, Buchbinder R et al. Corticosteroid injections for lateral epicondylitis: a systematic review. Pain 2002;96(1–2):23–40.
62. Smidt N, van der Windt DAWM, Assendelft WJJ, Deville WLJM, Korthals-de Bos IB, Bouter LM. Corticosteroid injections, physiotherapy, or a wait-and-see policy for lateral epicondylitis: a randomized controlled trial. Lancet 2002;359(9307):657–62.
63. Verhaar JA, Walenkamp GH, van Mameren H, Kester AD, van der Linden AJ. Local corticosteroid injection versus Cyriax-type physiotherapy for tennis elbow. J Bone Joint Surg Br 1996;78(1):128–32.
64. Korthals-de Bos IB, Smidt N, van Tulder MW, Rutten-van Mölken MPMH, Adèr HJ, van der Windt DAWM et al. Cost effectiveness of interventions for lateral epicondylitis: results from a randomised controlled trial in primary care. Pharmocoeconomics 2004;22(3):185–95.
65. Stahl S, Kaufman T. The efficacy of an injection of steroids for medial epicondylitis: a prospective stud of sixty elbows. J Bone Joint Surg Am 1997;79(11):1648–52.
66. Stahl S, Kaufman T. Ulnar nerve injury at the elbow after steroid injection for medial epicondylitis. J Hand Surg 1997;22(1):69–70.
67. Richards RR, Regan WD. Medial epicondylitis caused by injury to the medial antebrachial cutaneous nerve: a case report. Can J Surg 1989;32(5):366–367, 369.
68. Marshall S. Carpal tunnel syndrome. Clin Evid 2002;(8):1060–74.
69. Agarwal V, Singh R, Sachdev A, Wiclaff, Shekhar S, Goel D. A prospective study of the long-term efficacy of local methyl prednisolone acetate injection in the management of mild carpal tunnel syndrome. Rheumatology 2005;44(5):647–50.
70. Celiker R, Arslan S, Inanici F. Corticosteroid injection vs. nonsteroidal antiinflammatory drug and splinting in carpal tunnel syndrome. Am J Phys Med Rehabil 2002;81(3):182–6.
71. O'Gradaigh D, Merry P. Corticosteroid injection for the treatment of carpal tunnel syndrome. Ann Rheum Dis 2000;59(11):918–9.
72. Richie CA, Briner WW Jr. Corticosteroid injection for treatment of de Quervain's tenosynovitis: a pooled quantitative literature evaluation. J Am Board Fam Pract 2003;16(2):102–6.
73. Anderson BC, Manthey R, Brouns MC. Treatment of De Quervain's tenosynovitis with corticosteroids. A prospective study of the response to local injection. Arthritis Rheum 1991; 34(7):793–8.
74. Richie CA, Briner WW Jr. Corticosteroid injection for treatment of de Quervain's tenosynovitis: a pooled quantitative literature evaluation. J Am Board Fam Pract 2003;16(2):102–6.
75. Anderson BC, Manthey R, Brouns MC Treatment of De Quervain's tenosynovitis with corticosteroids. A prospective study of the response to local injection. Arthritis Rheum 1991;34(7):793–8.

76. Witt J, Pess G, Gelberman RH. Treatment of de Quervain's tenosynovitis. J Bone Joint Surg Am 1991;73:219–22.
77. Apimonbutr P, Budhraja N. Suprafibrous injection with corticosteroid in de Quervain's disease. J Med Assoc Thai 2003;86(3):232–7.
78. Taras JS, Raphael JS, Pan WT, Movagharnia F, Sotereanos DG. Corticosteroid injections for trigger digits: is intrasheath injection necessary? J Hand Surg Am 1998;23(4):717–22.
79. Chodoroff G, Honet JC. Cheiralgia paresthetica and linear atrophy as a complication of local steroid injection. Arch Phys Med Rehabil 1985;66(9):637–9.
80. Murphy D, Failla JM, Koniuch MP. Steroid versus placebo injection for trigger finger. J Hand Surg Am 1995;20(4):628–31.
81. Benson LS, Ptaszek AJ. Injection versus surgery in the treatment of trigger finger. J Hand Surg Am 1997;22(1):138–44.
82. Nimigan AS, Ross DC, Gan BS. Steroid injections in the management of trigger fingers. Am J Phys Med Rehabil 2006;85(1):36–43.
83. Anderson B, Kaye S. Treatment of flexor tenosynovitis of the hand ("trigger finger") with corticosteroids. A prospective study of the response to local injection. Arch Intern Med 1991;151(1):153–6.
84. Nimigan AS, Ross DC, Gan BS. Steroid injections in the management of trigger fingers. Am J Phys Med Rehabil 2006;85(1):36–43.
85. De Wolf AN, Mens JM. Localized corticosteroid injections for the "rigger finger": good short-term results, but with a great likelihood of recurrence. Ned Tijdschr Geneeskd 1998; 142(20):1168–9 (Dutch).
86. Van Ijsseldijk AL, de Wilt JH, Lameris TW, Brouwer KJ. Topical corticosteroid injection for trigger finger: good short-term results, but fairly high risk of recurrence. Ned Tijdschr Geneeskd 1998;142(20):1168–9.
87. Shbeeb MI, O'Duffy JD, Michet CJ Jr, O'Fallon WM, Matteson EL. Evaluation of glucocorticosteroid injection for the treatment of trochanteric bursitis. J Rheumatol 1996;23(12):2104–6.
88. Ege Rasmussen KJ, Fano N. Trochanteric bursitis: treatment by corticosteroid injection. Scand J Rheumatol 1985;14(4):417–20.
89. Hofmeister E, Englehardt S. Necrotizing fasciitis as complication of injection into greater trochanteric bursa. Am J Orthop 2001;30(5):426–7.
90. Shrier I, Matheson GO, Kohl HW(III). Achilles tendonitis: are corticosteroid injections useful or harmful? Clin J Sport Med 1996;6(4):245–50.
91. Linke E. Achilles tendon ruptures following direct cortisone injection. Hefte Unfallheilkd 1975;121:302–3 German.
92. Gill SS, Gelbke MK, Mattson SL, Anderson MW, Hurwitz SR. Fluoroscopically guided low-volume peritendinous corticosteroid injection for Achilles tendinopathy. A safety study. J Bone Joint Surg Am 2004;86A(4):802–6.
93. Crawford F, Atkins D, Edwards J. Interventions for treating plantar heel pain. Cochrane Database Syst Rev 2000;3:CD000416.
94. Crawford F, Thomson C. Interventions for treating plantar heel pain. Cochrane Database Syst Rev 2003;3:CD000416.
95. Sellman JR. Plantar fascia rupture associated with corticosteroid injection. Foot Ankle Int 1994;15(7):376–81.
96. Tsai WC, Hsu C-C, Chen CPC, Chen MJL, Yu T-Y, Chen Y-J. Plantar fasciitis treated with local steroid injection: comparison between sonographic and palpation guidance. J Clin Ultrasound 2006;34(1):12–16.
97. Tsai WC, Wang C-L, Tang F-T, Hsu T-Z, Hsu K-H, Wong M-K. Treatment of proximal plantar fasciitis with ultrasound-guided steroid injection. Arch Phys Med Rehabil 2000; 81(10):1416–21.
98. Stitik TP, Foye PM, Chen B, Nadler SF. Joint and soft tissue corticosteroid injections: a practical approach. Consult Prim Care 2000;40(8):1469–75.
99. Peller JS, Bardana EJ Jr. Anaphylactoid reaction to corticosteroid: case report and review of the literature. Ann Allergy 1985;54(4):302–5.

100. Ijsselmuiden OE, Knegt-Junk KJ, van Wijk RG, van Joost T. Cutaneous adverse reactions after intra-articular injection of triamcinolone acetonide. Acta Derm Venereol 1995;75(1):57–8.

101. Mace S, Vadas P, Pruzanski W. Anaphylactic shock induced by intraarticular injection of methylprednisolone acetate. J Rheumatol 1997;24(6):1191–4.

102. Pollock B, Wilkinson SM, MacDonald Hull SP. Chronic urticaria associated with intra-articular methylprednisolone. Br J Dematol 2001;144(6):1228–30.

103. Sener O, Caliskaner Z, Yazicioglu K, Karaayvaz M, Ozanguc N. Nonpigmenting solitary fixed drug eruption after skin testing and intra-articular injection of triamcinolone acetonide. Ann Allergy Asthma Immunol 2001;86(3):335–6.

104. Preuss L. Allergic reactions to systemic glucocorticoids: a review. Ann Allergy 1985;55(6): 772–5.

105. Millard RS, Dillingham MF. Peripheral joint injections. Phys Med Rehabil Clin North Am 1995;3:841–849.

106. Gottlieb NL, Riskin WG. Complications associated with locally injected microcrystalline corticosteroid esters. JAMA 1980;243:1547.

107. George WM. Linear lymphatic hypopigmentation after intralesional corticosteroid injection: report of two cases. Cutis 1999;64(1):61–4.

108. Kumar P, Adolph S. Hypopigmentation along subcutaneous veins following intrakeloid triamcinolone injection: a case report and review of literature. Burns 1998;24(5):487–8.

109. Canturk F, Canturk T, Avdin F, Karagoz F, Senturk N, Turanli AY. Cutaneous linear atrophy following intralesional corticosteroid injection in the treatment of tendonitis. Cutis 2004;73(3):197–8.

110. Corazza M, Capozzi O, Virgilit A. five cases of livedo-like dermatitis (Nicolau's syndrome) due to bismuth salts and various other non-steroidal anti-inflammatory drugs. J Eur Acad Dermatol Venereol 2001;15(6):585–8.

111. KaCherasse Ahn MF, Mistrih R, Maillard R, Maillard H, Strauss J et al. Nicolau's syndrome after local glucocorticoid injection. Joint Bone Spine 2003;70(5):390–2.

112. Wicki J, Droz M, Cirafici L, Vallotton MB. Acute adrenal crisis in a patient treated with intraarticular steroid therapy. J Rheumatol 2000;27:510–1.

113. Cahill BR. Atraumatic osteolysis of the distal clavicle. A review. Sports Med 1992;13:214–22.

114. Kay NR, Marshall PD. A safe, reliable method of carpal tunnel injection. J Hand Surg 1992;17A:1160–1.

115. Reid DM, Eastmond C, Rennie JAN. Hypothalamic-pituitary adrenal axis suppression after repeated intra-articular steroid injections. Ann Rheum Dis 1986;45:87.

116. Kumar S, Singh RJ, Reed AM, Lteif AL. Cushing's Syndrome after intraarticular and intra-dermal administration of Triamcinolone Acetonide in three pediatric patients. Pediatrics 2004;113(6):1820–4.

117. Robinson DE, Harrison- Hansley E, Spencer RF. Steroid pyschosis after an intra-articular steroid injection. Ann Rheum Dis 2000;59:927.

118. Gray RG, Tenenbaum J, Gotlieb NL. Local corticosteroid treatment in rheumatic disorders. Semin Arthritis Rheum 1981;10:231–54.

119. O'Sullivan MM, Rumfeld WR, Jones MK, Williams BD. Cushing syndrome suppression of hypothalamic–pituitaryadrenal axis after intraarticular steroid injection. Ann Rheum Dis 1985;44:561–3.

120. Gray RG, Gottlieb NL. Rheumatic disorders associated with diabetes mellitus: literature review. Semin Arthritis Rheum 1976;6:19–34.

121. Slotkoff AT, Clauw DJ, Nashel DJ. Effects of soft tissue corticosteroid injection on glucose control in diabetics, Arthritis Rheum 1994;37:S347.

122. Romanski B, Pawlik K, Wilewska-Klubo T. The use of triamcinolone acetonide in the treat-ment of severe intrinsic bronchial asthma. Allergol Immunopathol 1978;6:321–4.

123. Willey RF, Fergusson RJ, Godden DJ, Crompton GK, Grant IW. Comparison of oral prednisolone and intramuscular depot triamcinolone in patients with severe chronic asthma. Thorax 1984;39:340–4.

124. Cunningham GR, Goldzieher JW, de la Pena A, Oliver M. The mechanism of ovulation inhibition by triamcinolone acetonide. J Clin Endocrinol Metab 1978;46:8–14.
125. Mens JM, Nico De Wolf A, Berkhout BJ, Stam HJ. Disturbance of menstrual pattern after local injection with triamcinolone acetonide (letter). Ann Rheum Dis 1998;57:700.
126. Jansen TL, Van Roon EN. Four cases of a secondary Cushingoid state following local triamcinolone acetonide(Kenacort) injection. Neth J Med 2002;60(3):130–2.
127. Cuchacovich M, Tchernitchin A, Gatica H, Wurgaft R, Valenzuela C, Cornejo E. Intraarticular progesterone: effects of a local treatment for rheumatoid arthritis. J Rheumatol 1988;15: 561–5.
128. Brann DW, McDonald JK, Putnam CD, Mahesh VB. Regulation of hypothalamic gonado-tropin-releasing hormone and neuropeptide Y concentrations by progesterone and corticos-teroids in immature rats; correlation with luteinizing hormone and follicle-stimulating hormone release. Neuroendocrinology 1991;54:425–32.
129. Berger RG, Yount WJ. Immediate "steroid flare" from intraarticular triamcinolone hexac-etonide injection: case report and review of the literature. Arthritis Rheum 1990;33: 1284–6.
130. McCarty DJ, Hogan JM. Inflammatory reaction after intrasynovial injection of microcrystal-line adrenocorticosteroid esters. Arthritis Rheum 1964;7:359.
131. Kahn CB, Hollander JL, Schumacher HR. Corticosteroid crystals in synovial fluid. JAMA 1970;211:807.
132. Emkey RD, Lindsay R, Lyssy J, Weisberg JS, Dempster DW, Shen V. The systemic effect of intra-articular corticosteroid on markers of bone formation and bone resorption in patients with rheumatoid arthritis. Arthritis Rheum 1996;39:277–82.
133. Birrer RB. Aspiration and corticosteroid injection. Practical pointers for safe relief. Phys Sports Med 1992;20:57–71.
134. Kive P. The etiology and conservative treatment of humeral epicondylitis. Scan J Rehabil Med 1982;15:37–41.
135. Gordon GV, Schumacher HR. Electron microscopy study for depot corticosteroid crystals with clinical studies after intra-articular injection. J Rheumatol 1979;6:7–14.
136. Chakravarty K, Pharoah PDP, Scott DGI. A randomized controlled study of post-injection rest following intra-articular steroid therapy for knee synovitis. Br J Rheumatol 1994;33:464–8.
137. Neustadt DH. Intra-articular corticosteroids and other agents: aspiration techniques. In Katz W, ed. The Diagnosis and Management of Rheumatic Diseases. Second ed. Philadelphia, PA: J.B. Lippincott; 1988:812–25.
138. Sweetnam DR, Mason RM, Murray R. Steroid arthropathy of the hip. Br Med J 160;1:1392–4.
139. Murray RO. Steroids and the skeleton. Radiology 1961;77:729–43.
140. Steinberg CL, Duthric RB, Piva AE. Charcot-like arthropathy following intraarticular hydro-cortisone. JAMA 1962;181:851–2.
141. Alarcon-Segovia D, Ward LE. Marked destructive changes occurring in osteoarthritic finger joints after intraarticular injection of steroids. Arthritis Rheum 1966;9:443.
142. Miller RT, Restifo RA. Steroid arthropathy. Radiology 1966; 86:652–7.
143. Hollander JL, Jessar RA, Brown EM. Intrasynovial corticosteroid therapy: a decade of use. Bull Rheum Dis 1961;11:239.
144. Mankin HJ, Conger KA. The acute effects of intraarticular hydrocortisone on articular carti-lage in rabbits. J Bone Jt Surg 1966;48A:1383–8.
145. Annefeld M. The dose dependent effect of glycosaminoglycan peptide complex on corticosteroid-induced disordered metabolism in cartilage tissue of rats. [English] Der dosi-sabhangige Effekt vom Glycosaminoglycan-Peptid-Komplex auf den durch Corticosteroide gestorten Stoffwechsel in Knorpelgeweben von Ratten. [German] Zeitschrift fuer Rheumatologie 1989;48(4):188–93.
146. Robion FC, Doize B, Boure L, Marcoux M, Ionescu M, Reiner A et al. Use of synovial fluid markers of cartilage synthesis and turnover to study effects of repeated intra-articular administration of methylprednisolone acetate on articular cartilage in vivo. J Orthop Res 2001;19(2):250–8.

147. Celeste C, Ionescu M, Robin Poole A, Laverty S. Repeated intraarticular injections of triamcinolone acetonide alter cartilage matrix metabolism measured by biomarkers in synovial fluid. J Orthop Res 2005;23(3):602–10. Epub 2004 Dec 21.
148. Chandler GM, Jones DT, Wright V, Hartfall SJ. Charcot's arthropathy following intraarticular hydrocortisone. British Med J 1959;1:952–3.
149. Pelletier JP, Martel-Pelletier J. Protective effects of corticosteroids on cartilage lesions and osteophyte formation in the pond-nuki dog model of osteoarthritis. Arthritis Rheum 1989; 32:181–93.
150. Beary JP. Osteoarthritis. In Beary JP, Christian CL, Johanson NA, eds. Manual of Rheumatology and Outpatient Orthopedic Disorders: Diagnosis and Therapy. Boston, MA: Little, Brown and Company; 1987:187–98.
151. Raynauld JP. Safety and efficacy of long-term intra-articular steroid injections in osteoarthritis of the knee. Arthritis Rheum 2003;48(2):370–7.
152. Neustadt DH. Intraarticular steroid therapy. In Moskowitz RW, Howell DS, Goldberg VM, Mankin HJ, eds. Osteoarthritis: Diagnosis and Medical/Surgical Management. Philadelphia, PA: WB Saunders; 1992:493–510.
153. Hochberg MC, Altman RD, Brandt KD, Clark BM, Dieppe PA, Griffin MR et al. Guidelines for the medical management of osteoarthritis. Arthritis Rheum 1995;38(11):1535–46.
154. Mazanec DJ. Pharmacology of corticosteroids in synovial joints. Phys Med Rehabil Clin North Am 1995;6:815–21.
155. Rodnan GP, Schumacher HR, Zvaifler NJ, eds. Osteoarthritis. In Primer on the Rheumatic Diseases. Eighth edition. Atlanta, GA: The Arthritis Foundation; 1983:104–8.
156. Hollander JL. Intrasynovial corticosteroid therapy in arthritis. Maryland State Med J 1972; 19:62–6.
157. Miller RT, Restifo RA. Steroid arthropathy. Radiology 1966;86:652–7.
158. Murray RO. Steroids and the skeleton. Radiology 1961;77:729–43.
159. McCarty DJ, Hogan JM. Inflammatory reaction after intrasynovial injection of microcrystalline adrenocorticosteroid esters. Arthritis Rheum 1964;7:359.
160. Hardin JG. Controlled study of the long term effects of "total hand" injection (abstract). Arthritis Rheum 1979;22:619.
161. Balch HW, Gibson JMC, El Ghobarey AF, El-Ghobarey AF, Bain LS, Lynch MP. Repeated corticosteroid injections into knee joints. Rheumatol Rehabil 1977;16:137–40.
162. Jalava S. Periarticular calcification after intra-articular traimcinolone hexacetonide. Scand J Rheumatol 1980;9:190–2.
163. Owen DS Jr. Aspiration and injections of joints and soft tissues. In Kelly WN, ed. Text Book of Rheumatology. Philadelphia, PA: WB Saunders; 1981:553–67.
164. Acevedo JI, Beskin JL. Complications of plantar fascia rupture associated with corticosteroid injection. Foot Ankle Int 1998;19(2):91–7.
165. Acevedo JI, Beskin JL. Complications of plantar fascia rupture associated with corticosteroid injection. Foot Ankle Int 1998;19(2):91–7.
166. Pfenninger JL. Injections of joints and soft tissue I: general guidelines. Am Fam Physician 1991;44:1196–202.
167. Kasten SJ, Louis DS. Carpal tunnel syndrome: a case of median nerve injection injury and a safe and effective method for injecting the carpal tunnel. J Fam Pract 1996;43(1):79–82.
168. Glaser DL, Schildorn JC, Bartolozzi AR, Dennis R, Li Y, Amato TR et al. Do you know what is on the tip of your needle? The inadvertent introduction of skin in to the joint. Arthritis Rheum 2000; 43:S149.
169. Stefanich RJ. Intra-articular corticosteroids in treatment of osteoarthritis. Orthop Rev 1986; 15:65–71.
170. Greer III RB. Into the knee with needle and steroids [editorial]. Orthop Rev 1993;22(12):1302.
171. Hollander JL. Intrasynovial corticosteroid therapy in arthritis. Med J 1970;19:62.
172. Gray RG, Tenenbaum J, Gotlieb NL. Local corticosteroid treatment in rheumatic disorders. Semin Arthritis Rheum 1981;10:231–54.
173. Pal B, Morris J. Perceived risks of joint infection following intra-articular corticosteroid injections: a survey of rheumatologists. Clin Rheumatol 1999;18:264–5.

174. Seror P, Pluvinage P, Lecoq d'Andre F, Benamour P, Attuil G. Frequency of sepsis after local corticosteroid injection (an inquiry on 1 160 000 injections in rheumatological private practice in France). Rheumatology 1999;38:1272–4.

175. Frederick HA, Carter PR, Littler JW. Injection injuries to the median and ulnar nerves at the wrist. J Hand Surg (Am) 1992;17(4):645–7.

176. McConnell JR, Bush DC. Intraneural steroid injection as a complication in the management of carpal tunnel syndrome. A report of three cases. Clin Orthop Relat Res 1990;(250):181–4.

177. Iizuka M, Yao R, Wainapel S. Saphenous nerve injury following medial knee joint injection: a case report. Arch phys Med Rehabil 2005;86(10):2062–5.

178. Foye PM, Stitik TP. Fluoroscopic guidance during injections for osteoarthritis. Arch Phys Med Rehabil 2006;87(3):446–7.

179. Green S, Buchbinder R, Glazier R, Forbes A. Systematic review of randomised controlled trials of interventions for painful shoulder; selection criteria, outcome assessment and efficacy. Br J Gen Pract 1998; 316(7128):354–60.

180. Covino BG. Pharmacology of local anaesthetic agents. Br J Anaesth 1986 Jul;58(7): 701–16.

181. Kieffer SA, Binet EF, Dairs DO, et al. Lumbar myelography with iohexol and metrizamide: a comparative multicenter prospective study. Invest Radiol 1986;20:522–30.

182. Obermann WR, Gerard JK. Knee Arthrography: a comparison of iohexol, ioxaglate sodium meglumine, and metrizoate1. Radiology 1987;162:729–33.

183. Laerum F. Acute damage to human endothelial cells by brief exposure to contrast media in vitro. Radiology 1983;147:681–4.

184. Hall FM, Goldberg RP, Wyshak G, Kilcoyne RF. Shoulder arthrography: a comparison of morbidity after use of various media. Radiology 1985;154:339–41.

185. Kaplan PA, Lieberman RP, Chu WK. Comparison of omnipaque with hypaque in temporomandibular arthrography. Am J Roentgenol 1989;153:1225–7.

186. "Omnipaque™ (iohexol) Injection 240 300 350." Daily Med 24 May 2006. http://dailymed. nlm.nih.gov/dailymed/fdaDrugXsl.cfm?id=707&type=display 28 September 2006.

187. Almén T. Angiography with metrizamide. Animal experiments and preliminary clinical experiences. Acta Radiol (Suppl) 1977;355:419–30.

188. Skalpe IO. Adverse effects of water-soluble contrast media in myelography, cisternography and ventriculography. A review with special reference to metrizamide. Acta Radiol (Suppl) 1977;355:369–70.

189. Kieffer SA, Binet EF, Dairs DO et al. Lumbar myelography with iohexol and metrizamide: a comparative multicenter prospective study. Invest Radiol 1986;20:522–30.

190. Obermann WR, Gerard JK. Knee Arthrography: a comparison of iohexol, ioxaglate sodium meglumine, and metrizoate1. Radiology 1987;162:729–33.

191. Laerum F. Acute damage to human endothelial cells by brief exposure to contrast media in vitro. Radiology 1983;147:681–4.

192. Hall FM, Goldberg RP, Wyshak G, Kilcoyne RF. Shoulder arthrography: a comparison of morbidity after use of various media. Radiology 1985;154:339–41.

193. Kaplan PA, Lieberman RP, Chu WK. Comparison of omnipaque with hypaque in temporomandibular arthrography. Am J Roentgenol 1989;153:1225–7.

194. Almén T. Angiography with metrizamide. Animal experiments and preliminary clinical experiences. Acta Radiol (Suppl) 1977;355:419–30.

195. Skalpe IO. Adverse effects of water-soluble contrast media in myelography, cisternography and ventriculography. A review with special reference to metrizamide. Acta Radiol (Suppl) 1977;355:369–70.

196. Owen DS. Aspiration and injection of joints and soft tissues. In Kelly WN, Harris ED, Ruddy S, Sledge CB, eds. Textbook of Rheumatology. Fourth Ed. Philadelphia: PA: WB Saunders; 1993:545.

197. Caruso I, Montrone F, Fumagelli M, Patrono C, Santandrea S, Gandini MC. Rheumatoid knee synovitis successfully treated with intraarticular rifamycin SV. Ann Rheum Disease 1982;41:232–6.

Chapter 3
Viscosupplementation

Todd P. Stitik, Jong H. Kim, Gregory Gazzillo, and Charles Lee

Introduction

Viscosupplementation is the intra-articular (IA) injection of hyaluronic acid (HA, aka hyaluronans, sodium hyaluronans, or hyaluronates) into synovial joints for the relief of osteoarthritic pain. HAs are only FDA approved for the treatment of pain associated with knee osteoarthritis (OA). In contrast, outside the US, HAs are generally approved for the treatment of pain of OA in all joints. Because evidence is accumulating to support the use of HAs in joints in addition to the knee, FDA approval for use in other joints, particularly the hips, may be forthcoming.

Mechanism of Action

HAs play an important role in the extracellular matrix of virtually every organ system. Within synovial joints, they are the major component of synovial fluid and comprise part of the structure of hyaline cartilage. In the setting of OA, both the concentration and molecular weight (MW) of HAs decrease. This leads to a decrease in the beneficial effects of HAs within both the synovial fluid and within cartilage.

Synovial fluid has the important rheological (mechanical) properties of viscosity ("lubrication" such as with range of motion), elasticity ("shock absorption" or "cushioning" such as when one steps off of a curb), a mechanical barrier effect (by which HAs block nociceptor agonists by "coating" nociceptors to form a protective barrier, thereby preventing pain mediators from directly activating nociceptors [1]), and a mechanical sponge effect within a joint [2] (by binding or entangling particulate debris in the osteoarthritic joint). In the osteoarthritic joint, all four of these

T.P. Stitik (✉)
Department of Physical Medicine and Rehabilitation, New Jersey Medical School,
Newark, NJ, USA
e-mail: todd.stitik@gmail.com

properties (i.e., viscosity, elasticity, mechanical barrier effect, and mechanical sponge effect) are believed to be deficient. Definite proof of viscosity and elasticity reduction has in fact been shown in the OA joint [3]. Decreased absolute hyaluronan concentration as well as a decrease in the average MW of the native hyaluronan account for these reductions [4, 5]. The original term "viscosupplementation" was coined to describe the effect that restoration of the hyaluronan concentration would have on improving (i.e., supplementing) viscosity, thereby improving the lubricating and cushioning properties of the synovial fluid to a more healthy state. In addition, it is theorized that the rapid clearance of injected HA results in removal of these deleterious substances from the joint space by acting as a mechanical sponge. However, there is no direct evidence to support this hypothesis.

Loss of hyaluronans from the extracellular matrix of the cartilage impacts dramatically negatively on its structural integrity, with a resultant reduced ability to resist stress and shear forces. Cartilage then "breaks down" more readily and perhaps cannot reconstitute itself as well as it can in the non-OA joint.

The term "viscosupplementation," however, ignores the other important biological properties of synovial fluid, which are adversely affected in OA and improved with intra-articular administration of hylauronates. Evidence that these additional nonmechanical effects are playing a role in the analgesic effects of viscosupplementation comes from the simple fact that the viscosupplements have a residence time in the joint on the order of days before clearance out of the joint, but the clinical effect is often on the order of months.

Accordingly, there are two proposed broad categories of mechanism(s) of action by which HAs elicit pain relief: viscoelastic and biological (Table 3.1). There is a substantial body of evidence that a combination of both of these broad mechanisms is involved.

There are several different biological effects of HAs as shown in Table 3.2. Among these biological effects is a clinically significant anti-inflammatory effect. Some proof for this is a double-blind, saline-controlled study of 110 patients with knee OA who received four weekly intra-articular injections of Hyalgan® (Sanofi-Aventis, Bridgewater, NJ, USA) or saline [6]. At 4 weeks after the last injection, patients who received Hyalgan® had significantly less synovial effusions compared

Table 3.1 Proposed mechanisms of action of viscosupplements

Biological effects	Anti-inflammatory [6, 57, 76, 81–108]
	Antioxidant [85, 93–96, 109]
	Cartilage and chondrocytes [58, 110–112]
	Hyaluronate: Restoration of endogenous synthesis via a positive feedback mechanism [8–10, 113, 114]
	Immune cells: Favorable effects [78, 98–100, 102, 103, 115–117]
Viscoelastic properties	Anti-nociceptive effect [1, 118–121]
	"Mechanical spongy" trapping of immune complexes and inflammatory cells, thereby facilitating their removal [2]
	Restoration of synovial fluid viscosity and elasticity, both immediately and up to 3–7 days after the injection [13, 76, 122–131]

Table 3.2 FDA-approved viscosupplements

Viscosupplements trade name (US generic name)	Composition	Injections per cycle	Molecular weight (kDa)	Labeling Precaution on retreatment efficacy/safety
Hyalgan® (Sanofi-Aventis, Bridgewater, NJ, USA) (sodium hyaluronate)	Sodium hyaluronate, naturally derived, purified HA	3 or 5	500–730	No
Synvisc® (Genzyme Corporation, Cambridge, MA, USA) (hylan GF-20)	Hylan polymers derived from HA and chemically modified to enhance viscosity	3[a]	6,000 + gel	No
Supartz® (Smith & Nephew, London, UK) (sodium hyaluronate)	Sodium hyaluronate, naturally derived, purified HA	3 or 5	620–1,170	Yes
Orthovisc® (Anika Therapeutics, Inc., Bedford, MA, USA) (high molecular weight hyaluronan)	Sodium hyaluronate naturally derived, purified HA	3 or 4	1,100–2,900	Yes
Euflexxa® (Ferring Pharmaceuticals, Inc., Saint-Prex, Switzerland) (1% sodium hyaluronate)	Fermented, bacterial streptococcus derived HA	3	2,600–3,400	Yes

[a] At the time of this writing, an application was being considered by the FDA for a one injection cycle of Synvisc® (Synvisc-one)

with saline-control patients, suggesting a lesser degree of inflammation. This anti-inflammatory effect may be partly responsible for joint effusion resolution that is often seen during a viscosupplementation treatment cycle. Another potentially very important biological effect is a possible cartilage protective (chondroprotective) effect. A specific receptor (CD 44 receptor) has been identified that binds to exogenously administered HA and can distinguish between HAs of varying MW. One publication found that an HA of MW 500–730 kDa (i.e., Hyalgan®) may be more effective at inhibiting metalloproteinases (matrix metalloproteinases MMPs, enzymes produced by synovial cells and by chondrocytes that are involved in cartilage catabolism) associated with cartilage degradation [7].

The production of newly synthesized HA appears to be facilitated by exogenous HA in a dose-dependant fashion [8]. The mechanism appears to involve HA binding to chondrocytes via the CD44 receptor. This binding has been shown to mediate the function and proliferation of the chondrocytes [9]. Exogenous HA administered to arthritic cell cultures has been shown to lead to an increase in synovial membrane cells (synoviocytes) and to the production of HAs of near normal MW [10]. This finding of hyaluronan with a MW larger than that of the injected solution and in the range of normal synovial fluid hyaluronan in the synovial fluid of treated joints has been shown in both human and equine studies [11, 12]. This "re-education of the synovial cell" is most likely what is responsible for the perpetuated improvement in rheologic properties that has been demonstrated in spite of relatively rapid clearance of exogenous HA from the joint. Smith and Ghosh found that the efficacy of HA production by cultured fibroblasts was conditional upon the concentration and MW of the exogenous HA [8]. Both the very low (i.e., <500 kD) and very high (i.e., >4,000 kD) MW exogenous HA preparations were not as effective at stimulating endogenous HA production. A model to explain the above observation hypothesizes that there is weak binding to receptors by HA of very low MW, and that there is a limitation of the number of sites that can be occupied on the cell surface via steric hindrance from HA molecules of very high MW.

Efficacy

Prior to their use in humans, HAs were used in Europe to treat posttraumatic OA in racehorses. They are so efficacious for equine arthritis that they are considered to be the treatment of choice in this setting [13–18].

Proof of Overall Efficacy

In humans, there have been multiple clinical trials demonstrating the overall efficacy of hylauronates. Many of the more salient studies published during and prior to 2000 have been summarized elsewhere [19], whereas those studies after

2000 were summarized in a different publication [20]. There have also been several large meta-analyses that support the use of HAs for painful knee OA. At the time of this writing, the largest meta-analyses, the Cochrane meta-analysis, also concluded that the HA class was effective [21]. The effect size ranged from modest to large and equivalent to or superior to effect sizes historically reported for standard-of-care oral analgesics. HAs are also cited as a valid treatment option in the American College of Rheumatology (ACR) 2000 treatment guidelines for knee OA and by the Orthopedic Consensus Conference on the use of HAs [22, 23].

When Should HAs Be Used?

The issue of when to use an HA in a knee OA patient is a very practical clinical question with which a physician is often faced. Although physicians who are less familiar with HAs may choose to use them later on in the disease course, patients at all stages of OA have reported benefits of pain relief. Relatively, early use of HAs is consistent with the FDA-approved indication that states that, for OA knee pain, HAs should be used in patients who have failed to obtain adequate and sustained relief from nonpharmacologic treatment and simple analgesics such as acetaminophen (Tylenol®, McNeil-PPC, Fort Washington, PA, USA). For example, a patient with early stage knee OA who is still having pain despite attempts at exercise and weight loss and regular use of acetaminophen is considered to be a candidate for HAs. Because HAs appear to have distinct mechanisms of action, they can be used prior to prescription pain medications, as an adjunct therapy, or after failure of one or more courses of oral pain medications. At least one study suggests that early use may be best. Specifically, patients with symptoms of moderate to severe pain but less severe OA staging (modest or no joint space narrowing on standing X-rays) were the ones who were most successfully treated [24].

At the time of this writing, there are five HAs that have been approved under separate filings with the FDA (Table 3.2). While there are clear distinctions regarding manufacturing, dosing, MW, treatment regimens, approved labeling, and even biological activity in vitro, there is no consistent evidence from well-controlled clinical studies documenting a superiority of efficacy of one viscosupplement over another. However, the quantity and quality of the clinical evidence supporting each of these is distinct.

Long-Term Efficacy Studies

A prospective cohort study in a clinical rheumatology practice was conducted to evaluate the duration of efficacy of five weekly injections of Hyalgan® in patients with moderate to severe knee OA whose pain was not controlled by conventional measures [25]. Some patients reported a clinical response greater than 2 years after completion of their treatment. Almost 75% of patients who were considering total knee replacement (TKR) surgery before the study either no longer required the surgery or significantly delayed it. Of the patients who required a repeat treatment course, 67% had improvement at the completion of the second series. In terms of safety, there were only minor and infrequent local adverse events.

Kolarz and colleagues performed a multicenter, open-label observational study, evaluating the long-term benefits of Hyalgan® administered once weekly for 5 weeks [26]. Starting from 1 week after the last injection, significant improvements were noted with pain on movement and rest measured by the VAS and Likert scales, walking time, knee function, and global assessment of efficacy. Of the 108 enrolled patients, 59 (55%) improved enough whereby they did not require a second injection cycle during the 12-month study. The HA was found to be safe and well tolerated. Only 4 of 108 withdrew from the study because of AEs.

A prospective cohort study evaluated the long-term efficacy and safety of five weekly IA injections of Hyalgan® in patients with moderate to severe knee OA whose pain was not controlled by conventional measures. Total knee replacement surgery was avoided or significantly delayed in 15 of 19 patients who were considering surgery prior to the injections [25].

These two studies are consistent with the personal experience of one of the authors (TS) who agrees that patients who receive an HA often postpone the need for TKR. Some in fact have yet to undergo a TKR even years later and instead elect to continue to receive periodic cycles of viscosupplementation.

Another study that examined efficacy over 52 weeks found that, in direct comparison to saline for weeks 0–52, neither hyaluronan treatment (Supartz®, Smith & Nephew, London, UK) or Synvisc® (Genzyme Corporation, Cambridge, MA, USA) showed a significantly longer duration of clinical benefit than placebo [27]. However, when data for the two hyaluronan-treated groups were pooled, treatment with hyaluronan had a significantly longer duration of benefit compared with saline ($P = 0.047$).

A prospective open-label study evaluated the efficacy and tolerability of a second course of Synvisc® for the treatment of osteoarthritic knee pain over a 12-month period in patients who previously experienced a beneficial initial course of therapy [28]. All efficacy parameters significantly improved ($P < 0.001$) from baseline until the end of the 52-week study. Interestingly, the mean time between the first and second courses of Synvisc® was 19.6 months. Patients were administered the second course of Synvisc® when they requested it.

These two studies are also in keeping somewhat with both the personal experience of one of the authors (TS) and experience from a clinical trial in which many patients report pain relief for over 1 year from the time of a five injection cycle regimen [29]. However, in the senior author's experience with viscosupplementation since its FDA approval in 1997, a 19.6-month interval between cycles of viscosupplementation represents an uncharacteristically long time interval. This suggests that the patient population in this study was perhaps quite atypical in terms of its response to this treatment intervention.

Concomitant Use of HAs with Other Forms of Treatment

Appropriate Care with HAs vs. Appropriate Care Without HAs

Raynauld and coworkers performed a prospective, randomized open-label, 1-year, multicenter trial to evaluate the efficacy of "appropriate care with hylan G-F 20" compared to "appropriate care without Synvisc®" [30]. The appropriate care with HA group did significantly better in regards to WOMAC pain scale ($P = 0.0001$) than the appropriate care group alone. Significant improvements with appropriate care plus HA were also found with WOMAC, stiffness, and physical function as well as SF-36 aggregate physical component and Health Utilities Index Mark 3 overall health utility score (all $P < 0.0001$). This finding that adding viscosupplementation to other appropriate care provided additional benefit is consistent with the ACR 2000 Guidelines that recommend a combination of pharmacologic and nonpharmacologic treatment as the optimal way of managing patients with osteoarthritis.

Efficacy When Combined With Therapeutic Exercise

Both therapeutic exercise and viscosupplementation are generally recognized as effective interventions for knee OA. The concomitant use of these, however, has not been explored in detail. Bayramoglu and colleagues compared the efficacy of low MW HA plus physical therapy, vs. high MW HA plus physical therapy, vs. physical therapy alone in a pilot study of 37 patients with knee OA [31]. There was a significant reduction in the index of severity in all the three groups. This was not attributable to a strengthening effect, as there were no significant differences in pretreatment vs. post-treatment isokinetic muscle strength by the end of the 3-month study. While this study did not find an efficacy difference between a physical therapy program and IA HA, it did show that the combination of the two was effective. Another study of the combined effect of therapeutic exercise and HA administration examined the effects of a home exercise quadriceps strengthening program (HEP) consisting of quad sets and wall slides combined with IA HA [29]. A total of 60 patients were randomized into one of three groups as follows: 3 IA HA (Hyalgan®) and HEP group (3-HYL + HEP), 3 IA HA (Hyalgan®) group (3-HYL), and 5 IA HA (Hyalgan®) group (5-HYL). By the end of the 1-year study, the 3-HYL + HEP group significantly outperformed the 3-HYL group and performed almost as well as the 5-HYL with respect to pain relief. All three groups demonstrated significant improvements in pain compared to baseline. This study suggests that the addition of quadriceps strengthening exercises to HAs augments the benefit of HAs to the point where the efficacy of a three-injection regimen combined with exercise approaches that of a five-injection regimen.

This integrated approach to managing knee OA using a combination of therapeutic exercise and viscosupplementation as well as pulsed ultrasound was examined and compared to a control group and two other treatment groups that received either exercise only or exercise and pulsed ultrasound [32]. While all of the treatment groups showed improvements in various parameters compared to the control group and compared to their baseline values, the group that also received viscosupplementation did the best overall.

Although these studies are small, they are of potential major significance to musculoskeletal physiatrists. Therapeutic exercise is of obvious importance, and interventions that can possibly augment the effect of this intervention are of interest.

HAs Compared to Other Forms of Treatment

HA vs. Steroid

Bellamy and colleagues conducted a meta-analysis that reviewed intra-articular corticosteroids for the treatment of knee OA [33]. Within this review, there was a comparison made between IA HA and IA corticosteroids. The meta-analysis failed to show a statistically significant difference at 1–4 weeks after the injection. However, the HAs were found to be more effective than the corticosteroids between 5 and 13 weeks postinjection. The authors concluded that HA had a similar onset of action compared with corticosteroids but showed a more prolonged beneficial effect. These findings are quite consistent with known properties of both corticosteroid injections and HAs.

Effect of HAs on Muscle Strength

Tang and colleagues studied the effects of Supartz® on concentric and eccentric quadriceps muscle strength in patients with bilateral knee OA [34]. Knee muscle strength was recorded between 10° and 90° of knee flexion at angular velocities of 80° and 240° per second. Isokinetic eccentric muscle strength increased significantly at both speeds after HA injections ($P < 0.01$), while concentric flexion strength at the angular speed of 240° per second failed to reach statistical significance. The authors concluded that, in knee OA patients with an Ahlback grading scale of I or II, there may be an improvement in quadriceps muscle contraction strength (concentric and eccentric) after five weekly intra-articular knee injections of HA. Whether this increase in strength is clinically significant was not addressed by this study. Perhaps, however, a muscle strengthening effect from viscosupplementation in part explains its analgesic effect, as quadriceps weakness has been found to correlate with knee OA pain [35] and quadriceps strengthening has been found to lead to a reduction in knee pain [36–38].

As noted earlier, Bayramoglu and coworkers found no significant quadriceps or hamstring muscle strengthening effect from either PT alone or PT combined with HAs [31]. The finding of pain relief without a strengthening effect was also seen in the senior author's (TS) study of viscosupplementation and quad strengthening noted earlier [29]. It should be noted, however, that strength in both of these studies was measured isokinetically, whereas exercises were performed nonisokinetically. The discrepancy in how the exercises were performed compared to how strength was assessed may have accounted for the lack of demonstrable strengthening. Alternatively, the analgesic effect from viscosupplementation probably does not rely upon any strengthening that may occur from this treatment.

Effect of HAs on Knee Mechanics

Yavuzer and colleagues investigated the effects of a single course of three bilateral IA Synvisc® injections on the biomechanics of 12 patients with Kellgren and Lawrence grade II or III osteoarthritic knees [39]. At 1-week post-HA treatment, the total WOMAC score and pain subscore significantly improved. There were also significant improvements in sagittal plane excursions of the knee, extensor and adductor moments, and in scaled vertical forces. Given the improvement in these biomechanical characteristics, it was hypothesized by the authors of that study that the resultant decrease in excessive loads in the knees can "alter the natural history of the disease." While this hypothesis lacks confirmation, it perhaps serves as one possible explanation for the proposed chondroprotective effects of viscosupplements as discussed later in this chapter on the effect of HAs on articular cartilage quality.

Efficacy of HA With Lavage

Vad and colleagues evaluated the difference in efficacy between a single-needle knee lavage 1 week before the standard Synvisc® protocol of three injections vs. three injections of Synvisc® alone [40]. There was a significant improvement in outcomes favoring the group that received lavage prior to the viscosupplementation. These results were similar to those found in a study by Forster and Straw, which studied the effects of Hyalgan® [41]. While lavage is not routinely performed prior to HA administration, its beneficial effect does support the general recommendation of aspirating an effusion prior to administering an HA, as aspiration helps remove any inflammatory mediators that might be present within the joint and therefore might potentially diminish the effectiveness of the HA by degrading and diluting its concentration.

Repeat Cycles

There are no randomized controlled trials investigating the efficacy of intra-articular HAs used in repeated cycles. In general, however, intra-articular HAs are viewed by many as a potentially effective and safe long-term therapeutic option

[26, 28, 42]. The patients who are the most logically appropriate candidates for retreatment include those who had an initial beneficial response to the HA without any adverse effects. Although studies have been done with intervals spanning at least 4 months up to over 1 year from time of last treatment cycle, most insurance plans mandate a minimal duration between injections of 6 months [26, 28].

Repeat cycles of Hyalgan® were reported in a study by Scali [43]. This 30-month open design study to assess the efficacy and tolerability of repeated courses of treatment with HA every 6 months in 75 patients found that there was a 31% incremental mean spontaneous VAS over the five treatment cycles. In addition, neither local nor systemic adverse events were observed. This study is extremely relevant to clinical practice given the time course of this chronic disease process and the subsequent desirability to administer repeat treatment courses to those patients who respond.

Hyalgan® was trialed in 537 patients [42]. Of those patients, all but 21 returned for a second injection series. The authors interpreted this to mean that Hyalgan® was effective and acceptable enough to the patients that they would consider a repeat injection. The author concluded that intra-articular HA is an effective long-term therapeutic option for patients with knee OA. One author (TS) of this review also has had the personal experience in his clinical practice that patients who benefit from this treatment are generally willing to repeat it indefinitely as long as they continue to derive benefit from it. At the time of this writing, he has a patient in his practice who has received yearly injections with consistent efficacy for the last 8 years [44].

Waddell and colleagues conducted a prospective open label study to evaluate the efficacy of a repeat course of Synvisc® in patients who had already benefited from an initial course [28]. The average time until the second course was 19.6 months. The authors believed that repeated use of HA is supported by their study. Although this conclusion appears to be valid in this particular patient population, caution should be exercised so as to not overinterpret the findings from a patient population that had already responded to this intervention.

Prognostic Factors

Studies have been performed in order to attempt to determine which factors are related to a good clinical outcome after HA treatments [25, 40, 45, 46]. This is an important clinical management question, and additional data of this type may ultimately help to answer the frequently asked question by patients regarding the likelihood that they will improve.

Using Synvisc®, Conrozier and coworkers identified [45] factors that were significantly ($P < 0.5$) associated with good outcome. These included the physical exam finding of a moderate joint effusion, a lateral retropatellar injection approach, and the radiographic findings of joint space loss in a single compartment and meniscal calcinosis [45].

In addition to studying the effects of lavage prior to viscosupplementation, Vad and colleagues described factors associated with poor outcome. They found that moderate to severe patellofemoral arthritis and knee OA with radiological grade IV were negative prognostic factors [40].

Toh and coworkers performed a prospective cohort study to determine which radiographic changes were associated with a poor outcome after treatments with HA [46]. They used Orthovisc® (Anika Therapeutics, Inc., Bedford, MA, USA) for this study. A blinded observer rated the X-rays for general severity, alignment, severity of joint space narrowing, tibial spine morphology, sclerosis, osteophytes, and cyst formation at 12-weeks posttreatment. These changes were correlated to the WOMAC index for the respective subjects. Patients with only minor medial and lateral joint space narrowing demonstrated significant improvement. Patients in whom the osteoarthritic changes were moderate to severe did not significantly benefit from HA. In contrast, patients with moderate to severe knee osteoarthritis whose pain was not controlled by conventional measures had significant long-term benefit from one or two series of five weekly injections of Hyalgan® [25].

Side Effects

The safety of viscosupplementation has been well established throughout the years. This safety has been confirmed again by a very comprehensive (76 clinical studies with HAs) meta-analysis that concluded that the HA class was safe [21]. Iti, in fact, generally considered to be safer than other pharmacologic therapies for knee OA [47–50]. This is very clinically important, particularly in light of evidence that chronic use of some oral analgesics may be contraindicated in certain patient populations. Viscosupplements are inherently safe for a couple of important reasons. First, because HAs have no known hyaluronate-medication interactions, they are particularly appealing for those patients in whom the physician does not want to contribute to polypharmacy, often seen in elderly patients. Furthermore, they are a local therapy without systemic side effects, except in the extremely rare case of hypersensitivity to hyaluronates. The type and frequency of local side effects is dependent upon the chemical properties of the given viscosupplement. In brief, there are really two classes of viscosupplements: cross-linked and non-cross-linked. Non-cross-linked viscosupplements are simply sodium hyaluronate of differing MWs. In contrast, a cross-linked viscosupplement is comprised of sodium hyaluronate molecules that are chemically linked together by chemical bonds. In the case of the cross-linked viscosupplement Synvisc®, these chemical links are composed of formaldehyde and divinyl sulfone. Chemical cross-linking significantly increases the MW of the viscosupplement but also can lead to a unique local side effect known as a severe acute inflammatory reaction (SAIR) or pseudosepsis [47, 49, 51]. This reaction should not be confused with either an anaphylactoid or pseudogout-like reaction that can occur with any HA injections. In contrast, pseudosepsis presents similar to a septic knee, but synovial fluid and blood cultures are subsequently negative, hence the name pseudosepsis. The general requirement for a prior exposure as well as the development of antibodies to chicken proteins and Synvisc® suggest an immunologic mechanism for the SAIR [47, 52]. The typical scenario is that a patient who has been administered Synvisc® generally presents in 24–72 h complaining of pain, swelling, and stiffness in the injected knee(s). The differential diagnosis of this condition would then include an iatrogenic knee infection, crystalline deposition (particularly pseudogout), and a pseduoseptic reaction. The clinician can best make this distinction by aspirating the knee, visually inspecting the fluid, and sending it for laboratory analysis (including gram stain, culture, cell count, and crystal examination). Table 3.3 shows the fluid characteristics for the three scenarios. An SAIR will typically produce a very cloudy fluid (sometimes with a greenish discoloration). The treatment of a pseudoseptic reaction includes relative rest, ice, oral antiinflammatory medications, knee aspiration, and corticosteroid injection, once the clinician is certain that infection has been excluded.

Although the majority of SAIRs are temporary events, a report of six cases of chronic granulomatous inflammation after administration of IA Synvisc® has been published by Chen and colleagues [53]. Goldberg and Coutts felt that such granulomas represent a possible chronic sequelae after a pseudoseptic reaction and that these may require significant clinical intervention [51]. A case was also reported that initially confused a mass from a granulomatous reaction with a pseudosarcoma [54].

Other than SAIRs due to Synvisc®, local side effects including mild injection site pain and local soft tissue swelling are the most common adverse event associated in general with viscosupplements [55]. Rare cases of calcium pyrophosphate dehydrate (CPPD) arthritis or pseudogout episodes have been precipitated following both Hyalgan® and Synvisc® administration [47]. In such a case, patients usually present between 5 and 48 h after the injection with complaints of acute pain, signs of acute inflammation, and loss of knee function. CPPD crystals are generally present in the synovial fluid. It is usually transient and can be managed with NSAIDs. The exact mechanism of occurrence is unclear, but it has been suggested that the mechanical effect from the needle used during the injection can cause "strip mining" of crystals from the synovial lining, thus leading to an acute inflammatory reaction [56].

Table 3.3 Differences between a SAIR, pseudogout reaction, and a septic knee

Synovial fluid property	Adverse reaction type		
	SAIR	Pseudogout flare	Septic knee
Appearance	Slightly cloudy	Very cloudy, can be greenish	Very cloudy
Gram stain	WBCs	WBCs	WBCs, (+) organisms
Cell count	Very elevated WBCC with left shift	Somewhat elevated WBCC	Very elevated WBCC with left shift
Crystal exam	None	Negatively birefringent crystals	None

Safety of Repeat Cycles

It is likely that the clinician will encounter many patients who will respond favorably to an initial treatment cycle and then request an additional cycle when they become symptomatic again. Fortunately, repeat treatment cycles of HAs are well-tolerated for the long-term treatment of the pain of OA [26, 28, 42]. Both Hyalgan® and Synvisc®, the first two FDA-approved (1997) viscosupplements, are in fact also FDA-approved for retreatment. As more postmarketing surveillance data accumulate for the three other FDA-approved viscosupplements, it is likely that they will similarly become FDA approved for retreatment.

Finally, as is true of any musculoskeletal injection procedure, iatrogenic infection is possible. While intra-articular infections have been documented in clinical use, none have been reported within clinical viscosupplementation trials.

Evidence for Disease Modifying Properties

Certainly, an objective of any therapy is to treat the disease and not just the symptoms. Unfortunately, the therapies approved for the nonsurgical management of OA are all symptom relieving and not disease modifying, and some (i.e., corticosteroids and NSAIDs) have even been inferred to accelerate disease progression. Therefore, a topic of major clinical importance is whether HAs are chondroprotective and thereby alter disease progression. While disease modification models has been shown for several of the HAs in preclinical models of OA, it has proven challenging to definitively demonstrate chondroprotection in humans given the currently available tools [57–66]. These tools include biomarkers of cartilage turnover (i.e., cartilage breakdown products released into the serum and urine), histomorphology, and various imaging techniques, but they have inherent limitations. For example, there is uncertainty with choice of surrogate biologic markers for study, as this selection must obviously depend upon the likely mechanism of action of chondroprotection by viscosupplements. Diagnostic arthroscopy may provide definitive evidence but is highly invasive and cannot be uniformly adopted. Plain X-ray imaging as a method of assessing disease modification is limited by its insensitivity at detecting early cartilage changes and potential technical difficulties of reproducibility involved with taking standardized images. While some of the recently reported MRI techniques and perhaps sonography have shown great promise, MRIs remain rather costly and have not been uniformly accepted as a surrogate marker for OA [19].

Possible disease modification from HA theoretically can occur via two main mechanisms: promotion of cartilage repair and healing, and/or inhibition of cartilage destruction. As summarized in a review article by Goldberg and Buckwalter, stimulation of chondrocyte metabolism and growth, stimulation of synthesis of the cartilage matrix matter, and decreased chondrocyte apoptosis are methods by which healing and repair result from HAs [66]. In contrast, inhibition of cartilage destruction occurs via HAs' ability to inhibit activity and expression of degradative enzymes, chondrocytes proliferation, and programmed cell death (apoptosis), as well as by inhibition of the inflammatory process that induce degradative processes as described previously.

In addition to its direct effects upon the metabolism of hyaline cartilage, HA also appears to possibly alter disease progression through effects upon components of the extracellular matrix that play key roles in the structural integrity and function of hyaline cartilage. While type II collagen confers excellent tensile strength, the proteoglycans intercalate between the collagen fibrils and confer the compressibility and ability to resist shear. In the early stages of OA, the initial loss of proteoglycans contributes to the friability of the cartilage. There are three ways by which HAs have been reported to affect the proteoglycan content of cartilage (1) enhance the synthesis; (2) suppress or minimize damage; and (3) decrease the release or turnover of extracellular matrix components [58, 67–75].

Increased Synthesis of Extracellular Matrix Components of Cartilage

Ghosh and Guidolin reviewed in vitro and in vivo reports of the pharmacologic effects of HA in relation to their MW [76]. Experimental findings in light and electron microscopic studies of synovial membrane and cartilage biopsy specimens obtained from OA patients showed evidence that partial restoration of normal joint tissue metabolism was obtained after the administration of LMW HAs within the range of 500–1,000 kDa. Animal studies indicate that HAs with MW >2,300 kDa may be less effective in restoring synovial fluid rheology than HAs of half this size.

A review by Goldberg and Buckwalter found evidence of disease-modifying activity of HAs [66]. They concluded that these effects were secondary to both the complex biochemical effects of HAs in the synovium and extracellular matrix of the articular cartilage, i.e., interactions between exogenously administered HA and articular cartilage, subchondral bone, matrix proteoglycans, and collagens as well as clinical trials using sodium hyaluronate (MW 500–730 kDa) that evaluated joint-space width, chondrocyte density and vitality, and arthroscopic evaluation of chondropathy.

Other beneficial changes have also been observed with regards to the extracellular matrix components of cartilage. Chondroitin sulfate synthesis and chondrocyte cell counts significantly increased after treatment with HAs compared with pretreatment values [67]. HA has been found to decrease the release of PG from the cell matrix layer both in the presence and in the absence of interleukin-1, tumor necrosis factor alpha, or basic fibroblast growth factor [73]. In contrast, in an in vitro study, Stove and colleagues found that HA increased PG concentrations only in the presence of IL-1beta [69]. In regards to keratin sulfate, there was no statistically significant difference in synovial fluid keratin sulfate levels between the HA group and control groups [70]. Cartilage destruction caused by fibronectin fragments has been shown to diminish after administration of HA, both in vitro and in vivo [74, 77]. HA has been found to inhibit the fibronectin fragment-mediated reduction in PG in cartilage as well as to decrease the expression of MMPs and increase PG synthesis to above normal levels [75]. All of these factors provide evidence that could explain the benefit of HA use in knee·OA.

Animal Models of OA

Several OA animal models, especially the anterior cruciate ligament transection and meniscectomy models in rabbit, dog, and sheep, have been used to study the potential chondroprotective effect of HAs. This topic has been extensively reviewed elsewhere [66]. Using these models, HAs have been shown to be potentially chondroprotective by several different mechanisms.

Clinical Data Supporting Disease Modification Properties of HAs

The disease modifying effects of HAs have also been studied to a lesser degree in controlled clinical trials as reviewed by Goldberg and Buckwalter [66]. The majority of these clinical studies have been with Hyalgan®. The structural outcome parameters used for assessments have included arthroscopy, microscopy, weight-bearing X-rays, and morphologic assessment on biopsy.

A prospective, randomized, controlled study compared conventional therapy to intra-articular injections of Hyalgan®, with respect to cartilage effects [60]. There was significantly less chondropathy found in the HA group and a significant improvement noted with arthroscopic assessment. Both groups, however, had similar improvements in pain ($P = 0.13$) and function ($P = 0.66$), and improvements in joint space narrowing ($P = 0.39$).

In an open clinical trial by Frizziero and co-workers, the effect of HAs (Hyalgan®) on the synovial membrane and cartilage was assessed [57]. By 6 months after treatment, there was a statistically significant improvement in chondrocyte vitality and density, rebuilding of the superficial amorphous layer of the cartilage, and a decrease in synovial inflammation. Treatment also led to a reduction in joint effusions.

A randomized open-label clinical trial examined the arthroscopic and electron microscopic changes in knee cartilage 6 months after administration of Hyalgan® compared with methylprednisolone acetate treatment [78]. On arthroscopy, both groups had a significant decrease in inflammatory scores. Histologically, HA significantly reduced the number and aggregation of lining synoviocytes. The effects of HA were more pronounced in primary OA than in secondary OA.

Guidolin and colleagues also compared intra-articular injections of Hyalgan® with methylprednisolone acetate [62]. Biopsies of cartilage were taken and analyzed under an electron microscope both at baseline and 6 months after treatment. HA treatments were significantly better than methylprednisolone treatments in almost all morphometric assessments. There was a significant improvement in chondrocyte density, metabolism and territorial matrix appearance as well as a significant repair of the superficial layer after treatments with HA.

Cubukcu and coworkers examined the effects of intra-articular Synvisc® on symptoms, functional outcome, and changes in articular cartilage assessed by magnetic resonance imaging (MRI) in patients with knee OA [79]. Thirty patients were randomly assigned to treatment with HA ($n = 20$) or saline ($n = 10$). All patients were assessed by clinical evaluation (WOMAC, VAS pain) and MRI (patellofemoral articular cartilage) at baseline, and clinical assessments after the first, second, third, and eighth weeks (MRI as well). When compared to saline injections, a significant statistical difference was found in all clinical parameters. On MRI, although the difference in the PF joint cartilage quality in the HA group before and after the treatment was statistically significant ($P < 0.05$), this significance was not detected between the groups after the treatment ($P > 0.05$).

Jubb and colleagues investigated the effects of Hyalgan® on longitudinal differences in mean joint space width (JSW) of the medial compartment of the knee at 52 weeks in patients with mild to moderate knee (Kellgren grades 2–3) OA [59]. The patients received three courses of three weekly injections of the HA over a 12-month period. A standardized digital imaging analysis of JSW from weight-bearing X-rays was performed at baseline and at 1 year. Using a stratified data analysis, they found a significant difference in response to treatment. In patients with a JSW > 4.6 mm, the joint space narrowing was significantly reduced compared with placebo. In patients with a JSW < 4.6 mm, there was no difference noted between the treatment groups. This may suggest that patients with radiographically milder disease may respond better in terms of potential chondroprotection to intra-articular injection of HA into their osteoarthritic knee.

X-rays are an inexpensive, quick, and noninvasive tool commonly used to evaluate the severity and progression of OA. However, X-rays are not able to directly visualize articular cartilage, synovium, menisci, and other nonosseous structures that are often involved in of OA. Plain radiography is not sensitive for detecting early cartilage erosions, cracking, or fibrillations. MRI has been used to a limited degree in the evaluation of OA. Volumetric MRI is a newer imaging modality that may provide a more sensitive and accurate method of assessing potential chondroprotective effects of viscosupplementation. It is capable of studying cartilage with regards to cartilage volume, cartilage thickness, and degree of cartilage heterogeneity in patients with OA [80]. Although there have been no published RCTs to date using this diagnostic tool to assess potential chondroprotection from HAs, a four-center study is currently underway.

Summary and Conclusion

Overall, HAs are a safe and effective nonsurgical tool for clinicians who treat patients with symptomatic knee OA. They are especially important to consider in patients with concurrent diseases or on concomitant medications. Given the current knowledge of the precautions associated with chronic use of oral pain medications, HAs might be considered a first line therapeutic option after simple analgesics and nonpharmacologic interventions have failed. An integrated treatment algorithm should be considered for optimal clinical outcomes. Although the exact mechanisms of action are uncertain, clinical viscosupplementation trials overall have shown resultant pain relief and functional improvements. The issue of potential chondro-protection and disease modification is extremely important in light of the fact that all other nonsurgical treatments have only been proven to be of symptomatic benefit. HAs, particularly nonchemically modified HAs, have an excellent safety profile.

Acknowledgment   Special thanks to Michael J. Daly, PhD, who contributed to the content of this chapter.

References

1. Gotoh S. Miyazaki K, Onaya J, Sakamoto T, Tokuyasu K, Namiki O. Experimental knee pain model in rats and analgesic effect of sodium hyaluronate. Folia Pharm 1988;92:17–27.
2. Engstrom-Laurent A. Hyaluronan in joint disease. J Intern Med 1997;242:57–60.
3. Balazs EA. Sediment volume and viscoelastic behavior of hyaluronic acid solutions. Fed Proc 1966;25(6):1817–22.
4. Altman D. Laboratory Findings in Osteoarthritis. In Moskowitz, HD, Goldberg V, Mankin J, eds. Osteoarthritis-Diagnosis and Medical Surgical Management, Second ed. Philadelphia, PA: WB Saunders; 1992:313–28.
5. Balazs EA. The Physical Properties of Synovial Fluid and the Special Role of Hyaluronic Acid. In Helfet A, ed. Disorders of the Knee. Philadelphia, PA: Lippincott; 1974:61–74.
6. Dougados M. High molecular weight sodium hyauronate in Knee OA: 1-Year placebo-controlled trial. Osteoarthr Cartil 1993;1:97–103.
7. Greenberg DD, Stoker A, Kane S, Cockrell M, Cook JL. Biochemical effects of two different hyaluronic acid products in a co-culture model of osteoarthritis. Osteoarthr Cartil 2006; 14(8):814–22. Epub 2006 April 17.
8. Smith MM, Ghosh P. The synthesis of hyaluronic acid by human synovial fibroblasts is influenced by the nature of the hyaluronate in the extracellular environment.Rheumatol Int 1987;7(3):113–22.
9. Ishida O, Tanaka Y, Morimoto I, Takigawa M, Eto S. Chondrocytes are regulated by cellular adhesion through CD44 and hyaluronic acid pathway. J Bone Miner Res 1997;12:1657–63.
10. Vuorio E, Einola S, Hakkarainen S, Penttinen R. Synthesis of under-polymerised hyaluronic acid by fibroblasts cultured from rheumatoid and non-rheumatoid synovitis. Rheumatol Int 1982;2:97–102.
11. Peyron JG, Balazs EA. Preliminary clinical assessment of Na-hyaluronate injection into human arthritic joints. Pathol Biol 1976;22:731–6.
12. Balazs EA, Denlinger JL. Sodium hyaluronic acid and joint function. J Equine Vet Sci 1985;5:217–28.

13. Auer JA, Fackelman GE, Gingerich DA, Fetter AW. Effect of hyaluronic acid in naturally occurring and experimentally induced osteoarthritis. Am J Vet Res 1980;41:568–74.

14. Rydell NW, Butler J, Balazs EA. Hyaluronic acid in synovial fluid. VI: Effect if intra-articular injection of hyaluronic acid on the clinical symptoms of arthritis in track horses. Acta Vet Scand 1970;11:139–55.

15. Rydell N, Balazs E. Effect of intro-articular injection of hyaluronic acid on the clinical symptoms of osteoarthritis and on granulation tissue formation. Clin Orthop Rel Res 1971;80:25–32.

16. Asheim A, Lindblad G. Intra-articular treatment of arthritis in race-horses with sodium hyaluronate. Acta Vet Scand 1976;17(4):379–94.

17. Phillips MW. Clinical trial comparison of intra-articular sodium hyaluronate products in the horse. J. Equine Vet Sci 1989;9:39–40.

18. Gingerich DA, Auer JA, Fackerman CE. Effects of exogenous hyaluronic acid on joint function in experimentally induced equine osteoarthritis: dosage titration studies. Res Vet Sci 1981;30:192–7.

19. Peterfy C, Kothari M. Imaging osteoarthritis: magnetic resonance imaging versus x-ray. Curr Rheumatol Rep 2006;8(1):16–21.

20. Stitik TP, Levy JA. Viscosupplementation (biosupplementation) for osteoarthritis. Am J Phys Med Rehabil 2006;85(11 Suppl):S32–50.

21. Bellamy N, Campbell J, Robinson V, Gee T, Bourne R, Wells G. Viscosupplementation for the treatment of osteoarthritis of the knee. Cochrane Database Syst Rev 2006;19(2):CD005321.

22. Recommendations for the medical management of osteoarthritis of the hip and knee: 2000 update. American College of Rheumatology Subcommittee on Osteoarthritis Guidelines. Arthritis Rheum 2000 Sep;43(9):1905–15.

23. Kelly MA, Goldberg VM, Healy WL, Pagnano MW, Hamburger MI. Osteoarthritis and beyond: a concensus on the past, present, and future of hyaluronans in orthopedics. Orthopedics 2003;26:1064–81.

24. Neustadt DH. Long-term efficacy and safety of intra-articular sodium hyaluronate (Hyalgan) in patients with osteoarthritis of the knee. Clin Exp Rheumatol 2003;21(3):307–11.

25. Neustadt DH. Long-term efficacy and safety of intra-articular sodium hyaluronate (Hyalgan) in patients with osteoarthritis of the knee. Clin Exp Rheumatol 2003;21(3):307–11.

26. Kolarz G, Kotz R, Hochmayer I. Long-term benefits and repeated treatment cycles of intra-articular sodium hyaluronate (Hyalgan) in patients with osteoarthritis of the knee. Semin Arthritis Rheum 2003;32(5):310–9.

27. Karlsson J, Sjögren LS, Lohmander LS. Comparison of two hyaluronan drugs and placebo in patients with knee osteoarthritis. A controlled, randomized, double-blind, parallel-design multicentre study. Rheumatology (Oxford) 2002;41(11):1240–8.

28. Waddell DD, Cefalu CA, Bricker DC. A second course of hylan G-F 20 for the treatment of osteoarthritic knee pain: 12-month patient follow-up. J Knee Surg 2005;18(1):7–15.

29. Stitik TP, Foye PM, Nadler SF, Chen B, Stiskal DM, Schoenherr L. Intra-articular Hyaluronan therapy and concomitant home exercise strengthening – an additive therapeutic algorithm for osteoarthritis of the knee. Arch Phys Med Rehabil 2004;85(9):e9.

30. Raynauld JP, Torrance GW, Band PA, Goldsmith CH, Tugwell P, Walker V et al. A prospective, randomized, pragmatic, health outcomes trial evaluating the incorporation of hylan G-F 20 into the treatment paradigm for patients with knee osteoarthritis (Part 1 of 2): clinical results. Osteoarthr Cartil 2002 Jul;10(7):506–17.

31. Bayramoglu M, Karataş M, Cetin N, Akman N, Sözay S, Dilek A. Comparison of two different viscosupplements in knee osteoarthritis – a pilot study. Clin Rheumatol 2003;22(2):118–22.

32. Huang MH, Yang RC, Lee CL, Chen TW, Wang MC. Preliminary results of integrated therapy for patients with knee osteoarthritis. Arthritis Rheum 2005;53(6):812–20.

33. Bellamy N, Campbell J, Robinson V, Gee T, Bourne R, Wells G. Intraarticular corticosteroid for treatment of osteoarthritis of the knee. Cochrane Database Syst Rev 2006;2:CD005328.

34. Tang SF, Chen CPC, Chen MJL, Hong W-H, Yu T-Y, Tsai W-C. Improvement of muscle strength in osteoarthritic knee patients after intraarticular knee injection of hyaluronan. Am J Phys Med Rehabil 2005;84(4):274–7.

35. Felson DT. Nonmedical Therapies for Osteoarthritis. Bull Rheum Dis 1998;47(2):5–7.
36. Chamberlain MA, Care G, Harfield B. Physiotherapy in osteoarthritis of the knees: a controlled trial of hospital versus home exercises. Int Rehabil Med 1982;4:101–6.
37. Feinberg J, Marzouk D, Sokolek C, Katz B, Bradley J, Brandt K. Effects of isometric versus range of motion exercise on joint pain and function in patients with knee osteoarthritis (abstract). Arthritis Rheum 1992;35 (suppl 5):R28.
38. Jan MH, Lai JS. The effects of physiotherapy on osteoarthritic knees of females. J Formos Med Assoc 1993;90:1008–13.
39. Yavuzer G, Sonel B, Süldür N, Ergin S. Effects of intra-articular hylan G-F 20 injections on clinical and biomechanical characteristics of the knee in osteoarthritis. Int J Rehabil Res 2005;28(4):371–4.
40. Vad VB, Bhat AL, Sculco TP, Wickiewicz TL. Management of knee osteoarthritis: knee lavage combined with hylan versus hylan alone. Arch Phys Med Rehabil 2003;84(5): 634–7.
41. Forster MC, Straw R. A prospective randomised trial comparing intra-articular Hyalgan injection and arthroscopic washout for knee osteoarthritis. Knee 2003;10(3):291–3.
42. Petrella RJ. Hyaluronic acid for the treatment of knee osteoarthritis: long-term outcomes from a naturalistic primary care experience. Am J Phys Med Rehabil 2005;84(4):278–83.
43. Scali JJ. Intra-articular sodium hyaluronic acid in the treatment of osteoarthritis of the knee: a long term study. Eur J Rheumatol Inflamm 1995;15(1):57–62.
44. "Osteoarthritis" Filmed: Newark, N.J 5/17/07. "Healthy Body, Healthy Mind" Series on Public Broadcast System. http://www.itvisus.com/programs/hbhm/episode_412osteo.asp.
45. Conrozier T, Mathieu P, Schott A-M, Laurent I, Hajri T, Crozes P et al. Factors predicting long-term efficacy of Hylan GF-20 viscosupplementation in knee osteoarthritis. Joint Bone Spine 2003;70(2):128–33.
46. Toh EM, Prasad PS, Teanby D. Correlating the efficacy of knee viscosupplementation with osteoarthritic changes on roentgenological examination. Knee 2002;9(4):321–30.
47. Hamburger MI, Lakhanpal S, Mooar PA, Oster D. Intra-articular hyaluronans: a review of product-specific safety profiles. Semin Arthritis Rheum 2003;32(5):296–309.
48. Espallargues M, Pons JM. Efficacy and safety of viscosupplementation with Hylan G-F 20 for the treatment of knee osteoarthritis: a systematic review. Int J Technol Assess Health Care 2003;19(1):41–56.
49. Hammesfahr JF, Knopf AB, Stitik T. Safety of intra-articular hyaluronates for pain associated with osteoarthritis of the knee. Am J Orthop 2003;32(6):277–83.
50. Pagnano M, Westrich G. Successful nonoperative management of chronic osteoarthritis pain of the knee: safety and efficacy of retreatment with intra-articular hyaluronans. Osteoarthr Cartil 2005;13(9):751–61.
51. Goldberg VM, Coutts RD. Pseudoseptic reactions to hylan viscosupplementation: diagnosis and treatment. Clin Orthop 2004;419:130–7.
52. Hamburger M, Settles M, Teutsch J. Identification of an immunogenic candidate for the elicitation of severe acute inflammatory reactions (SAIRs) to hylan G-F 20. Osteoarthr Cartil 2005;13(3):266–8.
53. Chen AL, Desai P, Adler EM, Di Cesare PE. Granulomatous inflammation after Hylan G-F 20 viscosupplementation of the knee: a report of six cases. J Bone Joint Surg Am 2002;84-A: 1142–7.
54. Jones KB, Patel PP, Deyoung BR, Buckwalter JA. Viscosupplementation pseudotumor. A case report. J Bone Joint Surg Am 2005;87:1113–9.
55. Sodium hyaluronate (MW 500–730 kDa) product labeling.
56. Personal communication with Roland J. Moskowitz, MD.
57. Frizziero L, Govoni E, Bacchini P. Intra-articular hyaluronic acid in the treatment of osteoarthritis of the knee: clinical and morphological study. Clin Exp Rheumatol 1998;16(4):441–9.
58. Kikuchi T, Yamada H, Shimmei M. Effect of high molecular weight hyaluronan on cartilage degradation in a rabbit model of osteoarthritis. Osteoarthr Cartil 1996;4:99–110.

59. Jubb RW, Piva S., Beinat L, Dacre J, Gishen P. A randomised, placebo (saline)-controlled clinical trial of the structure modifying effect of 500–730 KDa sodium hyaluronate (Hyalgan) in osteoarthritis of the knee. Int J Clin Pract 2003;57:467–74.

60. Listrat V, Ayral X, Patarnello F, Bonvarlet JP, Simonnet J, Amor B. Arthroscopic evaluation of potential structure modifying activity of hyaluronan (hyalgan) in osteoarthritis of the knee. Osteoarthr Cartil 1997;5:153–60.

61. Carrabba M, Paresce E, Angelini M, Re KA, Torchiaa EEM, Perbellini A. The safety and efficacy of different dose schedules of hyaluronic acid in the treatment of painful osteoarthritis of the knee with joint effusion. Eur J Rheumatol Inflamm 1995;15:25–31.

62. Guidolin DD, Ronchetti IP, Lini E, Guerra D, Frizziero L. Morphological analysis of articular cartilage biopsies from a randomized, clinical study comparing the effects of 500–730 kDa sodium hyaluronate (Hyalgan) and methylprednisolone acetate on primary osteoarthritis of the knee. Osteoarthr Cartil 2001;9:371–81.

63. Jubb RW, Piva S, Beinat L, Dacre J, Gishen P, for the UK Hyalgan study group. Clinical trial to examine the effect of HA on articular cartilage through changes in radiological joint space. Presented at: Annual European Congress of Rheumatology European League against Rheumatology. June 13–16, 2001. Prague, Czech Republic.

64. Marshall KW, Manolopoulos V, Mancer K, Staples J, Damyanovich A. Amelioration of disease severity by intraarticular hylan therapy in bilateral canine osteoarthritis. J Orthop Res 2000;18:416–25.

65. Shimizu C, Yoshioka M, Coutts RD, Harwood FL, Kubo T, Hirasawa Y et al. Long-term effects of hyaluronans on experimental osteoarthritis in a rabbit knee. Osteoarthr Cartil 1998;6:1–9.

66. Goldberg VM, Buckwalter JA. Hyaluronans in the treatment of osteoarthritis of the knee: evidence for disease-modifying activity. Osteoarthr Cartil 2005;13(3):216–24.

67. Kawasaki K, Ochi M, Uchio Y, Adachi N, Matsusaki M. Hyaluronic acid enhances proliferation and chondroitin sulfate synthesis in cultured chondrocytes embedded in collagen gels. J Cell Physiol 1999;179:142–8.

68. Fukuda K, Dan H, Takayama M, Kumano F, Saitoh M, Tanaka S. Hyaluronic acid increases proteoglycan synthesis in bovine articular cartilage in the presence of interleukin-1. J Pharmacol Exp Ther 1996;277(3):1672–5.

69. Stove J, Gerlach C, Huch K, Gunther KP, Puhl W, Scharf HP. Effects of hyaluronan on proteoglycan content of osteoarthritic chondrocytes in vitro. J Orthop Res 2002;20:551–5.

70. Ghosh P, Holbert C, Read R, Armstrong S. Hyaluronic acid (hyaluronan) in experimental osteoarthritis. J Rheumatol Suppl 1995;43:155–7.

71. Creamer P, Sharif M, George E, Meadows K, Cushnaghan J, Shinmei M et al. Intra-articular hyaluronic acid in osteoarthritis of the knee: an investigation into mechanisms of action. Osteoarthr Cartil 1994;2:133–40.

72. Yoshioka M, Shimizu C, Harwood FL, Coutts RD, Amiel D. The effects of hyaluronan during the development of osteoarthritis. Osteoarthr Cartil 1997;5:251–60.

73. Shimazu A, Jikko A, Iwamoto M, Koike T, Yan W, Okada Y et al. Effects of hyaluronic acid on the release of proteoglycan from the cell matrix in rabbit chondrocyte cultures in the presence and absence of cytokines. Arthritis Rheum 1993;36:247–53.

74. Homandberg GA, Hui F, Wen C, Kuettner KE, Williams JM. Hyaluronic acid suppresses fibronectin fragment mediated cartilage chondrolysis: I. In vitro. Osteoarthr Cartil 1997; 5(5):309–19.

75. Kang Y, Eger W, Koepp H, Williams JM, Kuettner KE, Homandberg GA. Hyaluronan suppresses fibronectin fragment-mediated damage to human cartilage explant cultures by enhancing proteoglycan synthesis. J Orthopaed Res 1999;17(6):858–69.

76. Ghosh P, Guidolin D. Potential mechanism of action of intra-articular hyaluronan therapy in osteoarthritis: are the effects molecular weight dependent? Semin Arthritis Rheum 2002;32(1):10–37.

77. Williams JM, Plaza V, Hui F, Wen C, Kuettner KE, Homandberg GA. Hyaluronic acid suppresses fibronectin fragment mediated cartilage chondrolysis: II. In vivo. Osteoarthr Cartil 1997;5(4):235–40.

78. Pasquali Ronchetti I, Guerra D, Taparelli F, Boraldi F, Bergamini G, Mori G et al. Morphological analysis of knee synovial membrane biopsies from a randomized controlled clinical study comparing the effects of sodium hyaluronate (Hyalgan) and methylprednisolone acetate (Depomedrol) in osteoarthritis. Rheumatology 2001; 40:158–69.
79. Cubukcu D, Ardic F, Karabulut N, Topuz O. Hylan G-F 20 efficacy on articular cartilage quality in patients with knee osteoarthritis: clinical and MRI assessment. Clin Rheumatol 2005;24(4):336–41. Epub 2004 Dec 14.
80. http://www.nmr.mgh.harvard.edu/fMRI/new/QTV.com/gif/OA.html.
81. Moreland LW. Intra-articular hyaluronan (hyaluronic acid) and hylans for the treatment of osteoarthritis: mechanisms of action. Arthritis Res Ther 2003;5(2):54–67. Epub 2003 Jan 14.
82. Punzi L, Schiavon F, Cavasin F, Ramonda R, Gambari PF, Todesco S. The Influence of intraarticular hyaluronic acid on PGE2 and cAMP of synovial fluid. Clin Exp Rheumatol 1989;7:247–50.
83. Tobetto K, Yasui T, Ando T, Hayaishi M, Motohashi N, Shinogi M et al. Inhibitory effects of hyaluronan on [14C]arachidonic acid release from labeled human synovial fibroblasts. Jpn J Pharmacol 1992;60:79–84.
84. Yasui T, Akatsuka M, Tobetto K, Hayaishi M, Ando T. The effect of hyaluronan on interleukin-1α induced prostaglandin-E_2 production in human osteoarthritis synovial cells. Agents Actions 1992;37:155–6.
85. Presti D, Scott JE. Hyaluronan-mediated protective effect against cell damage caused by enzymatically produced hydroxyl (OH) radicals is dependent on hyaluronan molecular mass. Cell Biochem Funct 1994;12:281–8.
86. Comer JS, Kincaid SA, Baird AN, Kammermann JR, Hanson RR Jr, Ogawa Y. Immunolocalization of stromelysin, tumor necrosis factor (TNF) alpha, and TNF receptors in atrophied canine articular cartilage treated with hyaluronic acid and transforming growth factor beta. Am J Vet Res 1996;57:1488–96.
87. Hirota W. Intra-articular injection of hyaluronic acid reduces total amounts of leukotriene C4, 6-keto-prostaglandin F1alpha, prostaglandin F2alpha and interleukin-1beta in synovial fluid of patients with internal derangement in disorders of the temporomandibular joint. Br J Oral Maxillofac Surg 1998;36:35–8.
88. Takahashi K, Goomer RS, Harwood F, Kubo T, Hirasawa Y, Amiel D. The effects of hyaluronan on matrix metalloproteinase-3 (MMP-3), interleukin-1beta (IL-1beta), and tissue inhibitor of metalloproteinase-1 (TIMP-1) gene expression during the development of osteoarthritis. Osteoarthr Cartil 1999;7:182–90.
89. Nonaka T, Kikuchi H, Ikeda T, Okamoto Y, Hamanishi C, Tanaka S. Hyaluronic acid inhibits the expression of u-PA, PAI-1, and u-PAR in human synovial fibroblasts of osteoarthritis and rheumatoid arthritis. J Rheumatol 2000;27:997–1004.
90. Goto M, Hanyu T, Yoshio T, Matsuno H, Shimizu M, Murata N et al. Intra-articular injection of hyaluronate (SI-6601D) improves joint pain and synovial fluid prostaglandin E2 levels in rheumatoid arthritis: a multicenter clinical trial. Clin Exp Rheumatol 2001;19:377–83.
91. Pellitier JP, Martel-Pelletier J. The pathophysiology oof osteoarthritis and the implication of the use of hyaluronan and hylan as therapeutic agents in viscosupplementation. J Rheumatol 1993;20(suppl 39):19–24.
92. Yasui T, Akatsuka M, Tobetto K, Umemoto J, Ando T, Yamashita K et al. Effects of hyaluronan on the production of stromelysin and tissue inhibitor of metalloproteinase-1 (TIMP-1) in bovine articular chondrocytes. Biomed Res 1992;13:343–8.
93. Fukuda K, Takayama M, Ueno M, Oh M, Asada S, Kumano F, Tanaka S. Hyaluronic acid inhibits interleukin-1-induced superoxide anion in bovine chondrocytes. Inflamm Res 1997;46:114–7.
94. Fukuda K, Oh M, Asada S, Hara F, Matsukawa M, Otani K, Hamanishi C. Sodium hyaluronate inhibits interleukin-1-evoked reactive oxygen species of bovine articular chondrocytes. Osteoarthr Cartil 2001;9:390–2.
95. Sato H, Takahashi T, Ide H, Fukushima T, Tabata M, Sekine F et al. Antioxidant activity of synovial fluid, hyaluronic acid, and two subcomponents of hyaluronic acid. Arthritis Rheum 1988;31:63–71.

96. Moseley R, Leaver M, Walker M, Waddington RJ, Parsons D, Chen WYJ, Embery G. Comparison of the antioxidant properties of HYAFF®-11p75 AQUACEL® and hyaluronan towards reactive oxygen species in vitro. Biomaterials 2002;23:2255–64.
97. Takahashi K, Hashimoto S, Kubo T, Hirasawa Y, Lotz M, Amiel D. Hyaluronan suppressed nitric oxide production in the meniscus and synovium of rabbit osteoarthritis model. J Orthop Res 2001;19:500–3.
98. Peluso G, Perbellini A, Tajana G. The effect of high and low molecular weight hyaluronic acid on mitogen-induced lymphocyte proliferation. Curr Ther Res 1990;47:437–43.
99. Darzynkiewicz Z, Balazs EA. Effect of connective tissue intercellular matrix on lymphocyte stimulation. 1. Suppression of lumphocyte stimulation by hyaluronic acid. Exp Cell Res 1971;66:113–23.
100. Corrado EM, Peluso GF, Gigliotti S, De Durante C, Palmieri D, Savoia M et al. The effects of intra-articular administration of hyaluronic acid on osteoarthritis of the knee: A clinical study with immunological and biochemical evaluations. Eur J Rheumatol Inflamm 1995;15(1):47–56.
101. Hakansson L, Hallgren R, Verge P. Regulation of granulocyte function by hyaluronic acid. In vitro and in vivo effects on phagocytosis, locomotion, and metabolism. J Clin Invest 1980;66:298–305.
102. Partsch G, Schwaarzer C, Neumuller J, Dunky A, Petera P, Bröll H et al. Modulation of the migration and chemotaxis of PMN cells by hyaluronic acid. Z Rheumatol 1989;48:123–8.
103. Pisko E, Turner R, Soderstrom L, Panetti M. Inhibition of neutrophils, phagocytosis and enzyme release by hyaluronic acid. Clin Exp Rheumatol 1983;1:1–14.
104. Forrester J, Balazs E. Inhibition of phagocytosis by high molecular weight hyaluronate. Immunology 1980;40:435–43.
105. Balazs EA, Darzynkiewicz Z. The Efffect of Hyaluronic Acid on Fibroblasts, Mononuclear Phagocytes and Lumphocytes. In Kulonen E, Pikkarainen J, eds. Biology of the Fibroblast. London: Academic; 1973:237–52.
106. Sezgin M, Demirel AC, Karaca C, Ortancil O, Ulkar GB, Kanik A et al. Does hyaluronan affect inflammatory cytokines in knee osteoarthritis? Rheumatol Int 2005;25(4):264–9.
107. Shimizu M, Yasuda T, Nakagawa T, Yamashita E, Julovi SM, Hiramitsu T et al. Hyaluronan inhibits matrix metalloproteinase-1 production by rheumatoid synovial fibroblasts stimulated by proinflammatory cytokines. J Rheumatol 2003; 30(6):1164–72.
108. Wiig ME, Amiel D, VandeBerg J, Kitabayashi L, Harwood FL, Arfors KE. The early effect of high molecular weight hyaluronan (hyaluronic acid) on anterior cruciate ligament healing: an experimental study in rabbits. J Orthop Res 1990;8(3):425–34.
109. Larsen N, Lombard K, Parent E, Balazs E. Effect of hylan on cartilage and chondrocyte cultures. J Orthoped Res 1992;10:23–32.
110. Hulmes DJS, Marsden ME, Strachan RK, Harvery RE, McInnes N, Gardner DL. Intra-articular hyaluronate in experimental rabbit osteoarthritis can prevent changes in cartilage proteoglycan content. Osteoarthr Cartil 2004;12:232–8.
111. Takahashi K, Hashimoto S, Kubo T, Hirasawa Y, Lotz M, Amiel D. Effect of hyaluronan on chondrocyte apoptosis and nitric oxide production in experimentally induced osteoarthritis. J Rheumatol 2000;27:1713–20.
112. Lisignoli G, Grassi F, Zini N, Toneguzzi S, Piacentini A, Guidolin D et al. Anti-fas-induced apoptosis in chondrocytes reduced by hyaluronan. Evidence for CD44 and CD54 (Intercellular Adhesion Molecule 1) involvement. Arthritis Rheum 2001;44:1800–7.
113. Swanstrom OG. Hyaluronate (hyaluronic acid) and its use. In Milne FJ, ed. Proceedings of the 24th Annual Meeting of the American Association of Equine Practioners. Lexington, KY: American Association of Equine Practitioners; 1978:345–8.
114. Nizolek DJ, White KK. Corticosteroid and hyaluronic acid treatments in equine degenerative joint disease. A review. Cornell Vet 1981;71(4):355–75.
115. Forrester JV, Lackie JM. Effect of hyaluronic acid on neutrophil adhesion. J Cell Sci 1981;50:329–44.
116. Tobetto K, Nakai K, Akatsuka M, Yasui T, Ando T, Hirano S. Inhibitory effects of hyaluronan on neutrophil-mediated cartilage degradation. Connect Tissue Res 1993;29:181–90.

117. Balazs E, Briller S, Denlinger J. Na-hyaluronate molecular size variations in equine arthritis and human arthritic synovial fluids and the effect on phagocytic cells. In Talbott J, ed. Seminars in Arthritis and Rheumatism. New York: Grune & Stratton; 1981: Vol. 11:141–3.
118. Pozo MA, Balazs EA, Belmonte C. Reduction of sensory responses to passive movements of inflamed knee joints by hylan, a hyaluronan derivative. Exp Brain Res 1997;116(1):3–9.
119. de la Peña E, Pecson B, Schmidt RF, Belmonte C. Effects of hylans on the response characteristics of mechanosensitive ion channels. Presented at the 9th World Congress on Pain, Vienna, Austria, 1999.
120. Aihara S, Murakami N, Ishii R, Kariya K, Azuma Y, Hamada K et al. Effects of sodium hyaluronate on the nociceptive response of rats with experimentally induced arthritis. Nippon Yakurigaku Zasshi 1992;100:359–65.
121. Moore AR, Willoughby DA. Hyaluronan as a drug delivery system for diclofenac: a hypothesis for mode of action. Int J Tissue React 1995;17:153–6.
122. Asheim A, Lindblad G. Intra-articular treatment of arthritis in run horses with sodium hyaluronate. Acta Vet Scand 1976;(Suppl 17):379–94.
123. Namiki O, Toyoshima H, Morisaki N. Therapeutic effect of intra-articular injection of high molecular weight hyaluronic acid on osteoarthritis of the knee. Int J Clin Pharmacol Ther Toxicol 1982;20:501–7.
124. Tew WP. Sodium hyaluronate and the treatment of equine joint disorders. In Milne FJ, ed. Proceedings of the 30th Annual Meeting of the American Association of Equine Practioners. Lexington, KY; 1984:67–86.
125. Cannon JH. Clinical evaluation of intra-articular sodium hyaloronate in the Thoroughbred race horse. J Equine Vet Sci 1985;5:147–8.
126. Irwin DHG. Sodium hyaloronate in equine traumatic arthritis. J S Afr Vet Assoc 1980;50:231–3.
127. Nizolek DJH, White KK. Corticosteriod and hyaluronic acid treatments in equine degenerative joint disease: a review. Cornell Vet 1981;71:355–75.
128. Galley RH. The use of hyaluronic acid in the race horse. In Milne FJ, ed. Proceedings of the 32nd Annual Meeting of the American Association of Equine Practioners, Lexington, KY; 1986:657–61.
129. Balazs E. The physical properties of synovial fluid and the specific role of hyaluronic acid. In Heflet AJ, ed. Disorders of the Knee. Philadelphia, PA: J B Lippincott; 1982:61–74.
130. Mensitieri M, Ambrosio L, Iannace S, Nicolais L. Viscoelastic evaluation of different knee osteoarthritis therapies. J Mat Sci Mat Med 1995;6:130–7.
131. Grecomoro G, La Sala F, Francavilla G. Rheologic changes in the synovial fluid of patients with gonarthritis induced by intraarticular infiltration of hyaluronic acid. Int J Tissue React 2001;23(2):67–71.

Chapter 4
Low Back Pain: Considerations of When to Refer Patients for Interventional Spine Procedures

Eric L. Altschuler, Brian F. White, Todd P. Stitik, and Jong H. Kim

Introduction

Although this textbook will not specifically address the details of lumbosacral region spinal injection procedures, the important issue of when to refer a patient for a possible lumbosacral spinal injection will be discussed. This is an important topic to physicians involved with musculoskeletal medicine given the frequency with which patients report low back pain and the morbidity associated with it.

Low back pain is a significant complaint in modern society and consumes a large proportion of health care resources in the process of diagnosis, treatment, and preventative care. In addition to these costs, there is a significant loss of productivity due to both lost work time and decreased ability to perform while at work [1]. This often general clinical complaint represents a large, heterogeneous array of pathophysiologic entities and may be classified according to both symptomatic and anatomic schemas.

Pain may be specific and associated with red flags that suggest organic disease such as infection, malignancy, or fracture, or much more commonly is nonspecific without such signs [2]. Patients may present with a complaint of focal low back pain, low back pain with a secondary radicular complaint, or of a primary radicular pain with secondary low back pain. Care for these problems may fall to a variety of physicians ranging from primary care physicians or internists to specialty care providers such as physiatrists, orthopedists, or neurosurgeons.

The diversity of medical specialties involved in the care of this clinical entity reinforces both the breadth of pathophysiologic processes involved and the lack of consensus regarding the definition of the problem, its diagnosis, and ultimately its appropriate care. This chapter will discuss one aspect of the care for patients with low back pain: when to refer a patient with low back pain for an interventional spine procedure.

E.L. Altschuler (✉)
Department of Physical Medicine and Rehabilitation, New Jersey Medical School,
Newark, NJ, USA
email: eric.altschuler@umdnj.edu

T.P. Stitik (ed.), *Injection Procedures: Osteoarthritis and Related Conditions*,
DOI 10.1007/978-0-387-76595-2_4, © Springer Science+Business Media, LLC 2011

Epidemiology

Low back pain is a common problem affecting a significant portion of the populations of western societies. A survey study of the US population, NHANES III, estimated that the prevalence of back pain lasting at least 1 month during a 12-month period is 17.8% [2]. An Australian survey study demonstrated a point prevalence of 26%, a 12-month prevalence of 67%, and a lifetime prevalence of 79% [3]. A literature review [4] indicated a point prevalence range from 12 to 33%, a one year prevalence range from 22 to 65%, and a lifetime prevalence range from 11 to 84%.

Conventional wisdom holds that, once present, 90% of all back pain resolves spontaneously within a month. This notion has more recently come under scrutiny and the natural course of low back pain may not be so straight forward or benign. Results of a literature review examining the long-term (>12 months) outcome of low back pain suggest a more chronic entity [5]. This review indicates that 62% of low back pain patients continue to have pain 12 months after presentation, 16% of study patients were sick listed 6 months after inclusion in the study, 60% of low back pain patients report relapses of pain, and 33% reported relapses of work absences. This study review demonstrates that low back pain does not resolve spontaneously, and the authors call for further delineation of low back pain with more specific definitions and treatments.

Not only is low back pain a common condition, but it is also among the more costly medical conditions. An Australian study [6] indicates that the total costs were 9.17 billion AU dollars (~$6.88 billion US) for the year 2001. This cost represents both direct costs for care and treatment, and indirect costs such as lost work days and productivity, with indirect costs being the much larger portion, representing 89% of total costs or 8.15 billion AU dollars ($6.11 billion US). Direct costs were estimated to be 1.02 billion AU dollars ($750 million US); of this figure, 71% or 724 million AU dollars ($540 million US) were for treatment by practitioners such as general practitioners, chiropractors, physiotherapists, and acupuncturists. Given the large proportion of indirect costs, the authors conclude that it is vital to identify cost-effective management strategies that maximize functional return and expedite return to duties.

In a 2003 US study, participants were asked to record lost productive time due to painful conditions during a 2-week period. This study indicated that 13% of the total workforce experienced a loss of productive time during a 2-week period. Of this 13%, 3.2% of respondents reported lost productive time due to back pain and lost an average of 5.2 h per week. Additional painful conditions resulting in lost productive time included headache, arthritis pain, and musculoskeletal pain. Total annual costs were estimated to be $61.2 billion in the US; the specific costs associated with the back pain subset were not evaluated in this study.

Differential Diagnosis of Low Back Pain

The differential diagnosis for low back pain is large and may include nonmusculo-skeletal conditions such as infectious, neoplastic, or inflammatory illnesses. But much more commonly, low back pain is either due to musculoskeletal problems such as muscular or myofascial strain, ligamentous injury, or referred pain from structures such as the sacroiliac joint, or due to spinal column disorders such as discogenic pain, posterior element disorders such as facet arthropathy, spondylolysis, and spondylolisthesis, and spinal canal stenosis.

Conditions specific to injury of the intervertebral disc are variously defined by authors. However, a common definitional paradigm is to refer to a posterior disc bulge without rupture of the annulous fibrosis fibers as a "disc protrusion." A disc bulge that tears through the inner fibers with only the outer most fibers retaining the displaced nucleus pulposus is termed a "disc prolapse." Further damage with complete disruption of the annular fibers and contiguous extension of nucleus pulposus into the epidural space is a "disc extrusion." Finally, if the extruded material forms separate fragments of free nuclear material, it is termed a "disc sequestration" [7].

When a patient presents with low back pain, generation of an accurate diagnosis rests upon a thorough history and a thorough physical examination. Additionally, imaging studies are often required as an extension of this evaluation and typically include plain film radiography, MRI, and electrodiagnostic evaluation with nerve conduction studies and needle electromyography (NCS/EMG) [8, 9].

Initial Treatment of Low Back Pain

Initial treatment of low back pain, as with any medical condition or problem, of course begins with a thorough history and a thorough physical examination. Often, it is primary care physicians who perform this initial examination. A typical history includes questions of the location, duration, quantity, quality of the low back pain, aggravating or alleviating factors for the pain, and associated symptoms such as numbness or weakness. Examination includes: evaluation of gait; inspection, palpation, and range of motion of the back; evaluation of strength (manual muscle testing) and range of motion of the legs; examination of reflexes and sensation in the legs; and tests for neural tension signs such as the straight leg raise.

The first task in the history and the physical is the obligation to look for and rule out any signs of red flags that might indicate a malignant cause of low back, for example: cancer (a primary or metastasis) or infection. Red flags on history and physical include history of fevers, chills, night sweats, bowel or bladder problems, history or high suspicion for cancer, pain that wakes a patient from sleep or signs of systemic infection. Imaging can be of great benefit if malignancy or infection is suspected as a cause of low back pain. In the great majority of cases, a "red flag" cause can be ruled out by a primary care physician in a straightforward manner, and the patient has a more benign cause of their low back pain. The history and the physical examination can then be helpful in developing an initial treatment plan for low back pain and generating indications and questions to pose when referring a patient for an interventional procedure.

First line treatment for non-"red flag" low back pain – often regardless of potential pain generator (e.g., poor biomechanics, acute or chronic disc herniation) – typically includes conservative measures such as expectant management, over-the-counter medications such as acetaminophen and nonsteroidal anti-inflammatory medications (NSAIDs), and prescription medications such as antispasmodic medications, antidepressants (e.g., tricyclic antidepressants), antiseizure medications (e.g., gabapentin), and chronic opiates [8, 9]. In addition to these medical methods for management, initial components to conservative management may also include physical therapy and orthosis such as a lumbosacral corset.

Unfortunately, these measures fail to provide relief in a significant number of patients. What should be the next step in a rationally designed treatment plan? The next step has become fluoroscopically guided injections [10]. As injections into the lumbar spine can and on occasion do [11] have catastrophic complications, it is crucial to understand and study the efficacy and safety of such procedures. Here we discuss indications for referral for the most common interventional spine procedures:

1. Fluoroscopically guided epidural steroid injections via a caudal, interlaminar, or transforaminal approach [12]
2. Procedures for pain presumed to due to low back facet joints
3. Fluoroscopically guided injections for presumed sacroiliac pain and dysfunction
4. Discography, a diagnostic interventional procedure

Because of concerns of a high placebo response in patients with low back pain, ideally when studying efficacy, one wants to look to randomized, controlled studies. For example, as a referring physician referring a patient for a fluoroscopically guided transforaminal epidural steroid injection for an L4 disc herniation, one might ask: what is the evidence in terms of safety and efficacy of this procedure from large double blind trials? When one looks for such studies, it is clear that the literature is still sparse. Future studies will clearly be welcome, but, given the prevalence of back pain, it is incumbent and worthwhile to see what information is available for the referring physician.

Epidural Steroid Injections for Low Back Pain

Low back pain thought to emanate from an acute or chronically herniated disc or spinal stenosis can be diagnosed, for example, by radicular symptoms, a positive straight leg raise, and/or other physical exam findings localized to one or more lumbar spinal levels. Evidence of radiculopathy in patients who have otherwise failed other conservative treatment attempts is a typical indication to generate a referral for an epidural steroid injection. What is the current evidence of the efficacy of such injections?

A large, randomized double-blind, placebo controlled trial by Arden and colleagues [13] compared lumbar epidural steroid injection (steroid + local anesthetic, active) to a saline injection (placebo) in patients with sciatica and found at 3 weeks benefit from the steroid injection in terms of decreased pain and disability. However, this study failed to find a benefit of steroid over control at weeks 6–52. There was no obvious difference in response of patients with more acute or chronic sciatica, and no obvious predictors of response. This study found no benefit of repeat steroid injections, or any difference between steroid and control in terms of need for surgery.

Another moderate-sized, randomized, double blind trial by Ng and colleagues [14] compared fluoroscopically guided periradicular infiltration of steroid + bupivacaine to infiltration of bupivacaine alone in patients with chronic radicular pain and found no statistically significant difference between the groups in terms of pain or disability at 12 weeks. On average (with wide variation), there was about a 25–30% decrease in leg pain sustained out to 12 weeks, but not much decrease in back pain. They found that chronicity of symptoms was a negative predictor of outcome.

Wilson-MacDonald and coworkers [15] examined 92 patients with lumbosacral nerve root pain, all of whom had MRI evidence of disc prolapse ($N = 43$), spinal stenosis ($N = 32$), or both ($N = 17$). These patients were randomized to either epidural steroid injection or intramuscular injection of local anesthetic and steroid. Analysis indicated a decrease in pain in the epidural group that became notable at 10 days and lasted approximately 1 month. There was no significant long-term difference between the two treatment groups out to a 2-year follow-up, including operative rate, nor were the authors able to find any difference in outcome between patients presenting with spinal stenosis or disc prolapse. The authors suggest that small sample size may not have allowed for differentiation between spinal stenosis and disc prolapse outcomes.

Rivest and colleagues [16] studied the effect at 2 weeks of a single epidural steroid injections on patients with spinal stenosis and herniated discs. Their results were that 38% of the spinal stenosis patients noted improvement from baseline on pain scores while 61% of the herniated disc patients noted pain improvement. The authors conclude that spinal stenosis patients have a worse response to epidural steroid injection than do herniated disc patients, and they felt that specific randomized clinical trials are needed to evaluate epidural steroid injections in spinal stenosis patients.

Fukusaki and colleagues [17] studied the effects of epidural injections on patients with pseudoclaudication of less than 20 m and degenerative spinal stenosis. These patients were randomized into three groups:

Group 1: Epidural saline injection ($N = 16$)
Group 2: Epidural injection of local anesthetic ($N = 18$)
Group 3: Epidural steroid and local anesthetic injection ($N = 19$)

End points and evaluation were based upon improvement in walking distance with follow-up at 1, 4, and 12 weeks. The authors noted a small early benefit in groups 2 and 3 compared to group 1, but no difference between group 2 and group 3. They conclude that epidural steroid injection has no beneficial effect on pseudoclaudication due to spinal stenosis.

Riew and coworkers [18] studied the ability of selective nerve root steroid injections to obviate the need for spinal surgery in patients with lumbar radicular pain, and radiographically confirmed disc herniation or central or foraminal spinal stenosis. Patients were randomized to receive either epidural anesthetic injection or epidural steroid and anesthetic injection, and could opt for up to four injections. End points and evaluations included spinal surgery (considered treatment failure), decrease of neurologic symptoms, and relief of low back pain. Twenty out of 28 patients in the steroid group had avoided surgery during the follow-up period, while only 9 out of 27 in the local anesthetic group avoided surgery. Subgroup analysis indicated that selective nerve root injection of steroid and local anesthetic had a statistically significant improvement in both neurologic symptoms and relief of low back pain in the spinal stenosis group as well as the herniated nucleus pulposus group.

Overall, these studies indicate that there is a modest decrease in pain and disability for a few months following an interventional spine procedure, more for leg pain than back pain, and that steroid component of the injection may confer specific benefit for about a month. More studies of efficacy are clearly welcome. In terms of safety, not only are large formal studies important, but it may prove helpful or even necessary to have databases of outcomes for specific providers available to referring physicians and possibly to patients as well.

Facet Syndrome

In addition to the potential sources mentioned thus far, back pain may also emanate from the facet joints, which may serve as a nidus for pain throughout the spine including cervical, thoracic, and lumbar regions. The facet joint is a diarthrodial joint with a synovial lining, articular cartilage, a joint capsule, and synovial fluid. These joints are located in the posterior spinal column and are a key player in "posterior element pain."

Authors vary on the reported prevalence of facet mediated pain as a subset of chronic spine pain. Review articles have suggested a range of prevalence for lumbar facet joint involvement in chronic low back pain from 15 to 52% depending upon study parameters [19, 20]. A study by Manchikanti and colleagues evaluated the presence of facet mediated pain in each region of the spine [21] and found that 55% of chronic cervical spinal pain, 42% of thoracic spinal pain, and 31% of lumbar spinal pain is facet mediated.

Determination of the involvement of the facet joint in back pain is made using various diagnostic strategies. The "gold standard" used in many clinical research studies and in some interventional practices is a positive result with a "diagnostic facet block." This procedure may be occasionally taken to mean either direct injection of anesthetic into the facet joint capsule under fluoroscopic guidance or nerve block of the medial branch of the dorsal rami of the spinal nerve supplying sensory afferent fibers to the facet, though the later meaning is more technically specific.

More recently, bone scintigraphy with single photon emission computed tomography (SPECT) has begun to show promise in identifying facet joints likely to benefit from injection therapy. In a study by Pneumaticos and coworkers [22], it was demonstrated that, when the SPECT scans of patients with chronic low back pain demonstrated facet joint abnormalities, injection of those noted joints produced much greater pain relief than did injection of facet joints at levels indicated by the referring physician.

Typically "facetogenic pain" is considered in the differential diagnosis of pain generators for patients with axial back pain exacerbated by hyperextension maneuvers. However, when Schwarzer and colleagues attempted to correlate clinical exam findings with joint block confirmed facet pain, they found a much more complex picture [23].

Multiple interventions have been proposed to address facet mediated pain; these include direct injection of steroid and an anesthetic agent into the facet capsule, radiofrequency ablation of the medial branch, and injection of hyaluronate or sclerotherapeutics into the facet joint. Radiofrequency ablation (RFA) of the medial branch of the dorsal rami is considered by many practitioners to be the primary means for definitive treatment of facet pain defined by prior confirmation with a concordant response to a comparative local anesthetic block paradigm in which the first procedure utilizes a short-acting local anesthetic (most commonly lidocaine), while the second procedure utilizes a longer-acting anesthetic (most commonly bupivacaine). However, a randomized, controlled study of facet mediated pain by van Wijk and colleagues in 2005 [24] found that, although there was a reduction in pain levels in both the RFA and a sham treatment group, there was not a significant difference between the two groups in combined outcome measures.

The study by Pneumaticos and coworkers evaluating the use of SPECT imaging in identification of facet joints likely to respond to injection demonstrated an improvement in pain scores at 1-month follow-up for facet joint injection in SPECT identified facets, but not in those identified clinically. A direct comparative study by Fuchs and colleagues to evaluate intraarticular hyaluronate vs. steroid injection [25] noted that, though both improved chronic nonradicular lumbar pain, there was no noted difference between the two groups.

A less widespread approach is the intra-articular injection of sclerotherapeutic agents into the facet joint. This was analyzed in a retrospective study by Hooper and Ding [26] that did not have controls, but their results did demonstrate improvement in pain, ADLs, and ability to work in a range consistent with those reported for other interventional techniques. In summary, spinal pain of facet origin may represent a nontrivial proportion of chronic back pain, but it is challenging to diagnose accurately with the clinical exam; there are multiple potential interventional treatment options, the literature supporting their use is still modest at best; and large and well-designed studies in the future are urgently needed.

Interventional Procedures for Sacroiliac Joint Pain

The sacroiliac (SI) joint, a true diarthrodial joint, is innervated by the L4-S2 levels and is important to consider as a source of pain in patients presenting with low back pain. However, even the ability to specifically isolate the SI joint as a source of pain by history, and physical examination is highly controversial [27, 28]. In a systematic review, McKensie-Brown and colleagues [29] found fluoroscopically guided interventional procedures for SI joint pain to have moderate specific diagnostic value and limited to moderate therapeutic value. Large, well-designed future studies on the utility of interventional procedures to diagnose and treat SI joint pain should be closely watched by referring physicians.

Discography

Discography is a *diagnostic* interventional spine procedure of which referring physicians should be aware. This procedure is performed in patients with suspected discogenic pain by injecting contrast dye into the nucleus pulposus of the presumed offending disc. The injection is continued until 2 cm^3 has been injected or until the intradiscal pressure reaches 90 pounds per square inch. A positive test is one in which dye provocation produces pain in concordance with the location, quantity, and quality of the patient's clinical pain.

Additionally, a positive test requires that provocation of pain from neighboring disc levels does not reproduce the patient's pain.

In theory, this technique has the potential to be invaluable in finding specific generators of a patient's pain and possibly to select patients for surgery. However, in practice, this goal has not yet been met. A prospective study [30] in patients who underwent spinal fusion following discography did not find discography highly predictive of isolated intradiscal lesions. Radiofrequency ablation of the SI joints is becoming performed more commonly in clinical practice. Evidence is beginning to accumulate regarding its efficacy.

Summary and Conclusion

Low back pain is one of the most common diseases or conditions in modern society, and its impact on society in terms of health and economic issues is significant. Many patients will get better simply with the passage of time. Others will require some intervention of the part of the physician such as nonpharmacologic measures like physical therapy or intermittent use of acetaminophen, NSAIDs, or low to moderate doses of opiates. However, some patients will not improve by these means, and, given the high prevalence of chronic back pain, the total number of patients with recalcitrant pain is large.

Fluoroscopically guided epidural steroid injections or other interventional spine procedures are an option for patients with resistant pain. There is evidence supporting the use of such procedures; however, this evidence is modest and points to the need for larger, prospective, randomized, double blind trials not only to confirm efficacy, but to delineate a subset of patients with low back pain most likely to benefit from these interventions as well as the clinical and/or radiologic indications defining those patients.

Such well-designed studies will also serve to answer other questions such as the optimal timing for intervention in a rational treatment paradigm and the number for repeat injections likely to provide clinical benefit. The answer to questions of the safety of these procedures will be advanced by large studies, but databases of individual practitioners' outcomes may be needed to fully understand and assess the question of safety. The efficacy of fluoroscopically guided injections for SI joint pain and discography as a diagnostic procedure is much less clear. Again, large, well-designed studies in the future should further clarify these issues.

References

1. Stewart WF, Ricci JA, Chee E, Morganstein D, Lipton R. Lost productive time and cost due to common pain conditions in the US workforce. JAMA 2003; 290: 2443–54.
2. Manek NJ, MacGregor AJ. Epidemiology of back disorders: prevalence, risk factors, and prognosis. Current Opinion in Rheumatology 2005; 17: 134–40.
3. Walker BF, Muller R, Grant WD. Low back pain in Australian adults: prevalence and associated disability. Journal of Manipulative Physiologic Therapy 2004; 27: 238–44.
4. Walker BF. The prevalence of low back pain: A systematic review of the Literature from 1966 to 1998. Journal of Spinal Disorders 2000; 13: 205–17.
5. Hestbaek L, Leboeuf-Yde C, Manniche C. Low back pain: what is the long-term course? A review of studies of general patient populations. European Spine Journal 2003; 12: 149–65.
6. Walker BF, Muller R, Grant WD. Low back pain in Australian adults: the economic burden. Asaia Pacific Journal of Public Health 2003; 15: 79–87.
7. Magee DJ. Orthopedic Physical Assessment. Philadelphia, PA: WB Saunders; 2002; 471.
8. Deyo RA, Weinstein JN. Low back pain. New England Journal of Medicine 2001; 344: 363–70.
9. Carragee EJ. Persistent low back pain. New England Journal of Medicine 2005; 352: 1891–98.
10. McLain RF, Kapural L, Mekhail NA. Epidural steroid therapy for back and leg pain: mechanisms of action and efficacy. Spine J 2005; 5: 191–201.
11. Houten JK, Errico TJ. Paraplegia after lumbosacral nerve root block: report of three cases. Spine J 2002; 2: 70–5.
12. Chen B, Stitik TP, Foye PM. Spinal injection procedures in Rehabilitation Medicine. In DeLisa JA, Gans BM, Walsh NE, Bockenek WL, Frontera WR, eds. Physical Rehabilitation and Medicine: Principles and Practice, 4th Edition. Philadelphia, PA: Lippincott Williams & Wilkins; 2004: 369–87.
13. Arden NK, Price C, Reading I, Stubbing J, Hazelgrove J, Dunne C et al. A multicentre randomized controlled trial of epidural corticosteroid injections for sciatica: the WEST study. Rheumatology 2005; 44: 1399–406.
14. Ng L, Chaudhary N, Sell P. The efficacy of corticosteroids in periradicular infiltration for chronic radicular pain: a randomized, double-blind, controlled trial. Spine 2005; 30: 857–62.
15. Wilson-Macdonald J, Burt G, Griffin D, Glynn C. Epidural steroid injection for nerve root compression. A randomized, controlled trial. Journal of Bone and Joint Surgery British 2005; 87: 352–5.
16. Rivest C, Katz JN, Ferrante FM, Jamison RN. Effects of epidural steroid injection on pain due to lumbar spinal stenosis or herniated disks: a prospective study. Arthritis Care Res 1998; 11: 291–7.

17. Fukasaki M, Kobayashi I, Hara T, Sumikawa K. Symptoms of spinal stenosis do not improve after epidural steroid injection. Clinical Journal of Pain 1998; 14: 148–51.
18. Riew KD, Yin Y, Gilula L, Bridwell KH, Lenke LG, Lauryssen C et al. The effect of nerve-root injections on the need for operative treatment of lumbar radicular pain. A prospective, randomized, controlled, double-blind study. Journal of Bone and Joint Surgery American 2000; 82-A: 1589–93.
19. Manchikanti L, Singh V. Review of chronic low back pain of facet joint origin. Pain Physician 2002; 5: 83–101.
20. Dreyer SJ, Dreyfuss PH. Low back pain and the zygapophysial (facet) joint. Archives of Physical Medicine and Rehabilitation 1996; 77: 290–300.
21. Manchikanti L., Boswell MV., Singh V, Pampati V, Damron KS, Beyer CD. Prevalence of facet joint pain in chronic spinal pain of cervical, thoracic, and lumbar regions. BMC Musculoskeletal Disorders 2004; 5: 15.
22. Pneumaticos SG, Chatziioannou SN, Hipp JA, Moore WH, Esses SI. Low back pain: prediction of short-term outcome of facet joint injection with bone scintigraphy. Radiology 2006; 238: 693–8.
23. Schwarzer AC, Aprill CN, Derby R, Fortin J, Kine G, Bogduk N. Clinical features of patients with pain stemming from the lumbar zygapophysial joints. Is the lumbar facet syndrome a clinical entity? Spine 1994; 19: 1132–7.
24. van Wijk RM, Geurts JW, Wynne HJ, Hammink E, Buskens E, Lousberg R et al. Radiofrequency denervation of lumbar facet joints in the treatment of chronic low back pain: a randomized, double -blind, sham lesion-controlled trial. Clinical Journal of Pain 2005; 21: 335–44.
25. Fuchs S, Erbe T, Fischer HL, Tibesku CO. Intraarticular hyaluronic acid verses glucocorticoid injections for nonradicular pain in the lumbar spine. J Vasc Interv Radiol 2005; 16(11): 1493–8.
26. Hooper RA, Ding M. Retrospective case series on patients with chronic spinal pain treated with dextrose prolotherapy. Journal of Alternative and Complementary Medicine 2004; 10: 670–4.
27. Laslett M, Williams M. The reliability of selected pain provocation tests for sacroiliac joint pathology. Spine 1994; 19: 1243–9.
28. Dreyfuss P, Michaelsen M, Pauza K, McLarty J, Bogduk N. The value of medical history and physical examination in diagnosing sacroiliac joint pain. Spine 1996; 21: 2594–602.
29. McKenzie-Brown AM, Shah RV, Sehgal N, Everett CR. A systematic review of sacroiliac joint interventions. Pain Physician 2005; 8: 115–25.
30. Carragee EJ, Lincoln T, Parmar VS, Alamin T. A gold standard evaluation of the "discogenic pain" diagnosis as determined by provocative discography. Spine 2006; 31: 2115–23.

Chapter 5
Adminstrative Aspects of Office-Based Injection Procedures

Charles Sara, Jeffrey J. Fossati, Gregory J. Mulford, and Lisa Schoenherr

Introduction

Some physicians who are still practicing medicine may remember the days when doctors could simply be doctors. Unfortunately, the days of medicine when doctors could treat the patient without the absolute burden of the endless administrative tasks that seemingly consume more manpower than brainpower appear to have ended. The delivery of healthcare services in this country has continued to change drastically since the inception of doctoring.

Administrative burdens, especially pertaining to documentation, have increased significantly. In addition, due to the rise in the number of medical malpractice cases, a physician must take into account the endless policies and procedures that should be followed to make sure that compliance is met in every regard. Although a doctor must first be a skilled and compassionate clinician, he/she must also remain informed regarding the everyday necessary administrative and regulatory challenges in order to be in charge of his/her medical career.

This chapter will focus on some of the nonclinical, administrative aspects of being a physician, with an emphasis on outlining some of the "do's" and "don'ts" of running a financially sound practice, particularly with respect to office-based injection procedures.

The Role of Medicare in Billing and Coding

A physician can receive guidance about proper billing and coding of office-based procedures from manuals that are published annually. However, during the course of the year, Medicare can institute various billing and coding policy changes, seemingly without providing sufficient notice. If the physician does not adhere to

C. Sara (✉)
Department of Physical Medicine and Rehabilitation, Northern NJ Pain & Rehab,
Newark, Hackensack, USA
e-mail: csara@nipainandrehab.com

T.P. Stitik (ed.), *Injection Procedures: Osteoarthritis and Related Conditions*,
DOI 10.1007/978-0-387-76595-2_5, © Springer Science+Business Media, LLC 2011

these Medicare changes, this will be considered to be noncompliance with Medicare policy. Physicians can even be lulled into a sense of complacency as Medicare will provide a good faith method of prompt payment.

In fact, Medicare will usually pay the physician within ten working days without requiring the documentation upfront to support a given CPT code. However, in the case of a Medicare audit, all of the required documentation to support performance of a given injection procedure must be made available. Another important administrative aspect of office-based injection procedures that particularly pertains to Medicare involves the level of coding of concomitant office visits and the proper use of billing modifiers. The physician or designee should be very careful not to over- or under-code as both can be considered for the big "F" word: *FRAUD*. In the world of Medicare, administrative fraud can result in treble damages, losing a medical license, and, in the worst-case scenario, jail time for the physician. If treble damages are awarded, the penalty is repayment of three times what was *initially billed*, rather than three times the amount that was actually paid by the carrier. For example, if a physician billed $500 to Medicare for an office-based injection procedure but Medicare paid only $55 of the claim, and if an award for treble damages is made against the physician who submitted this bill, the physician would have to pay $1,500 (i.e., $500 × 3) in damages and not $165 (i.e., $55 × 3). When a carrier makes a claim like this against a physician for alleged fraudulent charges, it usually results in a full blown audit.

If treble damages are subsequently awarded as a result of a Medicare audit, the possibility of a negligent misrepresentation claim can arise. This may happen if it is felt that the patient would not have proceeded with the injection procedure had they had been informed of the potential risks of the procedure. Furthermore, treble damages awarded as a result of Medicare audits can also secondarily result in malpractice claims against a physician since malpractice is based on general negligence principles. Medicare audits resulting in treble damages do not necessarily result in malpractice claims since the patient is not always notified of a Medicare audit and subsequently the results of that audit, unless the patient is the whistleblower initially.

However, the physician has malpractice liability if procedures were judged during the audit to have been performed unnecessarily or if other administrative problems were found. For example, if a Medicare audit reveals a failure to document informed consent prior to an injection procedure, the lack of informed consent can create a separate battery-based action if the doctor's actions were determined to be intentional or reckless. This subsequently opens the physician up to the possibility of punitive damages. Lack of informed consent increases liability; in the sense that a plaintiff need not prove that their injuries arose from substandard care by the doctor. In other words, the doctor could have done everything right and still lose the case based upon the case of lack of informed consent.

One solution for preventing this kind of situation lies in instituting a simple office-based system that ensures compliance with Medicare policies and procedures. Since turnover in lower-level positions, such as receptionists and billing clerks, is very common in today's industry and since the administrative process involved with office-based injection procedures often begins with the receptionist and ends with the billing clerk, it is important to make the system as simple as possible, as it may prove to be quite difficult to train new staff if the system involves an overly complex administrative process.

It is also important to have a compliance plan as well as internal and external quality review and quality assurance programs in place. Although this can be satisfied by an outside vendor, internal chart review can be completed by a staff member to assure that all notes are signed and all paperwork is properly completed. Figure 5.1 shows an example of a chart review checklist that is used for auditing all patient

a

	MET	NOT MET
QA/QI Committee **Medical Record Review Sheet** Northern NJ Pain and Rehabilitation Center, Inc. supports the practice of consistent and complete documentation in the facility medical record as an essential component of quality patient care. Reviewers use the guidelines to review a sample of charts for chart documentation. Chart standardization is not mandated, however, the guidelines were approved as a minimum. **Guidelines for chart documentation:**		
1. Each and every page in the record contains the Patients name or ID number		
2. Personal/biographical data includes name, address, home telephone number, and date of birth.		
3. All entries in the medical record contain the physician or therapist's name.		
4. All entries are dated.		
5. The record is legible to someone other than the writer. Any record judged liable by one physician/therapist Reviewer should be evaluated by a second reviewer.		
6. Examination performed matches the body of the report.		
7. Recommendations for a follow up examination is Indicated on the report by a physician. Specific time of Return is noted e.g. days, weeks, and months.		
Threshold for indicator: 6 out of 7 must be met.		
Reviewer and date: _____	PASS	FAIL

Fig. 5.1 Examples of a chart review checklist used for auditing all patient records within a practice (including Medicare patients) in an effort to be in compliance with documentation requirements

b

Long term care/Chronic condition			
☐ Physical Medicine & Rehabilitation	Yes	No	N/A
☐ Physical Therapy	Yes	No	N/A
☐ Occupational Therapy	Yes	No	N/A
☐ Speech Pathology	Yes	No	N/A
☐ Psychology/Social Services	Yes	No	N/A
Soap notes current			
☐ Physical Medicine & Rehabilitation	Yes	No	N/A
☐ Physical Therapy	Yes	No	N/A
☐ Occupational Therapy	Yes	No	N/A
☐ Speech Pathology	Yes	No	N/A
☐ Psychology/Social Services	Yes	No	N/A
Team meetings minutes	Yes	No	N/A
Identifies dx	Yes	No	N/A

Fig. 5.1 (continued)

records within a practice (including Medicare patients) in an effort to be in compliance with documentation requirements.

It is recommended that all physicians attend a coding seminar in order to be able to understand and follow Medicare's guidelines. Medicare Part B in fact has a provider education and training department designed to train physicians in properly coding for all aspects of their respective practices. In addition, specialty societies often offer and encourage physicians to attend educational courses on coding, billing, and documentation.

Practices that submit a high volume of billing to Medicare may want to consider retaining an attorney who specializes in health care law. This is particularly true if the billing is somewhat complex, as can be the case for musculoskeletal injection procedures that involve image-guidance (i.e., ultrasound or fluoroscopic guidance) using a practice's own equipment. A healthcare attorney can be essential for the correct interpretation of the law in order to implement policy and procedures. This will initially incur a cost to a practice, but in the long run it may prove to be well worth the investment.

A health care attorney can also help a practice to interpret complex legal concepts so that the practice can grow without fear of being in violation of Medicare regulations as well as federal fraud and abuse statutes. For example, a New Jersey Physical Medicine and Rehabilitation practice hired a New Jersey Health Care attorney to interpret and apply the Federal Fraud and Abuse statutes, particularly as they pertained to the word "intent." The following is a sample of some of the topics that were covered during that legal consultation:[1]

- *Anti-kickback Statute.* The intent requirement for a violation of this statute is "knowingly and willfully." 42 U.S.C.1320a-7b. The interpretation of "knowingly and willfully" however is unsettled in the courts: courts are split as to whether specific intent to violate the Anti-kickback statute is required or if intent to act with an unlawful purpose is enough.
- *Stark (physician self-referral law).* Stark is a strict liability law; no intent is needed to violate Stark. 42 U.S.C. 1395nn (a) (1) (A).
- *False Claims Act Statutes.* A defendant must act knowingly, or in deliberate ignorance of, or with reckless disregard for, the truth or falsity of the submission. Specific intent to defraud is not required. 31 U.S.C. § 3729(b).
- Treble damages are calculated based on the damage actually sustained by the government (times three). 31. U.S.C. 3729 (a) (7).

If a Medicare audit is performed on a practice, the practice's demonstration of good faith measures at attempted compliance such as those discussed previously (e.g., internal and external quality review, quality assurance program, proactive retention of a healthcare attorney in an attempt to understand healthcare policies, and/or attendance at educational courses on billing, coding, documentation, and compliance) can prove to be helpful. These actions show that efforts have been made to try to be compliant with applicable regulations and policies.

Diagnostic Testing: A Source of Generating Referrals for Office-Based Injection Procedures

In addition to seeing patients for evaluation and management services, the physician who is comfortable and competent in performing certain diagnostic tests and/or other related procedures can enhance his/her ability to optimize patient care and realize his/her earning potential by offering diagnostic and therapeutic procedures in the office setting. The ability to provide diagnostic and therapeutic injections within one's practice can greatly assist with a practice's financial viability, both directly via the billing income from these procedures and indirectly from the additional procedures that can result. For example, physiatrists who specialize in outpatient musculoskeletal medicine typically also perform traditional electrodiagnostic testing [i.e., nerve conduction studies (NCS) and needle electromyography (EMG)].

In addition to serving as an important diagnostic test that can assist with patient management, electrodiagnostic testing can logically and appropriately lead to additional office-based injection procedures both for those patients who are under the direct care of the electromyographer and for those patients who have been referred for electrodiagnostic testing. Primary care physicians often refer patients

---

[1] It should be noted that the explanations shown here as well as the information contained in this chapter do not constitute legal advice.

for electrodiagnostic testing but typically do not perform any or certain injection procedures. This is in part because of the volume of patients that they are expected to see in this era of managed care and also due to actual and perceived inadequate training in this area of medicine.

The electrodiagnostic report that is sent to the primary care physician can help with this source of referrals by suggesting the option of an injection procedure, when appropriately based upon the electromyographer's findings and clinical recommendations. For example, if electrodiagnostic testing revealed the presence of carpal tunnel syndrome, the report could mention the possibility of another referral for a carpal tunnel injection.

Alternatively, an EMG/NCS that was negative for radiculopathy, peripheral entrapment neuropathy, and peripheral polyneuropathy in a patient whom the electromyographer found to have a myofascial pain syndrome with active trigger points could reasonably lead to the suggestion within the report for possible referral for trigger point injections. It is important to use good judgment with the wording of suggestions so as not to give the false or misleading impression that the electrodiagnostic testing will invariably be followed by the suggestion for another referral.

The electromyographer should also keep in mind that primary care management should be left to the primary care physicians so as not to interfere with this aspect of a patient's care. A typical example would be the electrodiagnostic test findings of diabetic peripheral neuropathy. In this scenario, the electromyographer should probably resist the temptation of making specific suggestions regarding the dosing of the patient's insulin or oral hypoglycemic medicine.

Caution should also be exercised with making management suggestions to physicians who are likely to treat a given condition in a manner other than using office-based injection procedures. For example, findings consistent with focal median nerve compression at the wrist in a patient referred by a hand surgeon will likely result in surgical decompression of the carpal tunnel, and any suggestion on the part of the electromyographer to do otherwise may not be appreciated and could very well lead to losing this referral source.

A well-run medical practice with a strong administrative team and processes helps to further maximize the financial potential from all cognitive and procedural services offered within the practice. For example, modern electrodiagnostic instruments can enable a physician to quickly produce a detailed report even before the patient leaves the office. In addition to providing the immediate documentation that supports the particular CPT codes used for the testing, an immediate detailed report is also a big plus for the patient as well as the referring physician. This may be particularly important if the referring physician needs the information to plan an interventional pain management procedure. For those situations in which a patient cannot be provided with a written report at the time of the testing, establishing verbal contact with the referring physician, followed by a typewritten report, can often serve as a substitute.

The referral source should never be placed in the situation whereby a patient has returned to the referring physician for a follow-up visit but the physician has not been made aware of the test results. Timely reporting of test results and good communication with referral sources should give the physician who performs electrodiagnostic testing the edge against local competitors who also perform electrodiagnostic testing.

Office-Based Injection Procedures: The Effect on a Practice's Financial Viability

In addition to office-based diagnostic testing, office-based injection procedures can also greatly enhance a practice's financial situation. Practices that do not have the resources to lease or purchase fluoroscopic or ultrasound equipment and/or do not have the physicians who are capable of performing these profitable image-guided injection procedures or the patients in need of these procedures may want to consider offering other types of office based-injection procedures. For example, some outpatient musculoskeletal medicine practices treat a high volume of patients with myofascial pain who are in need of trigger point injections. Performance of this procedure requires a minimal financial investment in materials and can yield a steady, although somewhat modest, supplemental income. A somewhat potentially more profitable procedure is viscosupplementation, an office-based intraarticular injection procedure of hyaluronan products (aka visco-supplements) for patients with knee osteoarthritis. It has been FDA-approved in the United States since 1997 and has been used essentially worldwide for approximately the last 25+ years. Its safety and effectiveness have been extensively studied and established.

If a practice has decided to offer this procedure to patients, the office manager or practice administrator should consider contacting the local pharmaceutical sales representative as he/she can be a valuable resource for helping to arrange for physician education in knee osteoarthritis and training in knee injections, and for training the staff in proper billing and coding. The pharmaceutical representative can also provide patient education materials for the office waiting room. This can serve as an effective method of referrals for the procedure.

The initial capital outlay for this procedure is far less than that required to perform image-guided injection procedures. It does, however, require a greater financial commitment than trigger point injections depending upon the mechanism of obtaining the viscosupplement. Options for obtaining the viscosupplement include writing a prescription for patients whose insurance companies require or allow them to receive and fill a prescription at any pharmacy or through a designated pharmacy or wholesaler, obtaining the viscosupplement from a hospital-based pharmacy that then bills for it, buying and billing for the viscosupplement, or participating in the competitive acquisition program (CAP) for Medicare patients (described later in this chapter).

In order to best accommodate those patients whose insurances allow them to have a prescription filled, the physician's office can arrange for a local pharmacy to stock the viscosupplement. The physician should generally find the pharmacy, particularly smaller pharmacies that are grateful for the business, eager to stock the product. These pharmacies may even help to refer patients to the practice for viscosupplementation. For those patient's who prefer to use their own pharmacy from which to obtain the viscosupplement, it can be helpful to have a staff member call the patient's pharmacy to make sure this item is stocked or that it can be ordered.

If the physician is in a hospital-based practice, the need to purchase and stock viscosupplements might not be present because the hospital might keep this medication in stock. The hospital would then bill the J-code for it as the supplier of the medication.

Because the viscosupplements are relatively expensive to purchase, proper billing of the J-code is essential. If the practice chooses to routinely buy and bill for the viscosupplement, the small profit from the J-code reimbursement [e.g., Medicare reimburses at 106% of the average sales price (ASP)] can further increase practice revenue beyond the revenue gained from billing for the injection procedure. Although buying in bulk can save money, the viscosupplements have a somewhat limited shelf life; therefore, it is important to rotate the supply.

If the practice chooses not to buy in bulk, understanding the turn around time to receive the product from the manufacturer or wholesaler can ensure that it will be received in time for the prospective procedure date. The billing information contained within the following sections is very important in order for the physician to properly bill and code for viscosupplementation. Throughout these sections, the viscosupplement Hyalgan® (Sanofi-Aventis, Bridgewater, NJ, USA) will be used as the example, as the authors have the most experience with this viscosupplement, and, at the time of this writing, it is the most commonly prescribed viscosupplement throughout the world and has the most extensive research data supporting its use.

Medicare: Payer Coverage and Reimbursement for Viscosupplementation

Medicare is a federally funded program providing coverage for individuals age 65 and over, individuals who are disabled, and individuals with permanent kidney failure. In general, Medicare Part B covers physician-administered drugs and services that are medically necessary and accepted by the medical community as an appropriate standard of care. To be covered by Medicare in the physician's office, hyaluronan products must be administered incident to a physician's service. "Incident to a physician's services" means that the physician must purchase the drug or biological, administer it to the patient or directly supervise administration by a staff member, and then bill Medicare.

In addition, the drug or biological must be of a type that is not generally self-administered. Hyaluronans fall into this category as they are intended for administration by a healthcare professional only. Although hyaluronans are technically classified as a medical device, this is somewhat of a semantic issue as they are treated by Medicare in the same fashion as medications or other biologics.

Medications administered in the physician office setting are reimbursed separately from the administration service performed by the provider. Medicare payment for drugs and devices administered in the physician's office has undergone significant reform. As of January 1, 2005, Medicare has been reimbursing most drugs based on 106% of the ASP [1]. The Medicare reimbursement rates change each quarter. In terms of cost sharing, Medicare reimburses 80% of the established allowable, and the remaining 20% is the responsibility of the patient or a secondary insurer.

Medicare beneficiaries may elect to have their traditional Medicare benefits administered by a private insurer for additional coverage, such as a pharmacy benefit. Patients with a Medicare HMO plan may have coverage through their pharmacy benefit. Patients may obtain medications or devices at the pharmacy and present them to their medical provider. In this case, the provider would indicate a "zero bill" for the drug or device along with the billing for the administration services.

In many geographic areas, Medicare beneficiaries also have the opportunity to enroll in managed care plans. Most Medicare beneficiaries have some form of supplemental coverage that will cover the 20% coinsurance and deductibles required under Part B. Medicare patients who do not have any form of supplemental coverage are responsible for paying their deductible and coinsurance for services provided in the physician's office.

As mandated by the Medicare Modernization Act of 2003 (MMA), a new CAP was implemented nationally on July 1, 2006, offering physicians an option to acquire nonself-administered drugs from vendors who are selected in a competitive bidding process [2] Through CAP, physicians were allowed to obtain Part B covered drugs from a vendor without purchasing the drugs for a period of 1 year.

The vendor is to bill Medicare for the viscosupplement and also bill the patient or secondary insurer for any portion not covered under Medicare. BioScrip (Elmsford, NY, USA) was selected as the sole vendor for CAP. If the physician opted not to participate in CAP for the election year, then the physician was to continue to buy and bill for Part B covered drugs (Fig. 5.2).

Whether or not a physician participates in CAP, the physician is responsible to bill the Medicare program for professional services rendered in administering the drug. Medicare reimburses for a physician's professional services according to the Resource Based Relative Value System (RBRVS) fee schedule [3].The RBRVS fee schedule assigns an allowable to each current procedural terminology (CPT) code by geographic region.

Physicians may also bill the Medicare program if another professional service is provided in the same visit. Other professional services (such as an evaluation) will most likely be rendered on the date of the first injection. For an office visit (indicated by an evaluation and management code), Medicare reimburses 80% of the established payment amount, and the remaining 20% is the responsibility of the patient or the patient's secondary insurer.

Since Medicare coverage policies may vary as to the number of reimbursable office visits allowed during a course of treatment with hyaluronan products, it is important that the physician checks with his or her local carrier for the most current coverage information as well as information on reimbursement for drugs and professional services.

```
┌─────────┐
│  1500   │
└─────────┘
HEALTH INSURANCE CLAIM FORM
APPROVED BY NATIONAL UNIFORM CLAIM COMMITTEE 08/05
```

PICA	PICA
1. MEDICARE MEDICAID TRICARE CHAMPVA GROUP FECA OTHER	1a. INSURED'S I.D. NUMBER (For Program in Item 1)
CHAMPUS HEALTH PLAN BLK LUNG	
(Medicare #) (Medicaid #) (Sponsor's SSN) (Member ID#) [X] (SSN or ID) (SSN) (ID)	12345678A
2. PATIENT'S NAME (Last Name, First Name, Middle Initial)	3. PATIENT'S BIRTH DATE SEX	4. INSURED'S NAME (Last Name, First Name, Middle Initial)
DOE JOHN Q	MM 08 DD 15 YY 1931 M [X] F	DOE JOHN Q
5. PATIENT'S ADDRESS (NO., Street)	6. PATIENT RELATIONSHIP TO INSURED	7. INSURED'S ADDRESS (No., Street)
543 MADISON STREET	Self [X] Spouse Child Other	543 MADISON STREET
CITY STATE	8. PATIENT STATUS	CITY STATE
ANY CITY XX	Single [X] Married Other	ANY CITY XX
ZIP CODE TELEPHONE (Include Area Code)		ZIP CODE TELEPHONE (Include Area Code)
12345 ( )	Employed Full-Time Student Part-Time Student	12345 ( )
9. OTHER INSURED'S NAME (Last Name, First Name, Middle Initial)	10. IS PATIENT'S CONDITION RELATED TO:	11. INSURED'S POLICY GROUP OR FECA NUMBER
a. OTHER INSURED'S POLICY OR GROUP NUMBER	a. EMPLOYMENT? (Current or Previous) YES [X] NO	a. INSURED'S DATE OF BIRTH MM 08 DD 15 YY 1931 SEX M [X] F
b. OTHER INSURED'S DATE OF BIRTH SEX MM DD YY M F	b. AUTO ACCIDENT? YES [X] NO PLACE (State)	b. EMPLOYER'S NAME OR SCHOOL NAME
c. EMPLOYER'S NAME OR SCHOOL NAME	c. OTHER ACCIDENT? YES [X] NO	c. INSURANCE PLAN NAME OR PROGRAM NAME
d. INSURANCE PLAN NAME OR PROGRAM NAME	10d. RESERVED FOR LOCAL USE	d. IS THERE ANOTHER HEALTH BENEFIT PLAN? YES [X] NO If yes, return to and complete item 9 a-d.

READ BACK OF FORM BEFORE COMPLETING & SIGNING THIS FORM.

12. PATIENT'S OR AUTHORIZED PERSON'S SIGNATURE I authorize the release of any medical or other information necessary to process this claim. I also request payment of government benefits either to myself or to the party who accepts assignment below.

SIGNED **SIGNATURE ON FILE** DATE

13. INSURED'S OR AUTHORIZED PERSON'S SIGNATURE I authorize payment of medical benefits to the undersigned physician or supplier for services described below.

SIGNED **SIGNATURE ON FILE**

14. DATE OF CURRENT: ILLNESS (First symptom) OR INJURY (Accident) OR PREGNANCY(LMP) MM DD YY	15. IF PATIENT HAS HAD SAME OR SIMILAR ILLNESS GIVE FIRST DATE MM DD YY	16. DATES PATIENT UNABLE TO WORK IN CURRENT OCCUPATION FROM MM DD YY TO MM DD YY
17. NAME OF REFERRING PROVIDER OR OTHER SOURCE	17a. 17b. NPI	18. HOSPITALIZATION DATES RELATED TO CURRENT SERVICES FROM MM DD YY TO MM DD YY
19. RESERVED FOR LOCAL USE		20. OUTSIDE LAB? YES [X] NO $ CHARGES
21. DIAGNOSIS OR NATURE OF ILLNESS OR INJURY (Relate Items 1, 2, 3 or 4 to Item 24E by Line) 1. 715.16 3. 2. 4.		22. MEDICAID RESUBMISSION CODE ORIGINAL REF. NO.
		23. PRIOR AUTHORIZATION NUMBER

24. A. DATE(S) OF SERVICE		B. PLACE OF SERVICE	C. EMG	D. PROCEDURES, SERVICES, OR SUPPLIES (Explain Unusual Circumstances) CPT/HCPCS MODIFIER	E. DIAGNOSIS POINTER	F. $ CHARGES	G. DAYS OR UNITS	H. EPSDT Family Plan	I. ID QUAL	J. RENDERING PROVIDER ID. #
From MM DD YY	To MM DD YY									
01 01 08	01 01 08	11		J7321	1		2		NPI	
01 01 08	01 01 08	11		20610 50	1		1		NPI	
									NPI	
									NPI	
									NPI	
									NPI	

25. FEDERAL TAX I.D. NUMBER SSN EIN [X]	26. PATIENT'S ACCOUNT NO. 2474-1-2	27. ACCEPT ASSIGNMENT? (For govt. claims, see back) [X] YES NO	28. TOTAL CHARGE $	29. AMOUNT PAID $	30. BALANCE DUE $
31. SIGNATURE OF PHYSICIAN OR SUPPLIER INCLUDING DEGREES OR CREDENTIALS (I certify that the statements on the reverse apply to this bill and are made a part thereof.) SIGNED **04 25 08** DATE	32. SERVICE FACILITY LOCATION INFORMATION		33. BILLING PROVIDER INFO & PH # ( )		

NUCC Instruction Manual available at: www.nucc.org   APPROVED OMB-0938-0999 FORM CMS-1500 (08-05)

Fig. 5.2 Sample of Health Insurance Claim Form 1500: Bilateral knee injections of a hyaluronic acid derivative (e.g., Hyalgan®, Sanofi-Aventis, Bridgewater, NJ, USA)

Medicaid: Payer Coverage and Reimbursement for Viscosupplementation

Medicaid is a federally and state funded program providing coverage for low income individuals. In general, Medicaid programs will cover drugs and devices for their FDA-approved indications. However, each Medicaid agency determines its own coverage and reimbursement payment policies. Hyaluronans may be covered as a medical benefit, pharmacy benefit, or both. Whether covered as a medical or pharmacy benefit, state Medicaid programs may apply coverage restrictions such as prior authorization. The prior authorization requirements will vary depending on the Medicaid program. It is important that the physician checks with his or her state Medicaid program for the most current coverage information.

Medicaid programs typically reimburse physician services according to fee schedules. Fee schedules for drugs may be based on a percentage of average wholesale price (AWP), wholesale acquisition cost (WAC), or other payment calculation as determined by the state. Some states may also adopt the ASP-based payment methodologies. In other states, Medicaid may require that physicians order hyaluronans through a Medicaid participating pharmacy. The pharmacy will then be reimbursed by Medicaid on the basis of AWP less a certain percentage or WAC plus a certain percentage.

In addition, some states have enrolled some of their Medicaid beneficiaries in managed care plans. Typically, guidelines for coverage and reimbursement for a Medicaid patient are the same as for a privately insured patient in the same plan. Payment for services provided to these beneficiaries is determined by each managed care plan according to the provisions of their contract with the state Medicaid programs.

Private Insurance: Payer Coverage and Reimbursement for Viscosupplementation

Private insurance is obtained through employers or individuals. Each private insurer determines its own coverage policies for drugs. In addition, most insurers offer multiple insurance plans wherein coverage for procedures and/or drugs or devices may vary depending on the exact plan. For example, prior authorization may be required before coverage is allowed, or physician-administered drugs may not be a plan benefit. If the physician determines that the drug is medically necessary, the physician should contact the private insurer to verify patient's benefits and determine coverage requirements, including the need for prior authorization, deductible status, benefit caps, out-of-pocket maximum, and whether the drug is covered and paid for under the medical or pharmacy benefits.

Private insurers' reimbursement for professional services and drugs varies from plan to plan and from patient to patient. Typically, reimbursement rates depend on two considerations: the reimbursement arrangement outlined in the patient's policy and any contractual arrangement between the physician and the insurer. Some indemnity payers continue to reimburse physicians on the basis of charges or discounted charges, while managed care organizations are more likely to pay for services according to fee schedules or capitated rates. Private payers may also reimburse physicians for hyaluronan products based on a percentage of the AWP or invoice cost.

Coding for All Payers: Viscosupplementation

Medicare, Medicaid, and most private payers accept the Healthcare Common Procedure Coding Systems (HCPCS) for coding of procedures and physician-administered drugs in the physician office setting. Physician offices typically use CMS-1500 forms in order to submit a bill to payers. In addition, insurers typically accept ICD-9-CM diagnosis codes to indicate the patient's diagnosis. The following are possible diagnosis, procedure, and product codes that may be appropriate for billing. Some insurers, however, may require local codes for certain procedures.

ICD-9-CM Diagnosis Codes: Viscosupplementation

Typically, payers cover hyaluronans for treatment of knee OA. When filing claims, the physician's office must indicate an ICD-9-CM diagnosis code indicating the patient's condition. Codes that may be used to describe the treatment of knee OA are:

- 715.16: Osteoarthritis, localized, primary, lower leg
- 715.26: Osteoarthritis, localized, secondary, lower leg
- 715.36: Osteoarthritis, localized, primary/secondary unknown, lower leg
- 715.96: Osteoarthritis, generalized/localized unknown, lower leg

It is important to note that covered diagnosis codes may vary as different payers have different diagnosis codes for which treatment with hyaluronan products are covered.

HCPCS and CPT Codes: Viscosupplementation

HCPCS Level I codes, also known as CPT codes, are used to bill for professional services. For example, physicians administering Hyalgan® would use CPT codes to bill for professional services to administer the viscosupplement. The following CPT code describes the procedure typically used for the administration of hyaluronans:

- 20610: Arthroc entesis, aspiration, and/or injection; major joint or bursa (e.g., shoulder, hip, or knee joint, subacromial bursa)

HCPCS Level II codes, also simply known as HCPCS codes, are used to report medical services, drugs, and supplies not contained in the CPT. For example, physicians administering Hyalgan® would use a "J" code to bill for the product. For dates of service on or after January 1, 2008, providers should use the following HCPCS code to bill for Hyalgan®:

- J7321: HYALURONAN (SODIUM HYALURONATE) OR DERIVATIVE, (Hyalgan® or Supartz®) INTRA-ARTICULAR INJECTION, PER INJECTION

Some payers require that the modifier "RT" (right knee) or "LT" (left knee) be added after CPT code 20610, in Block 24, Column D of the CMS-1500 claim form, to indicate which knee was injected. For a bilateral injection, the modifier 50 indicates both knees were injected in one setting (Fig. 5.2)

Claims Support and Appeal Process: Viscosupplementation

Claims may be denied or underpaid for a variety of reasons. Common reasons for denial or underpayment include clerical errors such as misspellings and transposed number, questions about medical necessity, improper use of ICD-9-CM codes, incorrect procedure codes or modifier usage, missing information, and incorrect billing units.

Payers typically have a formal process that permits the provider to appeal denied claims or inadequate reimbursement for drugs and/or services. If a claim for a hyaluronan product is denied, the physician will receive an Explanation of Benefits (EOB) from the local insurance claims processor explaining the reasons for noncoverage. The physician may resubmit the claim asking for a redetermination of coverage.

Some insurers may require a letter of medical necessity (LMN) along with the package insert and/or reprints of clinical articles to consider coverage of hyaluronan products. Resubmitted claims should fully document the medical necessity for hyaluronan treatment for the patient in question and include any supplemental information that may not have been included with the original claim.

The LMN should include specific details of a patient's case history and clinical experience, and demonstrate the medical necessity of the hyaluronan product for each individual patient. In addition, the LMN can also serve as a prior authorization letter when required. Package insert and/or reprints of clinical articles are typically available through the manufacturer's product information services. See Fig. 5.3 for an example of a LMN for Hyalgan® viscosupplementation.

Reimbursement Hotlines: Viscosupplementation

Many pharmaceutical companies provide reimbursement hotlines as a resource to assist healthcare providers with denied or underpaid claims and to facilitate the filing of the appeals. In addition, reimbursement hotlines may provide billing, coding, and reimbursement information about third-party payer coverage. Reimbursement hotlines can work directly with the physician's office to determine specific payer requirements for the patient.

If the product is not covered under the patient's plan benefit and alternate sources of reimbursement are not identified, many drug manufacturers have patient assistance programs that provide products free of charge to patients who are uninsured and meet the income eligibility requirements. Other program criteria may

[Date]

[Name of Medical Director]

[Title]

[Name of Insurer]

[Address of Insurer]

[City, State, Zip Code]

Re: *[patient's name]*

  [Patient I.D. Number]

Dear *[Name of Medical Director]*:

I am writing to provide additional information regarding the medical necessity of treating *[patient's name]* with Hyalgan® (sodium hyaluronate). Hyalgan® was approved for marketing by the Food and Drug Administration on May 28, 1997. Hyalgan® is indicated for the treatment of pain in osteoarthritis of the knee in patients who have failed to respond adequately to conservative non-pharmacologic therapy and to simple analgesics, e.g. acetaminophen. This letter provides information about this patient's medical history, an explanation of the use of Hyalgan®, and my rationale for this course of treatment.

Patient's Diagnosis and History

The history and course of osteoarthritis of the knee for *[patient's name]* is as follows: *[insert information concerning the date and method of diagnosis, previous treatments, symptoms, and reprints of any relevant medical tests or dictations]*.

Treatment Description

Hyalgan® is a viscous solution of purified natural hyaluronate derived from rooster combs. A US multicenter study has demonstrated that a course of treatment—five weekly intra-articular injections of Hyalgan® (20 mg sodium hyaluronate in 2 mL of phosphate buffer) over 4 weeks—will relieve pain n the majority of patients for 6 months. Some patients may experience benefit with three injections given at week intervals. This has been noted in studies reported in the literature in which patients treated with three injections were followed for 60 days. Hyalgan® has been in clinical use for over 15 years. Approximately 12.5 million injections have been administered to patients in 39 countries, including the US, the UK, France, Germany, Belgium, Italy, Austria, and Canada. While the precise mechanism of action of Hyalgan® is not fully understood, current evidence suggests that Hyalgan® increases the viscoelasticity of synovial fluid, which plays a key role in cushioning and protecting the joint. In the US clinical trials the only adverse event showing statistical significance vs. placebo was injection-site pain.

Treatment Rationale

This patient has tried and not responded to the conservative therapies described above. Because of this I *[will treat/have treated]* *[him/her]* with a course of Hyalgan® order to avoid the systemic side effects that are associated with oral NSAID therapy.

or

NSAID therapy would not be appropriate for *[patient name]* because off *[his/her]* preexisting medical conditions. *[Describe patient's relevant comorbidities]* Therefore, I *[will treat/have treated]* *[patient's name]* with a course of Hyalgan®.

or

[Patient's name] has been treated with an NSAID (*[name of NSAID]*) for the past *[X]* months. This has not proven satisfactory because of *[insert medical rationale for patient]* . Therefore, I *[will treat/have treated]* *[patient name]* with a course of Hyalgan®.

or

[Patient's name] has widespread osteoarthritis, including osteoarthritis of the knee(s). *[He/She]* is receiving NSA therapy (*[name of NSAID]*). However the pain of *[his/her]* osteoarthritis of the knee is inadequately controlled. Therefore, I believe the appropriate next step is a course of Hyalgan®.

Enclosed you will a find a letter from Sanofi-Aventis' Product information Services summarizing clinical information about Hyalgan® for your review. The package insert is also attached for your review.

I hope this information is helpful to you in understanding why I have pursued treatment with Hyalgan®. If you require any additional information, please contact me.

Sincerely.

[Physician's Name], M.D. or D.O.

Enclosures:
    Supportive Medical Literature
    Medicare Remittance Notice
    Claim form
    Clinic notes

Fig. 5.3 Sample claims appeal letter for medical necessity for Hyalgan® (Sanofi-Aventis, Bridgewater, NJ, USA) viscosupplementation

apply depending on the patient assistance program. Typical turnaround time for insurance verification is 48 h. Other services such as problem claims assistance and patient assistance program eligibility assessment are initiated within 24 h. Due to the complexity of the billing requirements for Medicare, Medicaid, and private insurers, reimbursement hotlines are a useful resource for healthcare providers.

Administrative Keys to Implementing Successful Injection Procedures Within a Practice

Choosing and documenting a diagnosis that is compatible with both the patient's medical condition and the diagnostic coding requirements for a given injection procedure are important administrative steps. They increase the probability that the patient will be eligible to receive the injections and that the practice will be reimbursed for a medically necessary injection procedure.

Once this has been accomplished, the procedure can be tentatively scheduled pending insurance authorization. However, this approach runs the risk of a patient presenting to the office for a procedure prior to a determination being made on the part of the insurance company. There are advantages and disadvantages to both approaches (i.e., prescheduling pending insurance authorization or not scheduling until receiving actual insurance authorization). Alternatively, scheduling the patient can await receipt of the precertification. Practices that perform a high volume of a given type of injection procedure (e.g., viscosupplementation) may want to consider scheduling these patients during a specified time block as the procedure can often be performed most efficiently in that manner with ancillary staff being made available to help with the process. Although some patients will not be able to conform to this particular scheduling routine, these patients can then be placed elsewhere within the schedule. Block scheduling can prove to be a major time saver with respect to the reception time that would otherwise be needed to review and coordinate the patient's schedule and the physician's schedule. Block scheduling can also help patients remember appointments. For example, it can be an advantage for patients to know in advance that they have been scheduled for a series of five Hyalgan® injections on Tuesday mornings at a particular time, rather than being scheduled on different days and at different times each week.

Precertification issues can also be simplified with block scheduling since, for example, the staff would be aware that all precertifications for viscosupplementation must be received by Monday of the week in order to be prepared for the Tuesday schedule. By having the staff double check at least the day before the procedure, an opportunity to communicate with the insurance company and the patient has been created. If need be, the patient can be informed that precertification has not yet been received and the procedure will need to be rescheduled. While it is not ideal to reschedule a procedure on the day before it was to occur, this is preferable to inform the patient about the need to reschedule once they have arrived on the day of the procedure or to perform the procedure without precertification.

Block scheduling can also help with the setup time involved with performing a given procedure. For example, if multiple patients are scheduled to undergo the same procedure during a given time period, an appropriate amount of materials used for the procedure can already be taken out and set up in advance. On the day of the injection procedure, additional important administrative steps must be followed. For example, obtaining and documenting informed consent is an important administrative aspect of office-based injection procedures. It is essential that a physician review the proposed procedure with the patient before it is performed by the physician. He/she should explain the procedure in sufficient detail and use terminology that is appropriate so that the patient has a clear understanding of the procedure as well as alternate options, risks, and potential side effects of the injections. Perhaps the most common patient complaint is that the physician did not mention a particular potential adverse reaction. Therefore, the physician should explain and document in the informed consent that the most common potential complications were explained. If a patient then experiences a postprocedure complication, it is at least documented within the informed consent that the patient was advised of those particular and other side effects. The expected outcomes and goals of the specific injection procedure should also be discussed and documented. As a general rule, it should be explained that there is the possibility of more discomfort due to a given procedure. The patient ideally should be encouraged to ask questions. The physician should try to keep in mind that, although a given procedure may be routine to the physician, it is not routine to the patient. The patient is often still anxious and uncomfortable, no matter how comforting the physician may be. Allowing the patient to ask questions is important. Once the informed consent discussion has been completed and signed, it is important to document this in writing. The following is a list of important categories that should be addressed on the actual informed consent form (Fig. 5.4):

- Name of procedure
- Purpose and benefits of the procedure
- Risks of the procedure
- Risks of not undergoing the procedure
- Alternate treatment options
- Risks and benefits of alternative treatment options
- Consent for administration of anesthesia
- A statement that the patient was encouraged to ask questions
- Signatures and dates to include physician, patient, guardian (if applicable), and witness to the consent process
- No guarantee of outcome or assurance about results

After an injection, ice or heat can be placed on the injection site for approximately 20 min following the procedure. This can help keep the patient in the office so that they can be observed for potential complications or side effects, particularly if local anesthetic was administered, as maximum arterial plasma concentrations of anesthetics develop within 10–25 min [4].

Consent For Surgical, Diagnostic and Other Procedures	**Patient Information**

1. **Procedure:** I hereby authorize and consent to the performance of the following procedure: _____under the direction of Dr._____ or designee with the assistance and participation of resident physicians.

2. **Purpose and Benefits:** I understand that the purpose for and potential benefits of the procedure are:

_____

_____

3. **Risks:** This authorization is given with the understanding that any procedure involves some risks and hazards. The more common risks of some procedures include infection, bleeding, scarring, nerve injury, blood clots, injury to other organs or blood vessels, allergic reactions, drug reactions, and heart attack. Other procedures have their own risks which can be serious and possibly fatal. Other risks specific to me for the procedure above include:

_____

4. **Risks of not having not having procedure:**

_____

5. a) **Alternatives:** Alternative forms of care if any include:

_____

  b) **Risks and benefits of alternatives:**

_____

6. **Anesthesia:** The act of delivering anesthesia has the benefits of relief and protection from pain, but carries no guarantees.

7. I recognize during the course of the procedure, unforeseen conditions may necessitate additional or different procedures than those described in # 1 above.
Please check A, or A and B.

_____ (A) I therefore authorize and consent to the performance by the medical staff of any additional treatments, procedures or operations only as they may relate to the primary treatments, procedures or operations as indicated in # 1.

_____ (B) Should any other unforeseen non-emergency conditions become evident during the performance by the medical staff of any additional operations or procedures that may be necessary to treat them.

8. **Patient's Consent:** I certify that I have read and fully understand this consent form that I understand the reason and purpose of the operation or procedure, its risks, benefits and alternatives, and possible complications as explained to me by:

Fig. 5.4 An example of an informed consent form

_____
Physician or designee

I certify that all explanations referred to above were made, I was encouraged to ask questions and that all blanks and statements requiring insertion or completion were filled in before I signed the consent. I acknowledge and understand that no guarantee or assurance has been made as to the results of the procedure and that it may not cure my condition.

_____   _____   _____
Signature of patient   Date   Time

_____
If patient is unable to sign, signature of other legally responsible person.

_____   _____
Relationship to patient   Time

The procedure or operation stated on this form, including the possible risks, benefits, complications, alternative treatments (including non-treatment) and anticipated results, was explained by me to the patient or his/her representative.

_____   _____   _____
Signature of physician   Date   Time

8. Informed Consent by Telephone:
Date:_____   Time:_____

_____   _____
Name of person giving telephone consent   Relationship to patient

_____
Telephone # and address of person giving telephone consent

_____   _____
Print name of physician who obtained consent   Signature of physician who obtained consent

_____   _____
Print name of witness to telephone consent   Signature of witness to telephone consent

---

Fig. 5.4 (continued)

Having the patient remain in the office for this time period can also give the patient the sense of having spent a definite block of time in the physician's office, as opposed to being briefly seen for a quick procedure and then billed at a higher rate compared to a regular office visit, during which they may have had more direct contact with the physician. When used solely for the purposes of observing for side effects and as a way of promoting general patient satisfaction, ice or heat modalities should not be billed separately as they might if the modality was being used for definite therapeutic benefit.

Once the procedure has been performed, a follow-up visit should be scheduled if one is not already pending. Ideally, patients should be scheduled for a follow-up appointment before they leave the office or facility. In addition, a phone call should be made to the patient that evening or the next morning following the procedure to see how they are doing. This call can be made by an ancillary staff person such as a nurse, assistant, or receptionist. The only time the physician should make this call is if the patient specifically asks for the doctor or if the procedure was unusually difficult, complications occurred, or the physician has any other concerns. When the ancillary staff contacts the patient, they should reaffirm that the follow-up appointment has been scheduled. A short list of typical patient questions and standard answers can be created so that the office personal can provide concise and well-informed answers. If this approach is used, it should be emphasized to the staff that they should not attempt to answer medical questions or give medical advice beyond those contained in the prefabricated list. Depending upon the patient's preference, these additional questions should either be referred to the physician at that time or they can be addressed at the time of the follow-up visit.

The procedure itself should be documented in sufficient detail so that there is no room for others to interpret what was done. This is important in cases of alleged malpractice whereby the opposing side may use a sparsely documented note to its advantage in order to allege that a standard of care was violated. Detailed procedure documentation is also important for purposes of reimbursement, as submission of the actual procedure note may be required by the insurance company.

Even if precertification was obtained, the claim still might not be paid if the office note does not substantiate that the procedure was actually performed. The use of prefabricated forms for paper chart documentation or computerized templates for computerized medical records can greatly assist with the ease with which complete documentation of a procedure is performed. Ideally, the form or template should be easily modifiable to allow for communicating any additional details that are not otherwise obvious from reading the form. A sample procedure note for each of the injection procedures discussed in the book is contained in each chapter.

In addition to documenting the actual procedure, the physician should give serious consideration to ensuring that the following information is present in the patient's medical record:

- Summary of the history of present illness
- Other treatments (if any) that were attempted prior to or in conjunction with the injection procedure
- Results of relevant diagnostic tests
- Current physical examination findings
- Diagnostic impression including a discussion of why the procedure is felt to be medically necessary

Unfortunately, even when precertification has been obtained, it still may be necessary to document in such a way that medical necessity for a procedure is obvious to anyone reviewing the patient's medical record. One should not assume that the preceding office note has been made available to the reviewer who is giving an opinion on the medical necessity of the procedure. Therefore, the physician may want to use captured notes in order to be able to literally copy and paste the information contained in a previous office note into the actual procedure note.

Alternatively, a previous comprehensive office note can be modified to reflect any recent changes in symptoms, medications, test results, and physical examination, and the procedure template is added to the remainder of the note. The final product then consists of a fully documented office note along with the details of the procedure that was performed that day. This should provide enough documentation to support the medical necessity for the procedure and satisfy the CPT coding requirements. This level of documentation can also be very helpful in cases of alleged malpractice if it is argued by the plaintiff's attorney that the procedure was not necessary in the first place.

Billing and Coding for Office-Based Injection Procedures

Once the clinician part of the procedure has been successfully completed and documented, the services performed must be properly billed and coded. Accurate billing and coding is essential for maximum and timely reimbursement. The procedure must be coded using the proper CPT codes that are linked to a correct International Classification of Diseases (ICD-9 codes).

A correct match between ICD-9 and CPT codes is crucial as all payment for the procedure will be denied if the ICD-9 code does not meet the payer's criteria for medical necessity or reimbursement guidelines. A current list of CPT codes and modifiers, along with descriptions for their appropriate use, can be found in any updated CPT manual. It is important that physicians ensure that the manual they are using is current because CPT codes and modifiers change from year-to-year without specific notification from insurance carriers, and it is the responsibility of the provider to stay abreast of these changes. A list of the most commonly used CPT codes for office-based injection procedures is shown in Table 5.1. Physicians can utilize their specialty organizations and annual meetings to keep up with changes in CPT and ICD updates. For example, the American Academy of Physical Medicine and Rehabilitation (AAPM&R) and the American Association of Neuromuscular and Electrodiagnostic Medicine (AANEM) publish user-friendly CPT billing and coding manuals. Practical billing and general administration continuing education credits are another way to keep up with these business and administrative aspects of medicine. The AAPM&R also conducts a billing and coding course in which these topics are covered. Staying current with Medicare changes and Medicare regulation is particularly important since Medicare often sets the standard that other insurance companies follow. All insurance carriers, including Medicare, have local representatives. Physicians should encourage key personnel from their office staff to get to know these representatives on a personal level.

Table 5.1 Commonly used CPT Codes for office-based joint and soft tissue injection procedures

Injection type	CPT code	Examples/comments
Carpal tunnel	20526	Injection, therapeutic, carpal tunnel
Intramuscular injections	90772	Use for injections into muscle, other than trigger point injections (see below); e.g., corticosteroid injection into piriformis muscle belly; Toradol injection
Joint/bursa		
• Large	20610 (Must specify side)	See Table 5.2 for classification of joints
• Medium	20605	and bursae based upon size
• Small	20600	
Tendon insertion site	20551	For example, rotator cuff tendon insertion site
Tendon sheath	20550	For example, trigger finger, bicipital tendon sheath; deQuervain's injection
Trigger point		
• 1–2 areas	20552	Use for traditional trigger point injections with local anesthetics and/or corticosteroids, and pertains to dry needling of trigger points
• ≥3 areas	20553	

Insurance company representatives are often pleased that the physician's office "wants to do it the right way."

The internet, using both general search engines and Pub Med, can also be a valuable tool. It is surprising how many people, including physicians, are willing to share billing and coding information [5, 6]. Learning from others' mistakes is often much less painful than learning from one's own mistakes. Due to the difficulties often associated with accurate coding in the setting of changing coding guidelines, some suggest considering outsourcing a practice's coding [7].

Examples of Billing and Coding for Office-Based Injection Procedures

Example 1

CPT 20605 should be used for a medium size joint (e.g., ankle joint) or bursa (e.g., olecranon bursa) aspiration and/or injection. If an injection was performed, a separate medication charge in the form of a J-code should also be submitted. For example, J1030 is used to indicate that 40 mg of methylprednisolone was administered at the time of the injection procedure (Fig. 5.5).

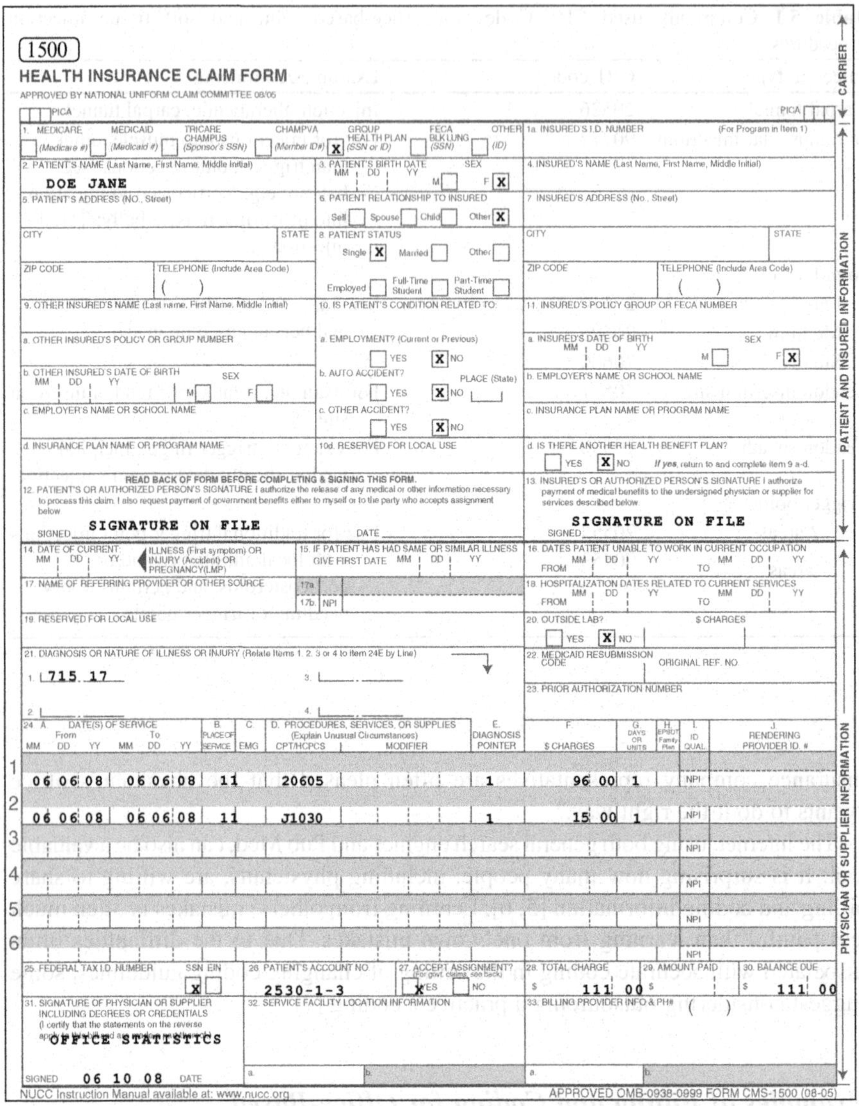

Fig. 5.5 Sample of Health Insurance Claim Form 1500: Unilateral injection of an intermediate size joint or bursa with methylprednisolone 40 mg

Example 2

If the injection was performed under fluoroscopic guidance, CPT code 77002 (fluoroscopic guidance for needle placement into a body region other than the spine) should be used in addition to the CPT code for the joint injection procedure and the J-code for the injectate.

Using Modifiers

Two-digit modifier codes are used to report that a given service or procedure has been "altered or modified by some specific circumstance." Depending on the particular circumstance, the two-digit modifier that best describes the situation should be used. The use of these two-digit modifiers is particularly relevant to office-based injection procedures as these procedures are sometimes conducted as part of an office visit, are sometimes performed bilaterally, are sometimes performed along with additional procedures, are sometimes discontinued due to extenuating circumstances, are sometimes performed along with other procedures that are not normally reported together, etc.

The most commonly applied modifiers in the setting of office-based injection procedures are discussed next. In order to facilitate use of these modifiers, a specific example for each of these modifiers has been provided.

Modifier 25: Significant, Separately Identifiable Evaluation and Management Service by the Same Physician on the Same Day of a Procedure or Other Service

If an office visit is also conducted at the time of an injection procedure, the appropriate Evaluation and Management (E/M) code should be used along with the 25 modifier. It is important to note that the physician should document within the note that the patient's overall condition required a significant, separately identifiable E/M service that was above and beyond the usual preprocedural and postprocedural care associated with the injection procedure.

Since the E/M service was provided due to a symptom or condition for which the injection procedure was performed, a separate ICD-9 code was not required for reporting the E/M service on the same day. Of note, for injection and/or aspiration procedures involving a major-sized joint or bursa such as a knee, hip, or shoulder, insurance carriers are requiring documentation on the HCFA 1500 claim form of the side(s) of the body on which the procedure was performed. Specifically, LT (left) or RT (right) should be used after the CPT code to indicate the side of the body on which the procedure was performed. Bilateral procedures are treated differently and are in the section on the 50 modifier.

Example 1

A patient is seen for left knee pain. The physician decides the patient could benefit from a corticosteroid knee injection on that visit. The physician should bill for the evaluation, and the procedure and related services using the modifier 25 applied to the E/M code. The J code for the corticosteroid should also be billed. Because both the E/M code and the joint injection were performed as a result of knee pain, only 1 ICD-9 code (i.e., knee pain = 715.16) is needed.

Example 2

An established patient is seen specifically for the purpose of undergoing a knee joint injection, but at the time of the procedure visit the patient is also complaining of lower back pain. The patient would also like his/her lower back pain addressed on this visit. The physician should bill for the procedure and a separate E/M service for the lower back pain evaluation using the modifier 25 applied to the E/M code. The physician must also add an additional diagnosis code for the back pain, which is linked to the E/M code but not to the procedure code.

Modifier 50: Bilateral Procedure

In contrast to the situations in which a patient underwent a left knee injection, modifier 50 should be used if an aspiration and/or injection procedure is performed bilaterally. This modifier should be applied for aspiration and/or injection of major, medium, and small sized joints or bursae (i.e., CPT 20610, 20605, and 20600, respectively).

In order to help the physician choose the proper CPT code based upon target structure size, Table 5.2 classifies joints and burse based upon size.

Modifier 51 vs. Modifier 59

Distinct Procedural Service

Under certain circumstances, the physician may need to indicate that a procedure or service was distinct or independent from other services performed on the same day. This code is used differently from the 51 multiple procedure modifier. One way to distinguish between these two modifiers as they pertain to injection procedures is to use the rule of thumb that the 51 modifier is used when the injection is through the same opening or body area, whereas the 59 modifier is used when the injections involve different body regions, as stated directly in the modifier description manual [8]. Rules regarding ICD-9 usage changed some time ago. There is no longer any requirement for two different ICD-9 codes per AMA coding guidelines. Medicare also follows this update.

Multiple Procedures

When the same provider performs multiple procedures (other than E/M services) at the same visit, the primary procedure or service may be reported as listed. Depending on the type of procedures, the 51 or 59 modifier can be used by appending these to the additional procedure(s). Modifier 59 identifies that add-on codes are being used. Add-on codes are codes that have a "+" by them in the CPT book. Some

Table 5.2 Size classification of joints and bursae

Body region	Specific structure	Major size (CPT 20610)	Medium size (CPT 20605)	Small size (CPT 20600)
Shoulder	AC joint		X	
	Glenohumeral joint	X		
	Subacromial bursa	X		
	Sternoclavicular joint		X	
Elbow	Elbow joint		X	
	Radiocapitellar joint		X	
	Olecranon bursa		X	
Wrist/hand	Wrist joint		X	
	Distal radioulnar joint		X	
	Triangular fibrocartialge complex (TFCC) region		X	
	1st carpometacarpal (CMC) joint			X
	Other carpometacarpal joint			X
	MCP joint			X
	PIP joint			X
	DIP joint			X
Hip region	Hip joint	X		
	Trochanteric bursa	X		
	Gluteus medius bursa	X		
	Iliopsoas bursa	X		
Knee region	Knee joint	X		
	Suprapatellar bursa	X		
	Prepatellar bursa	X		
	Infrapatellar bursa	X		
	Pes anserine bursa	X		
Ankle/foot region	Ankle joint		X	
	Subtalar joint		X	
	Sinus tarsi		X	
	Retrocalcaneal bursa		X	
	1st metatarsophalangeal (MTP) joint			X
	Other MTP joint			X
	PIP joint			X
	DIP joint			X

of the listed procedures are commonly carried out in addition to the primary procedure performed. These additional or supplemental procedures are designated as add-on codes. Add-on codes are not routinely used for office injection procedures. They are mainly used in interventional pain management procedures and are not covered in this chapter.

Here is an example. A patient with pain due to deQuervain's tenosynovitis comes to the office for a scheduled visit to have a right wrist corticosteroid tendon sheath injection, and this procedure is performed. At the time of the visit, he also reports complaints

PLEASE
DO NOT
STAPLE
IN THIS
AREA

HEALTH INSURANCE CLAIM FORM

PICA			PICA	

1. MEDICARE   MEDICAID   CHAMPUS   CHAMPVA   GROUP HEALTH PLAN   FECA BLK LUNG   OTHER   1a. INSURED'S I.D. NUMBER   (FOR PROGRAM IN ITEM 1)

(Medicare #)   (Medicaid #)   (Sponsor's SSN)   (VA File #) XX   (SSN or ID)   (SSN)   (ID)

2. PATIENT'S NAME (Last Name, First Name, Middle Initial)
DOE JANE

3. PATIENT'S BIRTH DATE   MM   DD   YY   M   SEX XX

4. INSURED'S NAME (Last name, First name, Middle Initial)

5. PATIENT'S ADDRESS (No., Street)

6. PATIENT RELATIONSHIP TO INSURED
Self   Spouse   Child   Other X

7. INSURED'S ADDRESS (No., Street)

CITY   STATE

8. PATIENT STATUS
Single X   Married   Other

CITY   STATE

ZIP CODE   TELEPHONE (Include Area Code) (   )

Employed   Full-Time Student   Part-Time Student

ZIP CODE   TELEPHONE (INCLUDE AREA CODE) (   )

9. OTHER INSURED'S NAME (Last Name, First Name, Middle Initial)

10. IS PATIENT'S CONDITION RELATED TO:

11. INSURED'S POLICY GROUP OR FECA NUMBER

a. OTHER INSURED'S POLICY OR GROUP NUMBER

a. EMPLOYMENT? (CURRENT OR PREVIOUS)
YES X NO

a. INSURED'S DATE OF BIRTH   MM   DD   YY   M   SEX X F

b. OTHER INSURED'S DATE OF BIRTH   MM   DD   YY   M   SEX   F

b. AUTO ACCIDENT?   PLACE (State)
YES X NO

b. EMPLOYER'S NAME OR SCHOOL NAME

c. EMPLOYER'S NAME OR SCHOOL NAME

c. OTHER ACCIDENT?
YES X NO

c. INSURANCE PLAN NAME OR PROGRAM NAME

d. INSURANCE PLAN NAME OR PROGRAM NAME

10d. RESERVED FOR LOCAL USE

d. IS THERE ANOTHER HEALTH BENEFIT PLAN?
YES X NO   If yes, return to and complete item 9 a-d.

READ BACK OF FROM BEFORE COMPLETING & SIGNING THIS FORM.
12. PATIENT'S OR AUTHORIZED PERSON'S SIGNATURE I authorize the release of any medical or other information necessary to process this claim. I also request payment of government benefits either to myself or to the party who accepts assignment below.   SIGNATURE ON FILE

SIGNED   DATE

13. INSURED'S OR AUTHORIZED PERSON'S SIGNATURE I authorize payment of medical benefits to the undersigned physician or supplier for services described below.   **AUTHORIZATION ON FILE**

SIGNED

14. DATE OF CURRENT: ILLNESS (First symptom) OR INJURY (Accident) OR PREGNANCY(LMP)   MM   DD   YY

15. IF PATIENT HAS HAD SAME OR SIMILAR ILLNESS GIVE FIRST DATE   MM   DD   YY

16. DATES PATIENT UNABLE TO WORK IN CURRENT OCCUPATION   MM   DD   YY   FROM   TO   MM   DD   YY

17. NAME OF REFERRING PHYSICIAN OR OTHER SOURCE

17a. I.D. NUMBER OF REFERRING PHYSICIAN

18. HOSPITALIZATION DATES RELATED TO CURRENT SERVICES   MM   DD   YY   FROM   TO   MM   DD   YY

19. RESERVED FOR LOCAL USE

20. OUTSIDE LAB?   YES X NO $ CHARGES

21. DIAGNOSIS OR NATURE OF ILLNESS OR INJURY. (RELATE ITEMS 1, 2, 3 OR 4 TO ITEM 24E BY LINE)

1. **719 24**   3.
2. **844 9**   4.

22. MEDICAID RESUBMISSION   CODE   ORIGINAL REF. NO.

23. PRIOR AUTHORIZATION NUMBER

24.

A. DATE(S) OF SERVICE From			To			B. Place of Service	C. Type of Service	D. PROCEDURES, SERVICES, OR SUPPLIES (Explain Unusual Circumstances) CPT/HCPCS	MODIFIER	E. DIAGNOSIS CODE	F. $ CHARGES		G. DAYS OR UNITS	H. EPSDT Family Plan	I. EMG	J. COB	K. RESERVED FOR LOCAL USE
MM	DD	YY	MM	DD	YY												
10	18	2006	10	18	2006	11	1	99205	25	1 2	250	00	1				
10	18	2006	10	18	2006	11	1	20550	59	1 2	140	00	1				
10	18	2006	10	18	2006	11		J1030		1 2	15	00	1				

25. FEDERAL TAX I.D. NUMBER   SSN EIN XX

26. PATIENT'S ACCOUNT NO.   **1694-1-16**

27. ACCEPT ASSIGNMENT? (For govt. claims, see back) X YES   NO

28. TOTAL CHARGE $ **405 00**

29. AMOUNT PAID $

30. BALANCE DUE $ **405 00**   **201-968-1200**

31. SIGNATURE OF PHYSICIAN OR SUPPLIER INCLUDING DEGREES OR CREDENTIALS (I certify that the statements on the reverse apply to this bill and are made a part thereof.)
OFFICE STATISTICS

SIGNED   **10 18 2006**   DATE

32. NAME AND ADDRESS OF FACILITY WHERE SERVICES WERE RENDERED (If other than home or office)

33. PHYSICIAN'S, SUPPLIER'S BILLING NAME, ADDRESS, ZIP CODE & PHONE #
214 STATE STREET
HACKENSACK, NJ 07601

PIN#   GRP#

(APPROVED BY AMA COUNCIL ON MEDICAL SERVICE 8/88)   **PLEASE PRINT OR TYPE**   APPROVED OMB-0938-0008 FORM CMS-1500(12-90)   FORM RRB 1500

CARRIER

PATIENT AND INSURED INFORMATION

PHYSICIAN OR SUPPLIER INFORMATION

Fig. 5.6 Sample of Health Insurance Claim Form 1500: High complex initial evaluation office visit and unilateral injection of tendon sheath or with methylprednisolone 40 mg.

of knee pain, which was also evaluated by the physician. Since the patient was seen for both the tendon sheath injection and knee pain, an E/M service for the knee pain would also be deemed medically necessary in addition to the injection CPT code 20550. An actual HCFA-1500 claim form for this very situation is shown in Fig. 5.6.

In contrast, if the patient were returning only for the tendon injection and for no other reason, an E/M service would not be deemed medically necessary as this was a visit that was scheduled for purposes of undergoing a tendon sheath injection.

Most payers do not pay for the cost of local anesthetics that are administered as part of the procedure. They consider these to be medications that are incidental to the procedure.

Modifier 53: Discontinued Procedure

Under certain circumstances, the physician may elect to terminate a therapeutic or diagnostic injection procedure. This usually involves procedural termination due to extenuating circumstances or those that threaten the well-being of the patient. For example, if a patient has a vasovagal episode during a carpal tunnel injection procedure but before the physician has had a chance to complete the procedure, the physician may choose to terminate the procedure at that point.

This circumstance may be reported by adding modifier 53 to the CPT 20526 procedure code reported by the physician. In contrast, if a patient comes to the office for a planned procedure but elects not to undergo the procedure before the procedure was begun, the 53 modifier is not appropriate. The physician may instead choose to bill for an E/M code at the appropriate level of care that was provided in lieu of the procedure.

Other Required Coding Information for Office-Based Injection Procedures

Insurance carriers are routinely asking that LOT numbers (aka MDC #s) located on the medication vial be entered onto the HICFA 1500 claim form. In addition, the dosage of the medication that was actually used should be documented in the office notes as well as on the HCFA 1500 claim form. Claims may be denied if any of this information has been omitted.

Appealing a Denied Claim for an Office-Based Injection Procedure

Payment for office-based injection procedures always carry the risk of being denied somewhere along the claims submission process. It is important to follow the designated guidelines that are set forth by the insurance carrier. These guidelines may require preauthorization or the burden of proof that the procedure was reasonable and necessary. Thorough documentation is the key to successful reimbursement. For procedures performed on patients with osteoarthritis, diagnostic test results such as X-ray reports should be kept in the chart in order to document the presence of osteoarthritis.

In addition, any other therapies that the patient has tried should also be documented. In case of a denial, one should not simply give up and accept the carrier's decision to deny payment. Instead, one can aggressively follow the available appeals mechanism as set forth by the insurance company, which every carrier is required by law to have in writing and make available to physicians and beneficiaries. The appeals process often involves submission of an appeal letter, but sometimes a simple phone call between the treating physician and the insurance company's medical director can result in successful reimbursement.

If an appeal letter is sent, consideration should also be given to submitting other key documents (e.g., imaging reports, electrodiagnostic testing reports, etc.) that may help the insurance company conclude that the injection procedure was medically necessary. Pursuing the appeals process is often worth the time, because it is a general rule that an appealed claim denial associated with proper documentation will often be paid.

Summary and Conclusion

Office-based injection procedures are a valuable service for meeting the medical needs of the patients served by physicians and can also strengthen the financial health of a medical practice. Mastering the administrative aspects of office-based injection procedures is vital in order to be properly reimbursed for these services and for the physician's skill and time needed to learn and perform them, for the potential liability to the physician that can arise in the event of an adverse outcome from these procedures, and for the office time required to precertify, bill, and collect for the procedures.

Perhaps the biggest mistake physicians make in this aspect of their practices is to delegate all responsibility to someone else in the belief that they do not have the time or knowledge necessary to be personally responsible. However, physician time spent on the administrative aspects of office-based injection procedures is time well spent.

References

1. http://www.cms.hhs.gov/McrPartBDrugAvgSalesPrice There are exceptions to this general reimbursement methodology.
2. http://www.cms.hhs.gov/CompetitiveAcquisforBios.
3. http://www.ama-assn.org/ama/pub/category/16392.html.
4. Essential equipment, safety precautions and emergency situations. Section I: Principles of musculoskeletal injections. In Kesson M, Atkins E, Davies I. Musculoskeletal Injection Skills. Philadelphia, PA: Butterworth-Heinemann;2003:10–7.
5. Mack AL. How to complete a medical insurance form. Funct Orthod 1997;14(5):18–9, 22, 24–7.

6. Lamothe HL. Clinical insights for office practice management. Orthop Nurs 1998; 17(1):23–6.
7. Miller J, Linberry J. Coding for effective denial management. Radiol Manage 2004; 26(1):18–21.
8. https://www.highmarkmedicareservices.com/refman/chapter-20.html#3.

Part II
Upper Limb Injection Procedures

Chapter 6
The Shoulder

Todd P. Stitik, Jong H. Kim, Michael J. Mehnert,
Mohammad Hossein Dorri, Jose Ibarbia, David J. Van Why,
Lisa Schoenherr, Naimish Baxi, Ladislav Habina, and Jiaxin J. Tran

Introduction

Shoulder region injection procedures collectively are one of the most frequently performed musculoskeletal injection procedures. A survey of primary care physicians determined that these represented the most common type of office-based injection procedure [1]. A study from an outpatient physiatric musculoskeletal practice found that the most commonly performed shoulder region injection procedure, injections into the subacromial space ($n = 114$; subacromial space $= 90$), represented 21% of the total injection procedures exclusive of trigger point injections performed during a 2-year time period [2]. Shoulder region injection procedures include those into joints, bursae, tendon sheaths, and tendon insertion sites as summarized in Table 6.1 and shown in Figs. 6.1 and 6.2.

Shoulder region injections can provide important diagnostic information, as the identification of a specific pain generator via traditional history and physical examination can be limited. An important reason for this limitation is the fact that a variety of different shoulder pathologies can cause very similar symptoms, including pain, loss of strength, decreased range of motion, and instability. In addition, the yield from the physical examination can be very limited due to factors such as pain-related guarding [60]. Furthermore, the degree of pathology may directly influence the yield of the physical examination. For example, Park and colleagues found the degree of impingement affected the diagnostic values of the commonly used clinical tests for demonstrating impingement [61]. Two other published studies have examined the accuracy of the physical examination for detecting AC joint pathology. With respect to the AC joint, some information is available on the relative accuracy of the physical examination in identifying patients who have AC joint pathology. For example, the senior author (TS) studied the positive predictive value for AC joint physical examination maneuvers (AC joint pain with

T.P. Stitik (✉)
Department of Physical Medicine and Rehabilitation, New Jersey Medical School,
Newark, NJ, USA
e-mail: todd.stitik@gmail.com

Table 6.1 Summary of shoulder region injection procedures

Injection type	Specific structure	Meta-analysis(es)	Prospective study(ies)	Case series/report(s) and/or retrospective studies	Described in general article(s) and/or injection textbook(s)
Articulation/joint	Acromioclavicular joint		[3–5]	[6]	[7–10, 11]
	Glenohumeral joint[a]	[12]	[13]		[7, 8, 10, 14]
	Sternoclavicular joint				[7, 8]
Bursa	Subacromial	[15]	[16]		[7, 8, 10, 17]
	Subscapularis				
Nerve block	Suprascapular nerve block		[18–22]	[23–48]	[7, 8, 49–52]
Tendon region injections	Supraspinatus tendon region		[53]		[7, 8, 10, 54, 55]
	Infraspinatus tendon region				[7, 8, 10, 56, 57]
	Teres minor tendon region				[10]
	Subscapularis tendon region				[7, 8, 58]
Tendon sheath	Bicipital tendon sheath				[7, 10, 59]

Listed within each injection type in order of descending amount of current evidence supporting its use. Representative references are provided for those procedures that are only described in general articles and/or textbooks
[a] Includes both simple corticosteroid injections and distension arthrography procedures

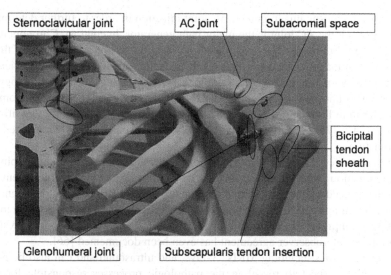

Fig. 6.1 Shoulder injection sites. Anterior view

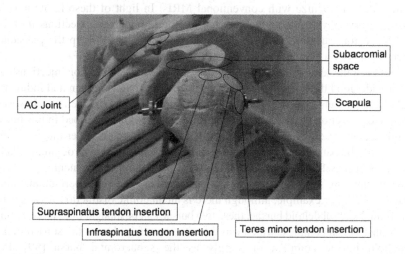

Fig. 6.2 Shoulder injection sites. Lateral/postolateral view

palpation, AC joint crepitus during passive abduction, AC joint region pain during active abduction, O'Brien's active compression test, passive crossed adduction-"Scarf test") in patients complaining of shoulder pain who then subsequently underwent a fluoroscopic-guided AC joint injection [62]. The study found that there was a very good positive predictive value for those patients who had three or more positive physical examination maneuvers. In contrast, the number of patients (i.e., three) who were studied who had only one or two positive physical examination maneuvers was too limited to draw any meaningful conclusions. Perhaps those patients with a limited number of positive physical examination maneuvers should undergo a diagnostic image-guided AC joint injection in order to further determine whether or not the AC joint is the major pain generator. In contrast, Chronopoulos and colleagues retrospectively calculated the sensitivities and specificities of three physical examination maneuvers (cross body adduction stress test, acromioclavicular resisted extension test, active compression test) for detecting AC joint pathology in patients who underwent subsequent distal clavicle excision for isolated acromio-clavicular joint lesions [63]. They concluded that these tests had utility (sensitivity range of 41–77%; specificity range of 79–92%), particularly when used in combination.

Further evidence suggestive of limitations in the accuracy of the shoulder physi-cal examination comes from the fact that newer physical examination maneuvers (e.g., the resisted supination external rotation test and the Kim test for the diagnosis of superior and posteroinferior labral tears, respectively) have been described in an attempt to improve examination efficacy [64, 65]. In addition, poor physical examination interobserver agreement has even been documented [66].

Imaging studies including MRIs, X-rays, and ultrasound and can also be non-specific with respect to revealing the pathologic processes responsible for the patient's pain [67, 68]. In addition, some shoulder pathology (e.g., labral tears) can be difficult to recognize with conventional MRIs. In light of these limitations in patient history, physical examination, and imaging, diagnostic injections into the shoulder region can potentially serve as an additional tool to help the physician correctly identify a given pain generator.

It has been the senior author's (TS) experience that shoulder region injections can also provide good therapeutic benefit, both directly by relieving pain and indirectly by allowing patients to more meaningfully participate in physical therapy. However, as is true of injection procedures into the other body regions described in this book, a combined approach of an injection and therapeutic exercise, either taught by the physician to the patient or as part of a structured physical therapy program, is likely to be more successful than an isolated injection without other treatment.

When planning shoulder region injections, there are several important anatomic considerations. For example, although there is an anatomic distinction between the subacromial and subdeltoid bursae, these two bursae can be thought of as representing one distinct bursal complex, which can therefore be referred to as the subacromial–subdeltoid bursae complex or simply as the subacromial bursa [69]. For simplification, these two structures will be collectively referred to in this book as the subacromial bursa. There is also often confusion between a subacromial injec-tion and a glenohumeral joint injection. Some texts in fact do not clearly make the distinction between these two separate structures [70]. If a patient has an intact rotator cuff, the subacromial space and the glenohumeral joint are anatomically distinct, and an injection can be performed into either structure with the injectate remaining only within the target structure. In the setting of a full-thickness rotator cuff tear, the two spaces are no longer anatomically separated. In fact, appearance of the injected contrast solution within the subacromial space after it has been injected into the glenohumeral joint was the basis behind shoulder arthrography when it was commonly used for the diagnosis of a rotator cuff tear, prior to the

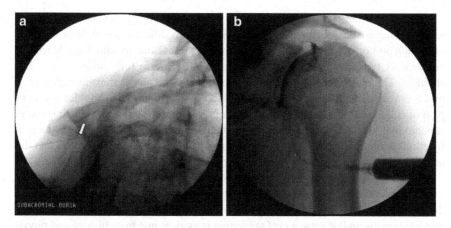

Fig. 6.3 Fluoroscopy guided injection into the subacromial space (**a**) and glenohumeral joint (**b**)

advent of MRI [69]. Although shoulder region injections into osteoarthritis patients have been previously described in some detail, fluoroscopic images of these injections have not been published within a book such as this (Fig. 6.3).

Subacromial Bursa (Subacromial Space) Injections

Although this injection is most commonly referred to as a subacromial bursa injection, this is likely a misnomer and should more accurately be referred to as a subacromial space or subacromial region injection unless ultrasound-guidance is used to visualize needle entry into the bursa. The senior author (TS) has begun using ultrasound guidance for some shoulder region injections procedures and has come to realize that, even in cases of acute subacromial bursitis, it is unlikely that non-image-guided injections are actually being placed into the bursa per se. Instead, the injections are more typically placed into the subacromial space, and at times are likely placed into the rotator cuff or into the deltoid muscle. This impression is supported by a study of ultrasound guidance for subacromial injections [71]. Precise placement of corticosteroid into the actual subacromial bursa led to a statistically significant improvement in range of abduction compared to blind injections, presumably into the subacromial bursa or subacromial space. For the purposes of this book, the injection will continue to be referred to using the classic terminology subacromial bursa injection.

It has been the senior author's (TS) clinical impression and experience that subacromial bursa injections comprise the vast majority of injections into the shoulder region in the outpatient musculoskeletal medicine setting. This injection is even more commonly used than a supraspinatus tendon insertion site injection because subacromial bursitis and supraspinatus tendonitis most commonly coexist, thus a subacromial bursa injection would probably be the logical first injection choice.

Subacromial bursa injections are performed for both diagnostic and therapeutic reasons. Diagnostic subacromial injections can help differentiate deficits in range of motion and/or strength due to impingement vs. those due to a high-grade rotator cuff tear. A typical scenario is a patient who is unable to fully abduct his or her shoulder. The patient's pain may be interfering with the physical examination such that it is very difficult to determine if the inability to abduct the shoulder is due to pain or is due to true weakness from a rotator cuff tear. In this setting, a diagnostic subacromial local anesthetic injection can help to immediately make the distinction by eliminating pain. Specifically, if the patient is able to essentially fully abduct the arm after the injection, then a large rotator cuff tear has likely been excluded.

In addition to their use as diagnostic tools, subacromial injections can also be used therapeutically, both as follow-up treatment in those patients with positive diagnostic injections and in those in whom the diagnosis of subacromial (aka subdeltoid) bursitis and/or rotator cuff tendonitis is evident just from history and physical examination. A therapeutic subacromial corticosteroid injection can be particularly helpful in those patients who might otherwise have difficulty participating in any meaningful way in physical therapy due to pain. Although adhesive capsulitis is another disorder for which subacromial injections are sometimes performed in patients with concomitant subacromial bursitis, most of the literature on corticosteroid injections for adhesive capsulitis pertains to glenohumeral joint injections.

AC Joint Injections

It has been the senior author's (TS) experience that the AC joint is the second most frequently injected shoulder region structure. This joint can be affected by a number of pathologic processes, including primary and posttraumatic secondary osteoarthritis, sprains, and osteolysis of the distal clavicle (aka bencher's shoulder or weightlifter's shoulder). It can be difficult to reliably make this determination based on history, physical examination, and imaging without performing a diagnostic injection for a number of reasons. First, there are several different potential pain referral patterns from the AC joint as was shown in a saline injection study [72]. Second, asymptomatic AC joint degeneration is frequently encountered and does not always correlate with the presence of symptoms [73]. In addition, AC joint and subacromial region pathology often coexist, especially because AC joint pathology is felt to frequently accompany chronic rotator cuff impingement syndrome [74]. Therefore, it can be virtually impossible to apportion the pain between the AC joint and the subacromial space without a diagnostic injection. The AC joint is also sometimes overlooked as a site of potential pathology because of certain radiographic issues. For example, in order to properly visualize the joint, an apical lordotic X-ray view is needed as this view positions the AC joint perpendicular to the X-ray beam. This view, however, is not routinely included in either a degenerative shoulder series or in a trauma shoulder series. The AC joint is also atypical in that erosions, rather than osteophytes, typically develop in osteoarthritis [75]. Therefore, radiographic evidence of "typical" osteoarthritis may be lacking on plain films, and therefore, the diagnosis of AC joint osteoarthritis might be simply overlooked. Finally, visualization of subtle AC joint separations requires weight-bearing stress views or use of dynamic ultrasound scanning.

AC joint corticosteroid injections are particularly important in the management of AC joint pathology, especially because therapeutic exercise has a very limited role in treating AC joint pathology. AC joint injections can also be helpful in patients who have received only partial benefit from subacromial corticosteroid injections. In retrospect, these patients were probably also apparently suffering from pathology in the AC joint. While injections in the AC joint are currently limited to corticosteroid injections, the senior author (TS) did conduct a double blinded randomized placebo controlled clinical trial on AC joint viscosupplementation with Hyalgan ® (Sanofi-Aventis, Bridgewater, NJ, USA) [3]. Fluoroscopic guidance was utilized to ensure injection accuracy. Use of image guidance for AC joint injection was found to be an important determinant of injection accuracy, as injection accuracy was only 39.4% in 66 shoulders when performed without image guidance [76]. A cadaveric study of injection accuracy found that the success rate for AC joint injection was only 67% in 16 shoulders [77]. The senior author (TS) also found that surface palpation by residents and fellows was inaccurate for identification of the underlying AC joint [78].

Glenohumeral Joint Injections

It has been generally taught that the glenohumeral joint is not a common site of primary osteoarthritis [79, 80]. However, secondary osteoarthritis can occur on a posttraumatic basis such as due to a previous humeral head fracture or due to a large rotator cuff tear (cuff arthropathy). Secondary osteoarthritis can also occur due to deposition of calcium hydroxyapatite crystals ("Milwaukee shoulder"). Glenohumeral joint injections are performed as a treatment for either primary or secondary osteoarthritis pain as part of the treatment of adhesive capsulitis and diagnostically in order to help determine if pathology within the joint (e.g., labral pathology) is acting as a pain generator. Although exact statistics are not readily available, it has been the senior author's (TS) impression that these injections are performed much less frequently compared to subacromial injections due to the higher frequency of subacromial pathology and the relative ease with which a subacromial injection can be performed compared to a glenohumeral injection.

Cochrane Database of Systematic Reviews examined the use of glenohumeral joint injections for adhesive capsulitis [12]. They found that the addition of glenohumeral joint corticosteroid injections to other treatments probably leads to improved pain and range of motion in the early stages of the disease process. However, since the natural history of adhesive capsulitis is generally good, there might not be any long-term differences among treatment approaches, including no specific treatment at all. There are fewer studies on their use in rotator cuff pathology, and their use in this setting is also questionable as one study found no difference in benefit from corticosteroid injections compared to ultrasound treatments, acupuncture, or even placebo treatment [81]. There have been several studies of intra-articular injections as one of the injection procedures for shoulder pain due to "mixed diagnoses" [82, 83]. However, due to the non-uniformity of diagnoses being treated and the combined injection procedures that were performed, it is difficult to draw conclusions. The senior author (TS) is particularly skeptical of nonimage-guided studies involving glenohumeral joint injections as he has an appreciation for how difficult it can sometimes be to place the needle into the joint, even using fluoroscopic or ultrasound guidance. Difficulty with accurate needle placement is particularly true in obese individuals. The senior author (TS) also believes that, even in nonobese individuals, the typical 1.5-in. needle length used for many other injections is inadequate to reach the actual glenohumeral joint.

The use of viscosupplementation for glenohumeral osteoarthritis has been studied. A nonfluoroscopic guided clinical trial was conducted, which compared Hylgan® to saline injections. The study found efficacy for those patients with glenohumeral osteoarthritis as the origin of their pain [84]. At this time, however, viscosupplements are not FDA-approved for shoulder osteoarthritic pain.

Rotator Cuff Tendon Region Injections

Depending upon the location of pathology, inflammation associated with rotator cuff tendinoses can theoretically be treated with injections into the rotator cuff tendon region, at the musculotendinous junction, or at the insertion sites of the tendons onto the corresponding bony structure (i.e., tenoperiosteal junction). As was stated in the introductory chapter, the use of autologous blood injections are not discussed in this book. For simplification, the term tendon region injection will be used in this book when referring to these injections. These procedures can at least be considered in the setting of rotator cuff tendonitis or partial tears in the acute setting when they are probably associated with inflammation. They are clearly different from subacromial injections in which the injections are performed into the subacromial space and inflammation associated with rotator cuff pathology is presumably treated by relieving the subacromial bursitis that may secondarily develop and/or by diffusion of the corticosteroid through the undersurface of the bursa and onto the underlying rotator cuff tendons. From the perspective of injection procedures, supraspinatus pathology should perhaps be considered as being somewhat unique compared to pathology of the other rotator cuff tendons, as the supraspinatus tendon and its insertion site are situated much closer to the subacromial bursa than the other three rotator cuff tendon insertion sites. Therefore, a subacromial injection procedure is logically more likely to help manage supraspinatus-related inflammation compared to pathology of the other rotator cuff tendons. The main site of pathology of supraspinatus tendonitis is usually in the rotator cuff critical zone of relative hypovascularity located 1 cm proximal to (rather than exactly at) its insertion site region on the greater tuberosity [85]. It is unclear as to whether injections at this site or into the subacromial space best treat the inflammation associated with supraspinatus pathology. Although it is generally believed that rotator cuff tendonitis and subacromial bursitis coexist, a supraspinatus tendon site injection has the advantage of placing the medication closer to the actual site of primary pathology in patients with rotator cuff tendonitis. This might only be of theoretical advantage, because corticosteroid perhaps diffuses out of the subacromial bursa and onto the rotator cuff tendon anyway. This might explain why patients who appear to primarily have supraspinatus tendonitis seem to respond at least in part to subacromial injections. A supraspinatus tendon insertion injection, however, is more difficult to perform than a subacromial injection. It is, therefore, still unclear as to the exact role of this injection procedure compared to the more traditionally used subacromial injection. The relatively recent use of ultrasound for injection guidance may lead to increased performance of injection procedures that are more targeted to specific sites of pathology along a rotator cuff tendon that have been visualized by an MRI and/or noted during the process of using ultrasound to guide the injection. Fluoroscopic guidance is of very limited value for these procedures, as the tendon cannot be visualized unless it is sufficiently calcified. The fluoroscope can help, however, to guide needle placement at the likely insertion site on the humeral head. The senior author (TS) has found that subsequent contrast dye injection is very unlikely to outline the actual tendon. Thus, the main use of contrast dye is to rule out inadvertent vascular injection, as this can occur even in the setting of a negative aspiration prior to injection. Although these injection procedures have been described in various texts and articles, very few studies have examined their efficacy and potential complications. The authors have limited collective experience in performing these procedures since they historically have preferred to treat rotator cuff tendonitis or acute partial rotator tears with a subacromial corticosteroid injection. Although the vast majority of pathology involves the supraspinatus in its critical zone, it is the consensus amongst the authors that most rotator cuff pathology is usually associated with a component of subacromial bursitis and therefore is adequately treated at least in part with a subacromial corticosteroid injection. The authors have preferred subacromial injections because they are easy to perform and there is an extremely limited body of literature on rotator cuff tendon region injections in general compared to subacromial injections. The authors' treatment approach, however, might be changing with the advent of ultrasound guidance and autologous blood injections, specifically PRP injections.

Supraspinatus Tendon Region Injection

A literature search found only one published study on this injection technique [51]. Withrington and colleagues compared supraspinatus tendon region corticosteroid injections with placebo injections in 25 patients with supraspinatus tendonitis [53]. The study found no difference in pain or analgesic consumption at 2 and 8 weeks follow-up.

Infraspinatus Tendon Region Injection

Isolated infraspinatus tendonitis is generally believed to be relatively rare compared to supraspinatus tendonitis. Infraspinatus tendonitis, however, has been described in certain individuals such as assembly line workers who perform activities such as installing brake pads, since this requires repetitive adduction and external shoulder rotation [54]. In contrast, two studies found that there was somatosensory alteration from injecting hypertonic saline into the infraspinatus muscle itself [86, 87].

Subscapularis Tendon Region Injection

Isolated subscapularis pathology is relatively rare compared to supraspinatus pathology. Subscapularis tendonitis, however, has been described in individuals such as assembly line workers who perform activities requiring repetitive adduction and internal shoulder rotation [56].

Although injections into the subscapularis tendon sheath or tendon insertion site have not been studied, the effect of botulism toxin injection into the subscapularis muscle has been reported [88]. In addition, the accuracy of injection into the subscapularis muscle during electromyography or botulism toxin, as well as subscapularis nerve injection accuracy have been repeated [89].

Teres Minor Tendon Region Injection

Isolated teres minor pathology is extremely rare, but the senior author (TS) has treated a patient with calcific tendonitis of this structure, probably due to chronic weightlifting activities. A search of the medical literature up until the time of this writing failed to reveal any studies on injections into the teres minor tendon sheath or insertion site.

Bicipital Tendon Sheath Injections

It has been traditionally taught that the long and short biceps head tendons are rarely involved in pathology without other concomitant shoulder pathology. In contrast, bicipital tendonitis is often present along with rotator cuff tendonitis and/or subacromial bursitis. As part of shoulder impingement syndrome, the long head of the biceps tendon is often impinged beneath the coracoacromial arch [90]. Increased use of diagnostic musculoskeletal ultrasound should help to more clearly define the frequency and extent of biceps tendon pathology.

There are no published actual studies on the efficacy, accuracy, or side effects associated with bicipital tendon sheath corticosteroid injections. A general statement appears throughout the literature that caution should be exercised with tendon sheath injections because inadvertent intratendinous injections have been associated with tendon rupture.

The authors have limited experience in performing bicipital tendon sheath injections as they believe that these injections are uncommonly needed in a typical outpatient musculoskeletal practice because bicipital tendonitis most often accompanies subacromial bursitis/rotator cuff tendonitis as a secondary pathologic process rather than as the primary pathology. An exception to this may be in patients who chronically overuse their anterior shoulder region structures, such as paraplegic patients who manually propel their wheelchairs. As such, an injection is often more logically performed into the subacromial space as this will directly treat the primary pathology and indirectly treat the secondary pathologic process. On occasion, an injection into both the subacromial bursa and the bicipital tendon sheath will be needed to optimally manage a patient's symptoms. This might change however, as ultrasound is being utilized more commonly in the senior author's (TS) practice.

The coracobrachialis muscle is rarely involved in pathology. Injury to this muscle was, however, described in a golfer who "grounded the club" (golf grounding syndrome aka "FOSTI FOYE" syndrome) [91]. There are no published reports on injection procedures of this structure.

Nerve Block Procedures: Suprascapular Nerve Block

Because the suprascapular nerve transmits sensation from the glenohumeral joint, the AC joint, and the shoulder capsule, a suprascapular nerve block at the supraspinatus notch region can, therefore, potentially relieve pain from all of these structures. However, this procedure also produces supraspinatus and infraspinatus weakness because the suprascapular nerve innervates these muscles. Although a generally accepted treatment algorithm for use of this injection procedure has not been published, this nerve block procedure can probably be considered as a second line injection procedure that is performed if a glenohumeral joint or AC joint injection was either not technically possible or not successful in alleviating a patient's pain. In addition, it can be used in cases of ongoing shoulder region pain with either multiple pain generators or without a specific known pain generator. Alternatively, the procedure can be performed to help diagnose and subsequently treat a patient with suprascapular nerve entrapment. There is also limited literature as described in the following text, which actually supports its use in the setting of ongoing pain due to subacromial or rotator cuff pathology.

Suprascapular nerve blocks and infusions have been studied alone and in combination with other procedures to varying degrees in the management of shoulder pain, for the prevention of referred shoulder pain after surgery, and as a diagnostic tool in hemiplegic shoulder pain. Painful conditions for which the nerve block and infusions have been used include adhesive capsulitis, osteoarthritis, rheumatoid arthritis, rotator cuff tendonitis and tears, acute shoulder dislocation, chronic shoulder pain presumptively from subacromial bursitis, shoulder pain after shoulder surgery, malignancy-associated shoulder pain, and referred shoulder pain. Despite the multitude of conditions for which this procedure has been used, there does not appear to be any consensus in the literature as to the exact indications for this procedure.

Suprascapular nerve blocks have been successful in limited trials in reducing shoulder pain associated with adhesive capsulitis [18, 19]. The use of suprascapular nerve blocks for adhesive capsulitis due to reflex sympathetic dystrophy (aka RSD or complex regional pain syndrome [CRPS]) has been described [23]. Suprascapular nerve blocks have also been studied in combination with stellate ganglion blocks and electroacupunture for adhesive capsulitis [24]. This study found that 50 patients who received the combination of a suprascapular nerve and stellate ganglion block along with electroacupuncture did significantly better than those 50 patients who only received electroacupuncture and those 50 who only underwent the two nerve block procedures. It was unclear from this study if the patients were felt to have adhesive capsulitis in association with RSD as a reason for including a stellate ganglion block.

Several small studies have been published on the use of this procedure for patients with rheumatoid arthritis (RA) or osteoarthritis (OA) affecting the shoulder region [25, 26]. There has only been one large randomized placebo controlled trial examining the efficacy of suprascapular nerve block for shoulder pain in arthritis and/or degenerative disease using pain and disability end points. Shanahan and colleagues conducted a randomized, double blind, placebo controlled trial of the efficacy of suprascapular nerve block for shoulder pain in RA and/or OA of the shoulder in 83 patients (108 shoulders). They found clinically and statistically significant improvements in all pain scores, all disability scores, and some range of movement scores in the shoulders receiving suprascapular nerve block compared with those receiving placebo at weeks 1, 4, and 12. In addition, there were no significant adverse effects in either group. The procedure has also been studied in combination with an axillary nerve block to treat pain associated with osteoarthritis and rheumatoid arthritis [27].

Vecchio and coworkers described the use of this block in rotator cuff tendonitis via a randomized controlled trial [28]. The authors concluded that a steroid/bupivacaine mixture was temporarily effective in reducing pain in rotator cuff tendonitis and tears, improving movement range in tendonitis, and is possible in an outpatient setting with little or no complication risk.

Case reports have been published on the successful use of suprascapular nerve blocks in the setting of acute shoulder dislocation [29]. However, when suprascapular nerve blocks were subsequently compared to intra-articular local anesthetic to relieve pain associated with acute shoulder dislocation, they were found to be inferior both in terms of efficacy and ease of administration [30].

Comments have been published on the use of this procedure for malignancy-associated shoulder pain [31]. Suprascapular nerve blocks have also been studied on a limited basis in the setting of reducing shoulder pain after nonarthroscopic shoulder surgery. It is believed to be a useful adjunct to general anesthesia and interscalene brachial plexus blocks for short-term postoperative analgesia, but there have been conflicting reports regarding its benefit at 24 h after surgery [32].

The procedure has been studied for referred shoulder pain after nonshoulder surgery but has not been found to be effective. For example, it did not prevent shoulder tip pain after laparoscopic surgery [33]. Another trial found that it did not offer pain relief of referred shoulder pain associated with thoracotomy [20]. Chronic shoulder pain, presumptively from the subacromial bursa, has been alluded to in the literature as a use for the procedure [34]. There have been no published studies, however, on its use in this setting.

In addition to its use in treating shoulder pain, suprascapular nerve blocks have been utilized in a study of painful shoulder in hemiplegic patients in order to help determine the etiology of the pain [35]. Using suprascapular nerve conduction studies along with the block procedure, it was concluded that a lesion of the suprascapular nerve was not responsible for the painful contracted shoulder of the hemiplegic patient, although such a lesion may exist incidentally.

In addition to single injection procedures, continuous suprascapular nerve blocks have been studied on a limited basis for chronic nonmalignant shoulder pain. This topic, however, is beyond the scope of this text.

The senior author (TS) has limited experience with this injection. This is in large part due to his willingness to perform and familiarity with glenohumeral joint and AC joint injections. The senior author considers suprascapular injections to be second line procedures because, in comparison with glenohumeral joint and AC joint injections, suprascapular nerve blocks are more technically difficult to perform, carry with them potentially greater morbidity, and can cause concomitant rotator cuff weakness, albeit transient.

The first paper describing a suprascapular nerve block appears to have been published in 1989 [36]. Since this time, several slight variations of this technique for suprascapular nerve blocks have been described [37–41, 49]. A PubMed literature search revealed only one study that compared the different injection techniques [41]. Specifically, a suprascapular nerve block technique using electromyography to localize the needle (aka near-nerve electromyography technique) was compared to a landmark-guided technique in patients with adhesive capsulitis. The near-nerve electromyography technique was felt to be more successful in providing and maintaining pain relief for the 60-min study time period. In this book, the authors describe a technique that combines the use of EMG-guidance and fluoroscopic guidance. Both forms of guidance are used in an effort to maximize accuracy and safety. More recently ultrasound-guided suprascapular nerve block procedures have been developed.

Sternoclavicular Joint Injection

The sternoclavicular (SC) joint is formed by articulations of the sternal end of the clavicle, the manubrium of the sternum, and the first rib cartilage. It is a true meniscus-containing synovial joint and is covered by a loose fibrous capsule that is reinforced by the anterior and posterior SC ligaments. It acts as a fulcrum for all shoulder girdle motions [49]. The joint is usually only a late and relatively mild site of osteoarthritic involvement despite relative excess use over a lifetime [92]. Although OA is the most common disorder of the SC joint, the osteoarthritic SC joint also generally does not cause significant functional impairment [93]. Injections and/or aspiration of the joint has been described in other settings such as in the rare occurrence of a traumatic SC joint dislocation [94]. Other pathologies that have be very rarely described but for which an injection might be required include infection [95], renal failure-related amyloid deposition, and Charcot joint in a patient with syringomyelia [96, 97].

Due to the relative scarcity of its involvement in pathology, it is not one of the more commonly injected structures about the shoulder-girdle. There are in fact no published studies on injections of the sternoclavicular joint.

The senior author (TS) does not have a significant amount of experience with this injection compared to other shoulder region injection procedures. His impression, however, is that it is a relatively easy injection to perform as the joint is quite superficial and readily palpable. A fluoroscopic guided approach to this injection is described in the book. Ultrasound guidance can also be used and to date the senior author (TS) has performed this on two occasions.

Summary and Conclusion

Shoulder injection procedures are powerful diagnostic and therapeutic tools for the care of patients with OA and other pathology of the shoulder-girdle region. While questions regarding many of the details of the specific procedures still need to be answered, a modest body of literature is available for some of these. The increased utilization of ultrasound within musculoskeletal medicine is likely to result in an increased performance and study of certain shoulder region injection procedures. Whatever the increased injection accuracy afforded with image guidance translates into, better efficacy remains to be seen.

References

1. Gormley GJ, Corrigan M, Steele WK, Stevenson M, Taggart AJ. Joint and soft tissue injections in the community: questionnaire survey of general practitioners' experiences and attitudes. Ann Rheum Dis 2003;62(1):61–4.
2. Stitik TP, Foye PM, Nadler SF, Chen B, Schoenherr L, Von Hagen S. Injections in patients with osteoarthritis and other musculoskeletal disorders: use of synthetic injection models for teaching physiatry residents. Am J Phys Med Rehabil 2005;84:550–9.
3. Stitik TP, Schoenherr L, Buttaci CJ, Foye PM, Yonclas PP, Kim JH. A randomized double-blinded crossover trial of acromioclavicular (AC) joint intra-articular sodium hyaluronate (Hyalgan®) for the treatment of chronic shoulder pain due to AC joint osteoarthritis. Arch Phys Med Rehabil 2006;87(11):e24.
4. Kurta I, Datir S, Dove M, Rahmatalla A, Wynn-Jones C, Maffulli N. The short term effects of a single corticosteroid injection on the range of motion of the shoulder in patients with isolated acromioclavicular joint arthropathy. Acta Orthop Belg 2005;71(6):656–61.
5. Jacob AK, Sallay PI. Therapeutic efficacy of corticosteroid injections in the acromioclavicular joint. Biomed Sci Instrum 1997;34:380–5.

6. Strobel K, Pfirrmann CW, Zanetti M, Nagy L, Hodler J. MRI features of the acromioclavicular joint that predict pain relief from intraarticular injection. AJR Am J Roentgenol 2003;181(3):755–60.

7. Stitik TP, Foye PM, Fossati J. Shoulder injections for osteoarthritis and other disorders. Phys Med Rehabil Clin N Am 2004;15(2):407–46.

8. Saunders S. Shoulder Treatments. In Law M, ed. Injection Techniques in Orthopaedic and Sports Medicine. Second edition. London: WB Saunders; 2002:30–45.

9. Waldman SD. Acromioclavicular Joint Pain. In Bralow L, Ross A, Carino M, eds. Atlas of Pain Management Injection Techniques. Philadelphia,PA: WB Saunders; 2000:40–2.

10. Kesson M, Atkins E, Davies I. The Shoulder. In Kesson M, Atkins E, Davies I, eds. Musculoskeletal Injection Skills. New York: Butterworth Heinemann; 2002:43–64.

11. Talia RF, Cardone DA. Diagnostic and therapeutic injection of the shoulder region. Am Fam Physician 2003;67(6):1271–8.

12. Buchbinder R, Green S, Youd JM. Corticosteroid injections for shoulder pain. Cochrane Database Syst Rev 2003;1:CD004016.

13. Miller SL, Cleeman E, Auerbach J, Flatow EL. Comparison of intra-articular lidocaine and intravenous sedation for reduction of shoulder dislocation: a randomized, prospective study. J Bone Joint Surg Am 2002;84-A(12):2135–9.

14. Waldman SD. Intra-articular Injection of the Shoulder Joint. In Bralow L, Ross A, Carino M, eds. Atlas of Pain Management Injection Techniques. Philadelphia, PA: WB Saunders; 2000:37–9.

15. Arroll B, Goodyear-Smith F. Corticosteroid injections for painful shoulder: a meta-analysis. Br J Gen Pract 2005;55(512):224–8.

16. Henkus HE, Cobben LP, Coerkamp EG, Nelissen RG, van Arkel ER. The accuracy of subacromial injections: a prospective randomized magnetic resonance imaging study. Arthroscopy 2006;22(3):277–82.

17. Waldman SD. Subdeltoid Bursitis Pain. In Bralow L, Ross A, Carino M, eds. Atlas of Pain Management Injection Techniques. Philadelphia, PA: WB Saunders; 2000:60–2.

18. Dahan TH, Fortin L, Pelletier M, Petit M, Vadeboncoeur R, Suissa S. Double blind randomized clinical trial examining the efficacy of bupivacaine suprascapular nerve blocks in frozen shoulder. J Rheumatol 2000;27(6):1464–9.

19. Jones DS, Chattopadhyay C. Suprascapular nerve block for the treatment of frozen shoulder in primary care: a randomized trial. Br J Gen Pract 1999;49(438):39–41.

20. Tan N, Agnew NM, Scawn ND, Pennefather SH, Chester M, Russell GN. Suprascapular nerve block for ipsilateral shoulder pain after thoracotomy with thoracic epidural analgesia: a double-blind comparison of 0.5% bupivacaine and 0.9% saline. Anesth Analg 2002;94(1): 199–202.

21. Di Lorenzo L, Pappagallo M, Gimigliano R, Palmieri E, Saviano E, Bello A et al. Pain relief in early rehabilitation of rotator cuff tendinitis: any role for indirect suprascapular nerve block? Eura Medicophys 2006;42(3):195–204.

22. Singelyn FJ, Lhotel L, Fabre B. Pain relief after arthroscopic shoulder surgery: a comparison of intraarticular analgesia, suprascapular nerve block, and interscalene brachial plexus block. Anesth Analg 2004;99(2):589–92.

23. Wassef MR. Suprascapular nerve block. A new approach for the management of frozen shoulder. Anaesthesia 1992;47(2):120–4.

24. Lin ML, Huang CT, Lin JG, Tsai SK. A comparison between the pain relief effect of electroacupuncture, regional never block and electroacupuncture plus regional never block in frozen shoulder Acta Anaesthesiol Sin 1994;32(4):237–42.

25. Emery P, Bowman S, Wedderburn L, Grahame R.Suprascapular nerve block for chronic shoulder pain in rheumatoid arthritis. BMJ 1989;299(6707):1079–80.

26. Brown DE, James DC, Roy S. Pain relief by suprascapular nerve block in gleno-humeral arthritis. Scand J Rheumatol 1988;17(5):411–5.

27. Shanahan EM, Ahern M, Smith M, Wetherall M, Bresnihan B, FitzGerald O. Suprascapular nerve block (using bupivacaine and methylprednisolone acetate) in chronic shoulder pain. Ann Rheum Dis 2003;62(5):400–6.

28. Vecchio PC, Adebajo AO, Hazleman BL. Suprascapular nerve block for persistent rotator cuff lesions. J Rheumatol 1993;20(3):453–5.
29. Edeland HG, Stefansson T. Block of the suprascapular nerve in reduction of acute anterior shoulder dislocation. Case reports. Acta Anaesthesiol Scand 1973;17(1):46–9.
30. Gleeson AP, Graham CA, Jones I, Beggs I, Nutton RW. Comparison of intra-articular lignocaine and a suprascapular nerve block for acute anterior shoulder dislocation. Injury 1997; 28(2):141–2.
31. Meyer-Witting M, Foster JM. Suprascapular nerve block in the management of cancer pain. Anaesthesia 1992;47(7):626.
32. Neal JM, McDonald SB, Larkin KL, Polissar NL Suprascapular nerve block prolongs analgesia after nonarthroscopic shoulder surgery but does not improve outcome. Anesth Analg 2003;96(4):982–6.
33. Hong JY, Lee IH Suprascapular nerve block or a piroxicam patch for shoulder tip pain after day case laparoscopic surgery Eur J Anaesthesiol 2003;20(3):234–8.
34. Carron H. Relieving pain with nerve blocks. Geriatrics 1978;33(4):49–57.
35. Lee KH, Khunadorn F. Painful shoulder in hemiplegic patients: a study of the suprascapular nerve. Arch Phys Med Rehabil 1986;67(11):818–20.
36. Granirer LW. A simple technic for suprascapular nerve block. N Y State J Med 1951; 51(8):1048.
37. Parris WC. Suprascapular nerve block: a safer technique. Anesthesiology 1990;72(3):580–1.
38. Risdall JE, Sharwood-Smith GH. Suprascapular nerve block. New indications and a safer technique. Anaesthesia 1992;47(7):626.
39. Dangoisse MJ, Wilson DJ, Glynn CJ. MRI and clinical study of an easy and safe technique of suprascapular nerve blockade. Acta Anaesthesiol Belg 1994;45(2):49–54.
40. Fournier R, Haller G, Hoffmeyer P, Gamulin Z. Suprascapular nerve block by a new anterior approach for perioperative analgesia during major scapular surgery in two patients. Reg Anesth Pain Med 2001;26(3):288–9.
41. Karatas GK, Meray J. Suprascapular nerve block for pain relief in adhesive capsulitis: comparison of 2 different techniques Arch Phys Med Rehabil 2002;83(5):593–7.
42. Kefalianakis F, Scriba K, Hoffmann M, Jung I, Kugler M. Incorrect positioning of a catheter for continuous block of the nervus suprascapularis. A case report. Anaesthesist 2003;52(6): 507–10.
43. Martinez J, Sala-Blanch X, Ramos I, Gomar C. Combined infraclavicular plexus block with suprascapular nerve block for humeral head surgery in a patient with respiratory failure: an alternative approach. Anesthesiology 2003;98(3):784–5.
44. Cesur M, Alici HA, Erdem AF, Dostbil A. A novel approach to locate the suprascapular nerve in a patient with a shoulder tumour: the specular symmetry technique. Anaesth Intensive Care 2006;34(1):121–3.
45. Eckert S, Hornburg M, Frey U, Kersten J, Rathgeber J. Frozen shoulder-MRI-verified continuous block of suprascapular nerve. Anasthesiol Intensivmed Notfallmed Schmerzther 2001;36(8):514–7.
46. Mercadante S, Sapio M, Villari P. Suprascapular nerve block by catheter for breakthrough shoulder cancer pain. Reg Anesth 1995;20(4):343–6.
47. Meyer-Witting M, Foster JM. Suprascapular nerve block in the management of cancer pain. Anaesthesia 1992;47(7):626.
48. Breen TW, Haigh JD. Continuous suprascapular nerve block for analgesia of scapular fracture. Can J Anaesth 1990;37(7):786–8.
49. Cailliet R. Shoulder Pain. Second edition. Philadelphia, PA: FA Davis;1989:64.
50. Waldman SD. Suprascapular Nerve Entrapment. In Ross A, Chappelle A, eds. Atlas of Uncommon Pain Syndromes: Philadelphia, PA: Saunders; 2003:63–6.
51. Waldman SD. Suprascapular Nerve Block. In Andjelkovic N, Chappelle A, eds. Atlas of Interventional Pain Management. Second edition. China: WB Saunders; 2004:163–5.
52. Waldman SD. Suprascapular Nerve Block. In Lampert R, Ross A, Ruzycka A, eds. Interventional Pain Management. Second edition. Philadelphia, PA: WB Saunders; 2001:388–9.

53. Withrington RH, Girgis FL, Seifert MH. A placebo-controlled trial of steroid injections in the treatment of supraspinatus tendonitis. Scand J Rheumatol 1985;14(1):76–8.
54. Waldman SD. Supraspinatus Tendinitis. In Bralow L, Ross A, Carino M, eds. Atlas of Pain Management Injection Techniques. Philadelphia, PA: WB Saunders; 2000:43–5.
55. Waldman SD. Supraspinatus Tendinitis. In Ross A, Chappelle A, eds. Atlas of Uncommon Pain Syndromes. Philadelphia, PA: WB Saunders; 2003:67–70.
56. Waldman SD. Infraspinatus Tendinitis. In Bralow L, Ross A, Carino M, eds. Atlas of Pain Management Injection Techniques. Philadelphia, PA: WB Saunders; 2000:46–8.
57. Waldman SD. Infraspinatus Tendinitis. In Ross A, Chappelle A, eds. Atlas of Uncommon Pain Syndromes. Philadelphia, PA: WB Saunders; 2003:71–4.
58. Waldman SD. Subscapularis Tendinitis. In Bralow L, Ross A, Carino M, eds. Atlas of Pain Management Injection Techniques. Philadelphia, PA: WB Saunders; 2000:49–51.
59. Waldman SD. Bicipital Tendinitis. In Bralow L, Ross A, Carino M, eds. Atlas of Pain Management Injection Techniques. Philadelphia, PA: WB Saunders; 2000:52–5.
60. McFarland EG, Kim TK, Savino RM. Clinical assessment of three common tests for superior labral anterior-posterior lesions. Am J Sports Med 2002;30(6):810–5.
61. Park HB, Yokota A, Gill HS, El Rassi G, McFarland EG. Diagnostic accuracy of clinical tests for the different degrees of subacromial impingement syndrome. J Bone Joint Surg Am 2005;87(7):1446–55.
62. Stitik TP, Butacci C, Foye PM, Yonclas P, Schoenherr L Predictive value of physical examination of the shoulder for diagnosing pain due to acromioclavicular joint osteoarthritis. Archives of PM&R 2005;86(9):E7.
63. Chronopoulos E, Kim TK, Park HB, Ashenbrenner D, McFarland EG. Diagnostic value of physical tests for isolated chronic acromioclavicular lesions. Am J Sports Med 2004; 32(3):655–61.
64. Myers TH, Zemanovic JR, Andrews JR. The resisted supination external rotation test: a new test for the diagnosis of superior labral anterior posterior lesions. Am J Sports Med 2005;33(9):1315–20. Epub 2005 Jul 7.
65. Kim SH, Park JS, Jeong WK, Shin SK. The Kim test: a novel test for posteroinferior labral lesion of the shoulder – a comparison to the jerk test. Am J Sports Med 2005;33(8):1188–92. Epub 2005 Jul 6.
66. Nørregaard J, Krogsgaard MR, Lorenzen T, Jensen EM. Diagnosing patients with longstanding shoulder joint pain. Ann Rheum Dis 2002;61(7):646–9.
67. Teefey SA, Middleton WD, Patel V, Hildebolt CF, Boyer MI. The accuracy of high-resolution ultrasound for evaluating focal lesions of the hand and wrist. J Hand Surg [Am]. 2004;29(3):393–9.
68. Dinnes J, Loveman E, McIntyre L, Waugh N. The effectiveness of diagnostic tests for the assessment of shoulder pain due to soft tissue disorders: a systematic review. Health Technol Assess 2003;7(29):iii, 1–166. Review.
69. Hazleman BL. The Shoulder. In Rheumatology examination and Injection Techniques. Philadelphia, PA: WB Saunders; 1992:36–7.
70. Akpinar S, Hersekli MA, Demirors H, Tandogan RN, Kayaselcuk F. Effects of methylprednisolone and betamethasone injections on the rotator cuff: an experimental study in rats. Adv Ther 2002;19(4):194–201.
71. Chen MJ, Lew HL, Hsu TC, Tsai WC, Lin WC, Tang SF et al. Ultrasound-guided shoulder injections in the treatment of subacromial bursitis. Am J Phys Med Rehabil 2006;85(1):31–5.
72. Gerber C, Galantay RV, Hersche O. The pattern of pain produced by irritation of the acromioclavicular joint and the subacromial space. J Shoulder Elbow Surg 1998;7(4):352–5.
73. Shaffer BS, Painful conditions of the acromioclavicular joint. J Am Acad Orthop Surg 1999;7(3):176–88.
74. Gurbuz H, Unalan H, Sarisaltik H, Sekhavat H, Candan L. The role of acromioclavicular arthritis in impingement syndromes. Yonsei Med J 1998;39(2):97–102.
75. Helms CA. Fundamentals of skeletal radiology. Second edition. WB Saunders, Philadelphia, PA; 1995:119.

76. Bisbinas I, Belthur M, Said HG, Green M, Learmonth DJ. Accuracy of needle placement in ACJ injections. Knee Surg Sports Traumatol Arthrosc 2006;14(8):762–5. Epub 2006 Feb 8.

77. Partington PF, Broome GH. Diagnostic injection around the shoulder: hit and miss? A cadaveric study of injection accuracy. J Shoulder Elbow Surg 1998;7(2):147–50.

78. Levy J, Stitik TP et al. AC Joint-Use of Fluoroscopic Feedback to Increase acromioclavicular (AC) Joint Palpation Accuracy &-Predictive Value of Physical Examination of the Shoulder for Diagnosing Pain due to Acromioclavicular Joint Osteoarthritis. Dept. of PM&R UMDNJ-NJMS: The 17th Annual Residents/Fellows Research Day 2006 Jun: 7.

79. Moskowitz RW, Altman RD, Hochberg MC, Buckwalter JA, Goldberg VM. Osteoarthritis: diagnosis and medical/surgical management. Fourth edition. Philadelphia, PA: Wolters Kluwer Health/Lippincott Williams & Wilkins; 2007.

80. Stitik TP, Ali A. Managing glenohumeral joint osteoarthritis. J Musculoskel Med 2005; 12: 674–88.

81. Berry H, Fernandes L, Bloom B, Clark RJ, Hamilton EB. Clinical study comparing acupuncture, physiotherapy, injection and oral anti-inflammatory therapy in shoulder-cuff lesions. Curr Med Res Opin 1980;7(2):121–6.

82. Richardson AT. Ernest Fletcher Lecture. The painful shoulder. Proc R Soc Med 1975;68(11): 731–6.

83. Winters JC, Sobel JS, Groenier KH, Arendzen HJ, Meyboom-de Jong B. Comparison of physiotherapy, manipulation, and corticosteroid injection for treating shoulder complaints in general practice: randomised, single blind study. BMJ 1997;314(7090):1320–5.

84. http://clinicaltrials.gov/ct/show/NCT00377624.

85. Rathbun JB, Macnab I. The microvascular pattern of the rotator cuff. J Bone Joint Surg [Br] 1970;52(3):540–53.

86. Leffler AS. Kosek E. Hansson P. Injection of hypertonic saline into musculus infraspinatus resulted in referred pain and sensory disturbances in the ipsilateral upper arm. Eur J Pain 2000;4(1):73–82.

87. Pasetti A, Sabbadini G. Hypesthesia caused by injection of irritatin substances into the infraspinatus muscle. Policlinico [PratP] 1956;63(20):686–9.

88. Yelnik AP, Colle FM, Bonan IV. Treatment of pain and limited movement of the shoulder in hemiplegic patients with botulinum toxin a in the subscapular muscle. Eur Neurol 2003;50(2): 91–3.

89. Chiodo A, Goodmurphy C, Haig A. Cadaveric study of methods for subscapularis muscle needle insertion. Am J Phys Med Rehabil 2005;84(9):662–5.

90. Patton WC, McCluskey GM 3rd. Biceps tendinitis and subluxation. Clin Sports Med 2001;20(3):505–29.

91. Fossati JJ, Stitik TP, Foye PM. Golf Club Grounding-Menace to the Coracobrachialis Muscle: A Case Series. AAPMR, 2003.

92. DePalma AF. Degenerative Changes in The Sternoclavicular and Acromioclavicular Joint in Various Decades. Springfield, IL:Charles C. Thomas, 1957.

93. Le Loet X, Vittecoq O. The sternocostoclavicular joint: normal and abnormal features. Joint Bone Spine 2002;69(2):161–9.

94. Ferrera PC, Wheeling HM. Sternoclavicular joint injuries. Am J Emerg Med 2000;18(1): 58–61.

95. Mousa AM, Muhtaseb SA, Al-Mudallal DS, Marafie AA, Habib FM. Brucellar sternoclavicular arthritis, the forgotten complication. Ann Trop Med Parasitol 1988;82(3):275–81.

96. Zingraff J, Drueke T, Bardin T. Dialysis-related amyloidosis in the sternoclavicular joint. Nephron 1989;52(4):367.

97. Chidgey LK, Szabo RM, Benson DR. Neuropathic sternoclavicular joint secondary to syringomyelia. A case report. Orthopedics 1988;11(11):1571–3.

Procedure Instructions

Injection Procedure: Acromioclavicular (AC) Joint Injection

1. Indications:
   (a) AC joint: diagnosis as pain generator [1]
   (b) AC joint osteoarthritis [1]
   (c) AC joint sprain: refractory to initial conservative management [1]
   (d) Osteolysis of the distal clavicle [2]

2. Contraindications especially pertinent to this procedure:
   (a) None documented

3. Side effects especially pertinent to this procedure:
   (a) Exacerbation of pain due to relative injectate pressure overload.
      • The AC joint is generally believed to have a relatively small capacity. Consistent with this general belief, it is the experience of the senior author (TS), from having conducted a fluoroscopic-guided clinical trial of 30 patients with AC joint osteoarthritis, each of whom received a minimum of four and a maximum of seven AC joint injections, and from having performed AC joint injection procedures on dozens of other patients with and without AC joint osteoarthritis, that the approximate maximal volume is just over 1 ml [2].
   (b) Potential joint damage from needle trauma
   (c) Potential trauma to underlying rotator cuff tendons, secondary to inadvertent injection through AC joint and into the tendons
   (d) Pneumothorax is also a potential, albeit unlikely, complication.

4. Technical details of note for this procedure (Fig. 6.4):
   (a) Preferred needle gauge; length; type: 25-gauge; 2-in.; spinal
      • Use of a 25-gauge, 1-in. or 1.5-in. straight needle has been suggested [3].
   (b) Need for image guidance: Optional
      • While fluoroscopic guidance is not essential (as some patients have an easily palpable AC joint), it is strongly preferred due to the variable anatomy [4, 5]. Even for individuals with readily palpable AC joints, the depth of injection can be difficult to judge without fluoroscopic guidance. In a study by Bisbinas and colleagues, only 26/66 (39.4%) injections by palpation were properly placed in the AC joint, as determined by follow-up fluoroscopy [6].
      • Image guidance has the added benefit of less pain and trauma from needle maneuvering, which makes the procedure more tolerable for the patient. In a cadaver study by Partington and Broome, only 16/24 (67%) of AC joint injections were placed correctly, with half of those entering other structures, particularly the subacromial bursa [7].
      • It has been the senior author's (TS) experience that fluoroscopic guidance is extremely helpful.

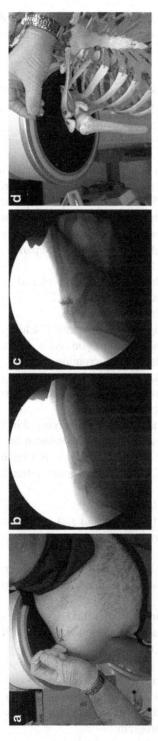

Fig. 6.4 Acromioclavicular (AC) joint injection (fluoroscopic-guided). (**a**) AC joint injection-human model. (**b**) Fluoroscopic image of needle entry into AC joint. (**c**) Fluoroscopic image of AC joint arthrogram. (**d**) Skeletal representation of AC joint injection

- Ultrasound guidance has also been described for this procedure and has been used on several occasions by the senior author (TS).

5. Step-by-step procedure:
   (a) Informed consent
   (b) Preprocedural testing: Identify and record the response to a physical examination preprocedural provocative maneuver if the procedure is a diagnostic injection.
   (c) Image guidance: Optional: Fluroscopic guidance
   (d) Patient positioning:
      - Have the patient in a seated position besides the fluoroscopy table, and angle the c-arm fluoroscope to provide an A-P lordotic view, at 10° of a cephalad tilt (Fig. 6.5). (This view helps to optimally visualize the joint by minimizing the appearance of overlying structures.)
      - The patient's shoulder should preferably be slightly extended (rather than flexed or in a neutral position), to help separate the acromion slightly from the distal clavicle.
      - If necessary, a weighted object may be placed in the patient's hand to further separate the acromion and clavicle.
   (e) Identification and marking of injection site.
      - Palpate laterally along the clavicle until reaching an anterior curvature. Move laterally beyond this until you feel a distinct depression between the end of the clavicle and the acromion.
      - Place a metallic marker over this site.
      - Shoot a fluoroscopic picture to assess if the proposed injection site correlates with the underlying AC joint.
      - Adjust as necessary, and mark the overlying skin by depressing it with a plastic needle cap or a marker with or without image guidance.
   (f) *Skin preparation.* Initial: Betadine® preparation using the no-touch technique
   (g) *Medication preparation.* 1 mL 2% preservative-free lidocaine
   (h) *Skin preparation.* Final: Alcohol prep
   (i) *Local anesthesia administration.*
      - Anesthetize the overlying skin and soft tissue using a *small amount of 1% lidocaine*, delivered via a *30-gauge, 1-in. needle*.
   (j) Needle placement:
      - Pierce the previously anesthetized skin and subcutaneous tissue site with the spinal needle and use intermittent fluoroscopic guidance for direction.
      - Attempt to aspirate any synovial fluid that might be present in the joint. (In the authors' collective experience, it is rare that synovial fluid can actually be aspirated from the AC joint.)
   (k) Contrast injection:
      - Inject the AC joint with a small amount of *Omnipaque*™ (generally less than 0.5 mL using a 1-mL syringe connected to the spinal needle via extension tubing). Adjust needle position, if necessary, in order to obtain a clearly defined arthrogram.

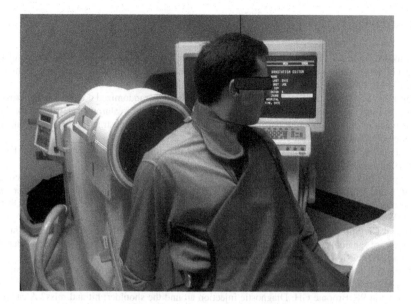

Fig. 6.5 Patient in a seated position besides the fluoroscopy table. C-arm fluoroscope angled to provide an A-P lordotic view, at 10° of a cephalad tilt

(l) Aspiration: Rule out intravascular entry, and confirm entry into target structure. Aspiration of a small amount of Omnipaque™ allows for a greater volume of subsequent injectate.

(m) Injection:
- Unclamp the syringe from the extension, and attach a *1-mL syringe containing the above-mentioned medication injectate.*
- Resistance
    - If resistance is encountered very early during the injection, rotate the needle as the needle bevel sometimes becomes lodged against the side of the joint.
    - If resistance is eventually encountered prior to delivering the entire injectate, this indicates that the capacity of the AC joint has been reached and the injection can be stopped.

(n) Postprocedural testing:
- Reassess the response to the same aforementioned preprocedural provocative maneuver.

(o) Repeat injection with therapeutic injectate:
- Repeat steps (d)–(f).
- Medication preparation: 20 mg of Depo-Medrol® with 0.5 mL of 1% preservative-free lidocaine
- Repeat steps (h)–(m).

(p) Apply adhesive *bandage* over the needle entry site

(q) Postprocedural care discussion

References

1. Stitik TP, Butacci C, Foye PM, Yonclas P, Schoenherr L. Predictive value of physical examination of the shoulder for diagnosing pain due to acromioclavicular joint osteoarthritis. Archives of PM&R 2005;86(9):E7.
2. Stitik TP, Schoenherr L, Buttaci CJ, Foye PM, Yonclas P. A randomized double-blinded crossover trial of acromioclavicular (AC) joint intra-articular sodium hyaluronate (Hyalgan) for the treatment of chronic shoulder pain due to AC joint osteoarthritis [abstract]. AAPM&R Annual Assembly 2006; Nov 9–12; New Orleans, LA.
3. Tallia AF, Cardone DA. Diagnostic and therapeutic injection of the shoulder region. Am Fam Physician 2003;67(6):1271–8.
4. Levy J, Stitik TP et al. AC Joint-Use of Fluoroscopic Feedback to Increase Acromioclavicular (AC) Joint Palpation Accuracy &-Predictive Value of Physical Examination of the Shoulder for Diagnosing Pain due to Acromioclavicular Joint Osteoarthritis. Dept. of PM&R UMDNJ-NJMS: The 17th Annual Residents/Fellows Research Day 2006 Jun: 7.
5. Buttaci CJ, Stitik TP, Yonclas PP, Foye PM. Osteoarthritis of the acromioclavicular joint: a review of anatomy, biomechanics, diagnosis, and treatment. Am J Phys Med Rehabil 2004;83(10):791–7.
6. Bisbinas I, Belthur M, Said HG, Green M, Learmonth DJ. Accuracy of needle placement in ACJ injections. Knee Surg Sports Traumatol Arthrosc 2006;8:1–4.
7. Partington PF, Broome GH. Diagnostic injection around the shoulder: hit and miss? A cadaveric study of injection accuracy. J Shoulder Elbow Surg 1998;7(2):147–50.

Injection Procedure: Bicipital Tendon Sheath Injection

1. Indications:
   (a) Bicipital tendonitis diagnosis as pain generator or treatment [1]

2. Contraindications especially pertinent to this procedure:
   (a) Previous injections. Repeat injections should be avoided due to the risk of tendon rupture [2]. The exact number of injections that increases the risk is not known with certainty.

3. Possible side effects especially pertinent to this procedure:
   (a) Iatrogenic injury to the tendon, including degeneration and rupture [3]

4. Technical details of note for this procedure (Fig. 6.6):
   (a) Preferred needle gauge; length; type: *25 gauge; 2-in.; spinal*
   (b) Need for image-guidance: Optional
      • Use of ultrasound has been described in 16 patients [3].
      • Use of fluoroscopy for image guidance during bicipital tendon sheath injection has not been described.
   (c) The tendon sheath is generally injected proximally, where the long head of the biceps traverses the bicipital groove, but an injection distally, at the insertion site, has also been described [2, 3].

5. Step-by-step procedure:
   (a) Informed consent
   (b) Pre-procedural testing: Identify and record the response to a physical examination pre-procedural provocative maneuver, if the procedure is a diagnostic injection.
   (c) Image guidance: Optional: Ultrasound or fluoroscopic-guidance
   (d) Patient positioning:
      • Place the patient in a seated position, generally with the affected arm hanging down to the side.
   (e) Identification and marking of injection site:
      • Palpate and locate the biceps tendon in the bicipital groove.
      • Mark the target using a marker or by depressing the skin with a plastic needle cap.
   (f) Skin preparation: Initial: Betadine® preparation using the no-touch technique.
   (g) Medication preparation:
      • Diagnostic injection:
         – 3 mL of 1% preservative-free lidocaine
      • Therapeutic injection:
         – 40 mg of Depo-Medrol® and ½ mL of 0.5% bupivacaine
   (h) Skin preparation: Final: Alcohol prep

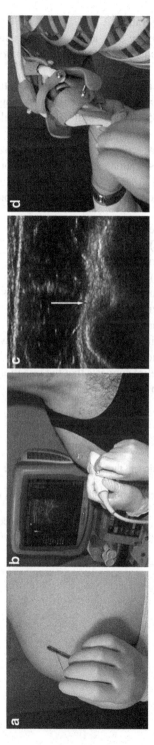

Fig. 6.6 Bicipital tendon sheath injection (ultrasound-guided). (**a**) Bicipital tendon sheath injection-human model. (**b**) Ultrasound transducer positioning for visualizing biceps tendon-human model. (**c**) Ultrasonogram corresponding to previous image. (**d**) Skeletal representation of bicipital tendon sheath injection

(i) Local anesthesia administration:
- Anesthetize the overlying skin and soft tissue using a *small amount of 1% lidocaine* delivered via a *25-gauge, 1½-in. needle.*

(j) Needle Placement:
- Pierce the previously anesthetized skin/and subcutaneous tissue site with a *25-gauge, 2-in. spinal needle.* Needle entry angle should be directed superiorly, at a 30–45° angle, essentially parallel to the tendon in the groove.

(k) Aspiration: Rule out intravascular entry and confirm entry into target structure.

(l) Injection: Unclamp the aspiration syringe and clamp on the injection syringe.

(m) Postprocedural testing:
- Reassess response to the aforementioned preprocedural provocative maneuver.

(n) Repeat injection with therapeutic injectate:
- Repeat steps (d) to (f).
- Medication preparation: 40 mg of Depo-Medrol®
- Repeat steps (h) to (l).

(o) *Adhesive bandage* application over the needle entry site

(p) Postprocedural care discussion

Note. For diagnostic injection:
- Improvement in pre-injection provocative maneuver (e.g., Speed's test) suggests bicepital tendinitis [2].
- Minimal or no pain relief suggests that the injection was not in the sheath or that another region is the source of pain.

References

1. Tallia AF, Cardone DA. Diagnostic and therapeutic injection of the shoulder region. Am Fam Physician 2003;67(6):1271–8.
2. Larson HM, O'Connor FG, Nirschl RP. Shoulder pain: the role of diagnostic injections. Am Fam Physician 1996;53(5):1637–47.
3. Sofka CM, Collins AJ, Adler RS. Use of ultrasonographic guidance in interventional musculoskeletal procedures: a review from a single institution. J Ultrasound Med 2001;20(1):21–6.

Injection Procedure: Glenohumeral Joint Capsule Distension Arthrography

1. Indications:
   (a) Adhesive capsulitis in patients who have had this diagnosis for at least 3 months without improvement, despite enrolling in a physical therapy program [1–3].

2. Contraindications especially pertinent to this procedure [3]:
   (a) Previous surgery resulting in an unpredictable altered anatomy
   (b) Rotator cuff tear (complete tear)

3. Possible side effects especially pertinent to this procedure:
   (a) Increased shoulder joint pain
   (b) Neurovascular bundle injury during needle advancement toward the glenohumeral joint if the injection approach is too medial [3, 4]

4. Technical details of note for this procedure (Fig. 6.7):
   (a) Preferred needle gauge; length; type: 22-gauge; *3½-in.; spinal*
   (b) Need for image guidance: Recommended: Fluoroscopic or ultrasound
     • In the authors' opinion, this injection cannot be done without imaging guidance.
   (c) Recommended dosage: Total volume of up to 100 mL have been injected [3], while some protocols limit the volume to 90 mL [2]. Buchbinder and colleagues performed a randomized, double-blind, placebo-controlled trial with an average of 43.3 mL of fluid injected into the shoulders of participants in the treatment group [1, 2].
   (d) The procedure is generally aborted if the patient experiences severe pain and requests termination or if a complete rotator cuff tear is appreciated (as the injectate will not distend the capsule but, instead, spread into the subacromial space) [2, 3].

5. Step-by-step procedure:
   (a) Informed consent
   (b) Pre-procedural testing: Identify and record the response to a physical examination pre-procedural provocative maneuver if the procedure is a diagnostic injection.
     • For example, have the patient perform active-assisted range of motion to assess pre-procedural shoulder mobility. This should then be compared with post-procedural range of motion.
   (c) Image guidance: Recommended: Fluoroscopic-guidance
   (d) Patient positioning:
     • For fluoroscopic-guidance procedures, the anterior approach is preferred. The patient should be positioned supine with the shoulder slightly externally rotated. It is easiest to simultaneously perform the fluoroscopy and interpret subsequent images when an anterior approach is used.

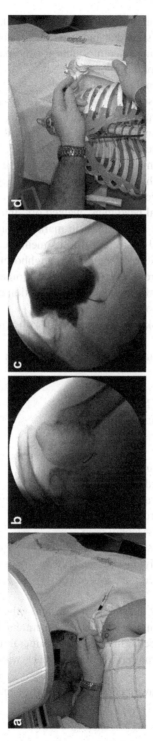

Fig. 6.7 Glenohumeral (GH) joint distension (fluoroscopic-guided). (**a**) GH joint distension-human model. (**b**) Fluoroscopic image of needle entry into GH joint. (**c**) Fluoroscopic image of GH joint distension arthrogram. (**d**) Skeletal representation of GH joint distension

- If necessary, a weighted object may be placed in the patient's hand to externally rotate the shoulder and increase the joint space, though this may eventually become uncomfortable for the patient and increase the tautness of the anterior capsule.

(e) Identification and marking of injection site:

- Aim the c-arm fluoroscope initially in a *posterior–anterior, contralateral oblique view*. Adjust as needed to clearly identify the joint space.
- Rotate the c-arm fluoroscope into a contralateral oblique orientation to best visualize the glenohumeral joint. Of note, however, rotating the c-arm or the patient may rotate the glenoid labrum into the path of the advancing needle, which subsequently increases the risk of iatrogenic injury [6] To minimize this possibility, the needle can be gently advanced to contact the humeral head then "walked off" into the joint space.
- Use fluoroscopy and a metallic skin marker to identify an area on the skin over the humeral head, lateral to its medial cortex. This will be the site of needle insertion; it should be neighboring the junction of the middle and lower thirds of the glenohumeral joint.
- Make adjustments in the metallic marker location and/or relative position of the c-arm fluoroscope as needed.
- Mark the overlying skin by depressing it with a plastic needle cap or a marker.

(f) Skin preparation: Initial: Betadine® preparation using the no-touch technique

(g) Medication preparation:

- Diagnostic injection: Not applicable.
- Therapeutic injection:
  - 10 mL of saline
  - 5 mL of lidocaine
  - 4 mL of Omnipaque™
  - 1 mL of Depo-Medrol® (40 mg/ml)

  (Higher volumes can and may be needed to achieve full capsular distension with or without rupture.)

(h) Skin preparation: Final: Alcohol prep

(i) Local anesthesia administration:

- Anesthetize the overlying skin and soft tissue using a *small amount of 1% lidocaine* delivered via a *25–gauge, 1½-inch needle*.

(j) Needle placement:

- Pierce the previously anesthetized skin and subcutaneous tissue with a 22-gauge, 3½-in. spinal needle. Use intermittent fluoroscopic guidance to direct the spinal needle into the glenohumeral joint.
- Advance the needle posteriorly until contact with the humeral head is made.

(k) Aspiration: Rule out intravascular entry and confirmentry into target structure.

(l) Contrast injection:
- Ensure adequate injection of *Omnipaque*™ into the joint, adjusting the needle position if necessary to obtain a well-defined arthrogram.

(m) Injection:
- Unclamp the syringe from the extension tubing. Attach a 20 mL syringe containing the previously mentioned medication mixture and proceed with injection. If resistance is encountered very early during the injection, rotate the needle to dislodge the bevel from either side of the joint.
- The capsule is distended with the above mixture, in 20 mL aliquots, until:
  - The patient requests termination secondary to pain
  - A rotator cuff tear is appreciated (by observing extravasation of dye from the glenohumeral joint into the subacromial space).
  - Loss of resistance is noted; this is consistent with capsular rupture. In other publications, contrast dye was injected after the procedure with capsular rupture determined by leakage of fluid outside of the capsule [1, 3].
  - A maximum volume is reached (90–100 mL maximum) [2, 3]. In order to avoid excessive corticosteroid dosing and/or local anesthetic toxicity, aliquots subsequent to the first 40 mL of injectate should not contain any corticosteroid and the proportion of local anesthetics should be decreased, as noted in the following chart:

20 mL aliquots	Depo-Medrol® (mL of 40 mg/mL)	Omnipaque® (mL)	Lidocaine (mL)	Saline (mL)
1st	1	4	5	10
2nd	1	4	5	10
3rd	0	5.5	1	13.5
4th	0	5.5	1	13.5

- Progressive resistance should be appreciated with continued injection (until rupture), and a distension pattern should be noted on repeat fluoroscopic views.

(n) Postprocedural testing:
- Reassess response to the aforementioned preprocedural provocative maneuver.

(o) Repeat injection with therapeutic injectate: Not applicable

(p) *Adhesive bandage* application over the needle entry site.

(q) Post-procedural care discussion
Note. For diagnostic injection:
- Improvement in range of motion is consistent with glenohumeral joint pathology. Adhesive capsulitis can then be confirmed by the shoulder capsular arthrographic appearance [5].

References

1. Buchbinder R, Green S. Effect of arthrographic shoulder joint distension with saline and corticosteroid for adhesive capsulitis. Br J Sports Med 2004;38:384–385.
2. Buchbinder R, Green S, Forbes A, Hall S, Lawler G. Arthrographic joint distension with saline and steroid improves function and reduces pain in patients with painful stiff shoulder: results of a randomized, double blind, placebo controlled study. Ann Rheum Dis 2004;63:302–309.
3. Hanchard N, Shanahan D, Howe T, Thompson J, Goodchild L. Accuracy and dispersal of subacromial and glenohumeral injections in cadavers. J Rheumatol 2006;33(6):1143–6.
4. Sethi PM, Kingston S, Elattrache N. Accuracy of anterior intra-articular injection of the glenohumeral joint. Arthroscopy 2005;21(1):77–80.
5. Vad VB, Sakalkale D, Warren RF. The role of capsular distension in adhesive capsulitis. Arch Phys Med Rehabil 2003;84:1290–2.

Injection Procedure: Glenohumeral Joint Injection

1. Indications:
   (a) Adhesive capsulitis diagnosis as pain generator [1]
   (b) Glenohumeral joint arthropathy (e.g., osteoarthritis, rheumatoid arthritis) [1, 2]
   (c) Glenohumeral joint diagnosis as a pain generator

2. Contraindications especially pertinent to this procedure:
   (a) None documented

3. Possible side effects especially pertinent to this procedure:
   (a) Increased shoulder joint pain
   (b) Neurovascular bundle injury during needle advancement toward the glenohumeral joint if the injection approach is too medial [3, 4]

4. Technical details of note for this procedure (Fig. 6.8):
   (a) Preferred needle gauge; length; type: 22-gauge; *3½-in.; spinal*
      • A 20-gauge, 3½-in. spinal needle has also been recommended [5, 6].
      • Unless the patient is very thin, it is unlikely for the joint to be reached with a needle shorter than 2 in.
   (b) Need for image guidance: Recommended
      • Literature reviews reported accuracy rates of 10–42% for glenohumeral injections. In a study by Sethi and colleagues, only 11/41 (26.8%) of anteriorly placed injections by an experienced musculoskeletal radiologist were intra-articular. Most common errors were due to too medial or superficial placement of injectate. The authors, therefore, do not recommend the anterior technique without radiologic guidance [4].
      • Image guidance could potentially avoid iatrogenic injury. A study of shoulder arthrography emphasized the importance to confirm intra-articular needle placement in order to avoid labral injury [6].
      • Sonography is an alternative to fluoroscopy for glenohumeral joint injections [7].

5. Step-by-step procedure:
   (a) Informed consent
   (b) *Pre-procedural testing.* Identify and record the response to a physical examination preprocedural provocative maneuver if the procedure is a diagnostic injection.
   (c) *Image guidance.* Recommended: Fluroscopic-guidance
   (d) Patient positioning:
      • For fluoroscopically guided procedures, the anterior approach is preferred. Patient should be positioned supine, with the shoulder slightly externally rotated. It is easiest to simultaneously perform the fluoroscopy and interpret the subsequent images when an anterior approach is used.
      • If necessary, a weighted object may be placed in the patient's hand to externally rotate the shoulder and increase the joint space, though this

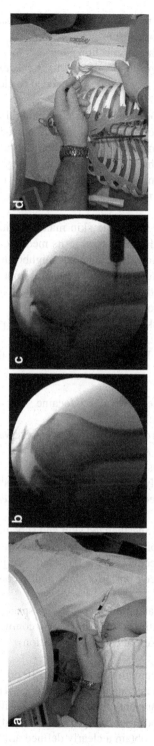

Fig. 6.8 Glenohumeral (GH) joint injection (fluoroscopic-guided). (**a**) GH joint injection-human model. (**b**) Fluoroscopic image of needle entry into GH joint. (**c**) Fluoroscopic image of GH joint arthrogram. (**d**) Skeletal representation of GH joint injection

may eventually become uncomfortable for the patient and increase the tautness of the anterior capsule.

(e) Identification and marking of injection site:

- Aim the c-arm fluoroscope initially in a *posterior–anterior, slightly contralateral oblique view*. Adjust as needed to clearly identify the joint space.
- Rotate the c-arm fluoroscope into a contralateral oblique orientation to best visualize the glenohumeral joint. Of note, however: rotating the c-arm or the patient may rotate the glenoid labrum into the path of the advancing needle, which subsequently increases the risk of iatrogenic injury [6]. To minimize this possibility, the needle can be gently advanced to contact the humeral head and then "walked off" into the joint space.
- Use fluoroscopy and a metallic skin marker to identify an area on the skin over the humeral head, lateral to its medial cortex. This will be the site of needle insertion; it should be neighboring the junction of the middle and lower thirds of the glenohumeral joint.
- Make adjustments in the metallic marker location and/or relative position of the c-arm fluoroscope as needed.
- Mark the overlying skin by depressing it with a plastic needle cap or a marker.

(f) Skin preparation: Initial: Betadine® preparation using the no-touch technique

(g) Medication preparation:

- Diagnostic injection:
  - 10 mL of 1% preservative-free lidocaine
- Therapeutic injection:
  - 80 mg Depo-Medrol® and 2 mL of 1% preservative-free lidocaine

(h) Skin preparation: Final: Alcohol prep

(i) Local anesthesia administration:

- Anesthetize the overlying skin and soft tissue using a *small amount of 1% lidocaine* delivered via a *25-gauge, 1-½ in. needle*.

(j) Needle placement:

- Pierce the previously anesthetized skin and subcutaneous tissue site with a 25-gauge, 1½-in. spinal needle. Use intermittent fluoroscopic guidance to direct the spinal needle into the glenohumeral joint.
- The needle is advanced posterior until gentle contact is made with the humeral head.
- The needle is then walked off into the joint space.

(k) Aspiration: Rule out intravascular entry and confirm entry into bursa (if enough bursal fluid is present to allow aspiration).

(l) Contrast injection:

- Inject the joint with enough contrast (up to 10 mL) to see an arthrogram. Extension tubing, connecting the constrate dye syringe and spinal needle, is recommended to prevent a shift in needle position during attachment and detachment to and from the spinal needle. Adjust needle position, if necessary, in order to obtain a clearly defined arthrogram.

(m) Aspiration: Rule out intravascular entry and confirm entry into target structure (if enough synovial fluid is present to allow aspiration).

(n) Injection:
- Unclamp the syringe from the extension tubing and attach the appropriately sized syringe containing the above-mentioned injectate.

(o) Postprocedural testing:
- Reassess the response to the same aforementioned preprocedural provocative maneuver.

(p) Repeat injection with therapeutic injectate:
- Repeat steps (d) to (f).
- Medication preparation: 80 mg of Depo-Medrol® and 2 mL of 1% preservative-free lidocaine bupivacaine
- Repeat steps (h) to (m).

(q) *Adhesive bandage* application over the needle entry site

(r) Postprocedural care discussion

Alternate approach *without* fluoroscopy: The joint can be injected from a posterior approach with the patient seated. The arm is positioned in front of the trunk and is medially (internally) rotated, with the forearm across the abdomen, in order to help open the posterior aspect of the joint space. The injection site can be localized by palpating the mediastinal posterolateral corner of the scapular spine; one can also identify the coracoid process anteriorly. After administering local anesthesia, pierce the skin just below the scapular spine insertion site and direct the needle toward the anterior coracoid process until it reaches the articular surfaces. Needle position can then be adjusted so that injection occurs without encountering resistance. If resistance is encountered, the needle is either (1) in the joint, but the opening is being occluded by labral cartilage or cartilage covering the humeral head or (2) the needle is located extra-articularly. A simple needle bevel rotation can help to distinguish between these two scenarios: gentle rotation would resume the flow of the injectate if the needle were lodged up against intra-articular cartilage.

References

1. Stitik TP, Foye PM, Fossati J. Shoulder injections for osteoarthritis and other disorders. Phys Med Rehabil Clin N Am 2004;15(2):407–46.
2. Tallia AF, Cardone DA. Diagnostic and therapeutic injection of the shoulder region. Am Fam Physician 2003;67(6):1271–8.
3. Hanchard N, Shanahan D, Howe T, Thompson J, Goodchild L. Accuracy and dispersal of subacromial and glenohumeral injections in cadavers. J Rheumatol 2006 Jun;33(6):1143–6.
4. Sethi PM, Kingston S, Elattrache N. Accuracy of anterior intra-articular injection of the glenohumeral joint. Arthroscopy 2005;21(1):77–80.
5. Depelteau H, Bureau NJ, Cardinal E, Aubin B, Brassard P. Arthrography of the shoulder: a simple fluoroscopically guided approach for targeting the rotator cuff interval. AJR Am J Roentgenol 2004;182(2):329–32.
6. Jacobson JA, Lin J, Jamadar DA, Hayes CW. Aids to successful shoulder arthrography performed with a fluoroscopically guided anterior approach. Radiographics 2003;23(2):373–8.
7. Zwar RB, Read JW, Noakes JB. Sonographically guided glenohumeral joint injection. AJR Am J Roentgenol 2004;183(1):48–50.

Injection Procedure: Infraspinatus Tendon Region Injection

1. Indications:
   (a) Infraspinatus tendinitis diagnosis as pain generator or treatment [1]

2. Contraindications especially pertinent to this procedure:
   (a) Previous injections. Repeat injections should be avoided due to the risk of tendon rupture [2]. The exact number of injections that increases the risk is not known with certainty.

3. Possible side effects especially pertinent to this procedure:
   (a) Potential damage from needle trauma/injection into the tendon, with possible tendon degeneration or rupture [3].

4. Technical details of note for this procedure (Fig. 6.9):
   (a) Preferred needle gauge; length; type: 22-gauge; *2½-in.; spinal*
   (b) Need for image guidance: Optional
      • In the authors' collective experience, ultrasound guidance should be used whenever available to better localize and inject the tendon insertion site.

5. Step-by-step procedure: [1]
   (a) Informed consent
   (b) *Preprocedural testing.* Identify and record the response to a physical examination preprocedural provocative maneuver if the procedure is a diagnostic injection.
   (c) Image guidance: Optional: Ultrasound guidance
   (d) Patient positioning: Have the patient in a seated position, with the arm held in an adducted position and the humerus slightly externally rotated. This arrangement exposes the infraspinatus tendon insertion site along the posterior aspect of the greater tuberosity of the humerus.[4]
   (e) Identification and marking of injection site:
      • If nonimage-guided: Locate the posterior aspect of the acromion. The infraspinatus tendon insertion will be lateral and inferior to this angle on the humerus. Have the patient activate the infraspinatus (i.e., externally rotate the humerus against resistance). Palpate this area to identify the posterior aspect of the greater tuberosity and the course of the tendon as it approaches/inserts onto this structure.
      • If image-guided: Locate the posterior aspect of the acromion. The infraspinatus tendon insertion will be lateral and inferior to this angle on the humerus. Have the patient activate the infraspinatus (attempt to externally rotate the humerus against resistance). Using ultrasound guidance, visualize the course of the tendon as it approaches/inserts onto the greater tuberosity.
      • Mark the skin over the site identified with a plastic needle cap or marker.
   (f) Skin preparation: Initial: Betadine® preparation using the no-touch technique.

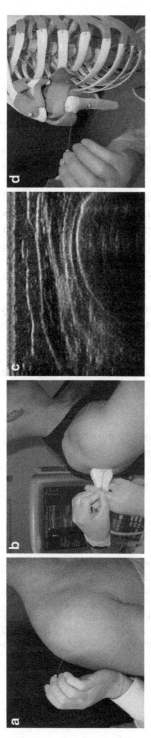

Fig. 6.9 Infraspinatus tendon injection (ultrasound-guided). (**a**) Infraspinatus tendon injection-human model. (**b**) Ultrasound transducer positioning for visualizing Infraspinatus tendon-human model. (**c**) Ultrasonogram corresponding to previous image. (**d**) Skeletal representation of Infraspinatus tendon injection

(g) Medication preparation:
  - Diagnostic injection:
    – 3 mL of 1% preservative-free lidocaine
  - Therapeutic injection:
    – 40 mg of Depo-Medrol® and 0.5 mL of 0.5% preservative-free bupivacaine
(h) Skin preparation: Final: Alcohol prep
(i) Local anesthesia administration: Optional
  - Anesthetize the overlying skin and soft tissue using a *small amount of 1% lidocaine* and delivered via a 25-*gauge, 1½-in. needle.*
(j) Needle placement:
  - Pierce the skin and subcutaneous tissue with a 22-gauge, 2½-in. needle.
  - Proceed the target until the needle impinges on bone.
(k) Aspiration: Rule out intravascular entry and confirm entry.
(l) Injection: Unclamp the aspiration syringe and clamp on the injection syringe.
  - Withdraw the needle slightly, out of the periosteum, and inject under slight resistance.
  - During injection, increased resistance to flow may indicate needle placement in the tendon itself as opposed to the peri-tendinous sheath and surrounding tissue.
(m) Postprocedural testing:
  - Reassess the response to the same aforementioned preprocedural provocative maneuver.
(n) Repeat injection with therapeutic injectate:
  - Repeat steps (d) to (f).
  - Medication preparation: 40 mg of Depo-Medrol
  - Repeat steps (h) to (m).
(o) Adhesive bandage application over the needle entry site.
(p) Postprocedural care discussion

References

1. Stitik TP, Foye PM, Fossati J. Shoulder injections for osteoarthritis and other disorders. Phys Med Rehabil Clin N Am 2004;15(2):407–46.
2. Tallia AF, Cardone DA. Diagnostic and therapeutic injection of the shoulder region. Am Fam Physician 2003;67(6):1271–8.
3. Sofka CM, Collins AJ, Adler RS. Use of ultrasonographic guidance in interventional musculoskeletal procedures: a review from a single institution. J Ultrasound Med 2001;20(1):21–6.
4. Saunders S. Injection techniques in orthopaedic and sports medicine. London: WB Saunders; 2002:50.

Injection Procedure: Sternoclavicular Joint Injection

1. Indications:
   (a) Degenerative sternoclavicular pathology [1, 2]
   (b) Sternoclavicular joint dislocation as pain generator [3]

2. Contraindications especially pertinent to this procedure:
   (a) None documented

3. Possible side effects especially pertinent to this procedure:
   (a) Brachiocephalic veins injury. These vessels are located immediately poste-
       rior to the sternoclavicular joint [3].
   (b) Pneumothorax or damage other mediastinal structures, particularly if the
       needle is pierced beyond the depth of the joint; these instances are not well-
       documented though.

4. Technical details of note for this procedure (Fig. 6.10):
   (a) Preferred needle gauge; length; type: 25-gauge; *1½-in.; straight.*
       • Needle limited to a maximum of 1½ in. should be used to prevent pos-
         sible iatrogenic trauma to the underlying structures.
   (b) Need for image guidance: Optional
       • There is no literature about the use of image guidance in sternoclavicular
         joint injections.

5. Step-by-step procedure:
   (a) Informed consent
   (b) Preprocedural testing: Identify and record the response to a pre-procedural
       provocative maneuver if the procedure is a diagnostic injection.
   (c) Image guidance: Optional
   (d) Patient positioning:
       • The patient should be positioned either seated or lying supine, with the
         affected arm laterally rotated in both instances.
   (e) Identification and marking of injection site:
       • Palpate medially along the clavicle to identify the medial aspect of the
         joint. Recall that the joint is not a true perpendicular joint, but instead
         runs superomediallyto inferolaterally.
       • The joint can be further identified by having the patient "shrug the shoul-
         ders" and perform protraction/retraction of the affected shoulder.
       • Mark the overlying skin by depressing the skin with a plastic needle
         cap.
   (f) Skin preparation: Initial: Betadine® preparation using the no-touch
       technique
   (g) Medication preparation:
       • Diagnostic injection:
         – 1 mL of 2% preservative-free lidocaine

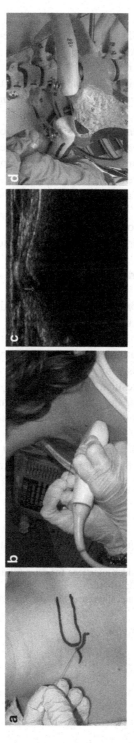

Fig. 6.10 Sternoclavicular (SC) joint injection (ultrasound-guided). (**a**) SC joint injection-human model. (**b**) Ultrasound transducer positioning for visualizing SC joint-human. (**c**) Ultrasonogram corresponding to previous image. (**d**) Skeletal representation of SC joint injection

- Therapeutic injection:
  - 40 mg Depo-Medrol® and 1 mL of 1% preservative-free lidocaine
(h) Skin preparation: Final: Alcohol prep
(i) Local anesthesia administration:
  - Anesthetize the overlying skin and soft tissue using a *small amount of 1% lidocaine* and delivered via a *30-gauge, 1-in. needle.*
(j) Needle placement:
  - Pierce the previously anesthetized skin and subcutaneous tissue site with a *25-gauge, 1-½ in. needle* and advance into the joint space.
(k) Aspiration: Rule out intravascular entry and confirm entry into target structure.
(l) Injection: Unclamp the aspiration syringe and clamp on the injection syringe.
(m) Postprocedural testing: Not applicable
  - Reassess the response to the same aforementioned preprocedural provocative maneuver.
(n) Repeat injection with therapeutic injectate:
  - Repeat steps (d) to (f).
  - *Medication preparation.* 40 mg of Depo-Medrol® with 1 mL of 2% preservative-free lidocaine
  - Repeat steps (h) to (m).
(o) *Adhesive bandage* application over the needle entry site
(p) Postprocedural care discussion:
  - Diagnostic Injection Results: [3]
    - Improvement in pain and range of motion (improvement in retraction, protraction) suggests the presence of sternoclavicular joint pathology.
    - Lack of or minimal pain relief suggests that the injection was not in the joint or that another region is the source of pain.

References

1. Le Loet X, Vittecoq O. The sternoclavicular joint: normal and abnormal features. Joint Bone Spine 2002;69:161–9.
2. Stitik TP, Foye PM, Fossati J. Shoulder injections for osteoarthritis and other disorders. Phys Med Rehabil Clin N Am 2004;15(2):407–46.
3. Lennard T. Physiatric procedures in clinical practice. Philadelphia, PA: Hanley & Belfus; 1995:18.

Injection Procedure: Subacromial Injection

1. Indications:
   (a) Adhesive capsulitis diagnosis as pain generator [1]
   (b) Differentiation of rotator cuff impingement vs. rotator cuff tear
   (c) Rotator cuff impingement [1]
   (d) Rotator cuff tendinitis, tendinosis [1]
   (e) Subacromial region: diagnosis as pain generator [1]
   (f) Subacromial bursitis [1] (sometimes referred to as subdeltoid bursitis)

2. Contraindications especially pertinent to this procedure:
   (a) None documented

3. Possible side effects especially pertinent to this procedure:
   (a) Iatrogenic injury of the deltoid muscle, subcutaneous tissue, acromioclavicular joint, glenohumeral joint, or rotator cuff with misplaced injections [2, 3]
   (b) Excessive subacromial corticosteroid injections have been shown to cause tendonopathy in rat studies; the implication of these results in human subjects is unknown [4].

4. Technical details of note for this procedure (Figs. 6.11 and 6.12): [4]
   (a) Preferred needle gauge; length; type: 21-gauge; *2-in.; straight* or comparable spinal needle
   (b) Need for image guidance: Optional
   - In a study by Henkus and colleagues, 13/17 (76%) of injections without imaging from a posterior approach and 10/16 (69%) of injections without imaging from an anteromedial approach were correctly placed into the subacromial bursa. MRI imaging was used after the procedure to confirm placement of injections. In the posterior approach, 9/13 69% of injections were given inadvertently into the deltoid muscle, glenohumeral joint, or rotator cuff. For the anteromedial approach, 5/10% of injections were misdirected into the deltoid muscle, subcutaneous tissue, acromioclavicular joint, glenohumeral joint, or rotator cuff. The overall injection accuracy using the posterior and anteromedial approaches was 60% [2]. As a result of this information and similar results from other studies, the authors of this book concluded that injection of the subacromial bursa without imaging might not have an acceptable level of accuracy.
   - Use of ultrasound guidance to increase the accuracy of subacromial bursa injections has been shown in the literature [5, 6]. However, whether or not increased accuracy that can be achieved with image-guidance leads to better outcomes remains to be studied [2].
   - The authors of this chapter have limited experience with the use of fluoroscopy- and ultrasound-guided subacromial injections.
   - A positive diagnostic injection can be immediately followed by repeating the injection procedure with corticosteroid if the clinician believes it is indicated. Alternatively, a therapeutic injection containing anesthetic and

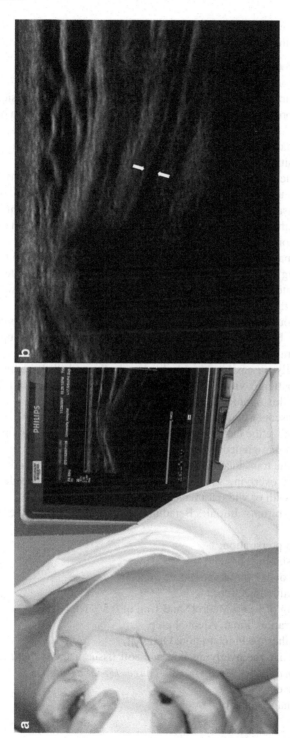

Fig. 6.11 Subacromial bursa injection (ultrasound-guided). (**a**) Ultrasound transducer positioning for visualizing subacromial bursa-human model. (**b**) Ultrasonogram corresponding to previous image

corticosteroid can be performed as a one-step procedure as well if it is not felt that a diagnostic injection is indicated.

5. Step-by-step procedure:
   (a) Informed consent
   (b) Preprocedural testing: Identify and record the response to a physical examination preprocedural provocative maneuver if the procedure is a diagnostic one.
   (c) Image guidance: Optional: Fluoroscopic or ultrasound guidance
   (d) Patient positioning:
     - The patient is seated on the exam table, with the affected arm hanging down to the side.
     - If necessary, a weighted object may be placed in the patient's hand to distract the humerus inferiorly and thus increase subacromial space.
   (e) Identification and marking of injection site:
     - If nonimage-guided: Identify the posterolateral corner of the scapula by palpating laterally along the scapular spine until the discrete corner is appreciated. Identify a point that is one-finger-breadth below this location (Fig. 6.13).
       - Although anterior and lateral injection approaches for this procedure have been described, the posterolateral approach is superior for several reasons. First, the posterolateral corner of the scapula is usually an easily palpable landmark. Second, the needle is out of the patient's view. Finally, the subacromial space is relatively wider with this approach.
     - If fluoroscopic-guided:
       - Visualize the target structure by positioning the c-arm fluoroscope.
     - If ultrasound-guided:
       - Use the transducer to image the underlying target structure.
     - Mark the overlying skin by depressing it with a plastic needle cap or a marker with or without image guidance.
   (f) Skin preparation: Initial: Betadine® preparation using the no-touch technique
   (g) Medication preparation:
     - Diagnostic injection:
       - 8 ml of 1% preservative-free lidocaine
     - Therapeutic injection:
       - 80 mg of Depo-Medrol® and 1 ml of 0.5% bupivocaine
   (h) Skin preparation: Final: Alcohol prep
   (i) Local anesthesia administration: Optional
     - Anesthetize the overlying skin and soft tissue using a *small amount of 1% lidocaine* delivered via a *25-gauge, 1½-in. needle.*
   (j) Needle placement:
     - If nonimage-guided:

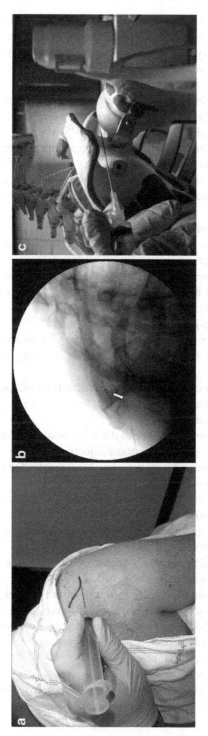

Fig. 6.12 Subacromial bursa injection (fluoroscopy-guided). (**a**) Human model. (**b**) Fluoroscopic image of needle placement. (**c**) Skeletal representation

- Pierce the previously anesthetized skin and subcutaneous tissue site with a *21-gauge, 2-in. needle* attached to an empty 10-mL syringe.
  - Needle entry angle should be directed superiorly and toward the anterior aspect of the subacromial bursa.
- If fluoroscopic-guided:
  - Use intermittent fluoroscopic-guidance to directly visualize needle entry into the subacromial space.
- If ultrasound-guided:
  - Use ultrasound to directly visualize needle placement into the subacromial bursa.

(k) Aspiration: Rule out intravascular entry and confirm entry into bursa (if enough bursal fluid is present to allow aspiration).

(l) Injection:
- If nonimage-guided:
  - Unclamp the syringe from the needle hub and attach the appropriately sized syringe containing the above injectate.
  - A lack of resistance should be appreciated during injection. If this sensation is not present or if there is significant resistance, the needle location may need to be adjusted.
- If fluoroscopic-guided:
  - Contrast injection: Inject the structure with an appropriate amount of Omnipaque™; connect the syringe to the spinal needle via extension tubing.
  - Medication injection: Use intermittent fluoroscopic guidance to visualize the change in dye pattern.
- If ultrasound-guided:
  - Use ultrasound-guidance to directly visualize the injection.

(m) Postprocedural testing: If diagnostic injection:
- Reassess the response to the same aforementioned preprocedural provocative maneuver.

(n) Repeat injection with therapeutic injectate:
- Repeat steps (d) to (f).
- Medication preparation for therapeutic injection:
- Repeat steps (h) to (m).

(o) Adhesive bandage application over the needle entry site

(p) Postprocedural care discussion:
- Educate the patient that the pain relief from a purely diagnostic procedure is only temporary. The pain will return, often to the same degree prior to the procedure. This does not indicate that there is a problem, but rather it is simply expected as the local anesthetic wears off and the corticosteroid has yet to take effect.
  Note. For diagnostic injection [7]:
- Improvement in pain with both active and passive range of motion suggests rotator cuff tendonitis/impingement.

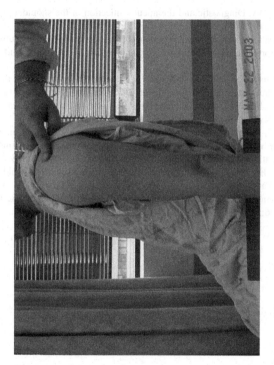

Fig. 6.13 Palpation of the posterolateral corner of the scapula

- Pain with passive range of motion improvement but persistent loss of active range of motion suggests a full-thickness rotator cuff tear.
- Improvement only in pain without active or passive range of motion improvement suggests a component of adhesive capsulitis.
- No or minimal pain relief suggests that the injection was not in the subacromial space or that the subacromial space or its contents is not a pain generator.

References

1. Tallia AF, Cardone DA. Diagnostic and therapeutic injection of the shoulder region. Am Fam Physician 2003;67(6):1271–8.
2. Henkus HE, Cobben LP, Coerkamp EG, Nelissen RG, van Arkel ER. The accuracy of subacromial injections: a prospective randomized magnetic resonance imaging study. Arthroscopy 2006;22(3):277–82.
3. Hanchard N, Shanahan D, Howe T, Thompson J, Goodchild L. Accuracy and dispersal of subacromial and glenohumeral injections in cadavers. J Rheumatol 2006;33(6):1143–6.
4. Stitik TP, Foye PM, Fossati J. Shoulder injections for osteoarthritis and other disorders. Phys Med Rehabil Clin N Am 2004;15(2):407–46.
5. Naredo E, Cabero F, Beneyto P, Cruz A, Mondéjar B, Uson J et al. A randomized comparative study of short term response to blind injection versus sonographic-guided injection of local corticosteroids in patients with painful shoulder. J Rheumatol 2004;31(2):308–14.
6. Chen MJ, Lew HL, Hsu TC, Tsai WC, Lin WC et al. Ultrasound-guided shoulder injections in the treatment of subacromial bursitis. Am J Phys Med Rehabil 2006;85(1):31–5.
7. Larson HM, O'Connor FG, Nirschl RP. Shoulder pain: the role of diagnostic injections. Am Fam Physician 1996;53(5):1637–47.

Injection Procedure: Subscapularis Tendon Region Injection

1. Indications:
   (a) Subscapularis tendinitis as a pain generator [1]
   (b) Treatment: Subscapularis tendinitis

2. Contraindications especially pertinent to this procedure:
   (a) Previous injections. Repeat injections should be avoided due to the risk of tendon rupture [2]. The exact number of injections that increases the risk is not known with certainty.

3. Possible side effects especially pertinent to this procedure:
   (a) Potential damage from needle trauma/injection into the tendon, with possible tendon degeneration or rupture [3]

4. Technical details of note for this procedure (Fig. 6.14):
   (a) Preferred needle gauge; length; type: 22-gauge; 2½-in.; *spinal*
   (b) Need for image guidance: Optional
      • In the authors' collective experience, ultrasound guidance should be used whenever available to better localize and inject the tendon insertion site.

5. Step-by-step procedure: [1, 4]
   (a) Informed consent
   (b) Preprocedural testing: Identify and record the response to a physical examination pre-procedural provocative maneuver if the procedure is a diagnostic injection.
   (c) Image guidance: Optional: Ultrasound-guidance
   (d) Patient positioning:
      • With the patient in a seated position, the arm is held in an adducted position (hanging down by the side) with the humerus externally rotated at 45°. This pose will expose the subscapularis tendon insertion site along the medial aspect of the humerus' lesser (anterior shoulder).
   (e) Identification and marking of injection site:
      • If nonimage-guided: Have the patient activate the subscapularis (internally rotate the humerus against resistance). Palpate for the medial aspect of the lesser tuberosity and the course of the subscapularis tendon, as it approaches/inserts onto this area.
      • If image-guided: Have the patient activate the subscapularis (internally rotate the humerus against resistance). Using ultrasound-guidance, visualize the course of the tendon as it approaches/inserts onto the lesser tuberosity.
      • Mark the overlying skin by depressing it with a plastic needle cap or a marker with or without image guidance.
   (f) Skin preparation: Initial: Betadine® preparation using the no-touch technique.
   (g) Medication preparation:

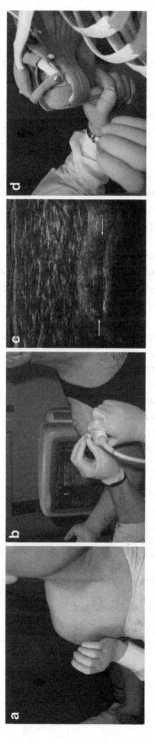

Fig. 6.14 Subscapularis tendon injection (ultrasound-guided). (**a**) Subscapularis tendon injection–human model. (**b**) Ultrasound transducer positioning for visualizing subscapularis tendon–human model. (**c**) Ultrasonogram corresponding to previous image. (**d**) Skeletal representation of subscapularis tendon injection

- Diagnostic injection:
  - 5 mL of 1% preservative-free lidocaine
- Therapeutic injection:
  - 40 mg of Depo-Medrol® and ½ cc of 0.5% bupivicaine in a 3 cc syringe
(h) Skin preparation: Final: Alcohol prep
(i) Local anesthesia administration: Optional
  - Anesthetize the overlying skin and soft tissue using a *small amount of 1% lidocaine* and delivered via a 25-*gauge, 1½-in. needle.*
(j) Needle placement:
  - Pierce the previously anesthetized skin and subcutancous tissue site with a 22-*gauge, 2½-in. spinal needle* until the needle impinges on bone.
  - During injection, increased resistance to flow may indicate placement in the tendon itself as opposed to the peri-tendinous sheath and surrounding tissue.
(k) Aspirate to rule out intravascular entry.
(l) Injection: Unclamp the aspiration syringe and clamp on the injection syringe.
  - Withdraw the needle slightly, out of the periosteum, and inject under slight resistance.
(m) Postprocedural testing:
  - Reassess the response to the same aforementioned preprocedural provocative maneuver.
(n) Repeat injection with therapeutic injectate:
  - Repeat steps (d) to (f).
  - Medication preparation:
  - Repeat steps (h) to (m).
(o) Apply adhesive bandage over the needle entry site
(p) Postprocedural care discussion

References

1. Stitik TP, Foye PM, Fossati J. Shoulder injections for osteoarthritis and other disorders. Phys Med Rehabil Clin N Am 2004;15(2):407–46.
2. Tallia AF, Cardone DA. Diagnostic and therapeutic injection of the shoulder region. Am Fam Physician 2003;67(6):1271–8.
3. Sofka CM, Collins AJ, Adler RS. Use of ultrasonographic guidance in interventional musculo-skeletal procedures: a review from a single institution. J Ultrasound Med 2001; 20(1):21–6.
4. Saunders S. Injection techniques in orthopaedic and sports medicine. London: WB Saunders; 2002:50.

Injection Procedure: Suprascapular Nerve Block

1. Indications:
   (a) Acute severe pain [1]
      - cancer
      - postoperative
      - trauma
   (b) Chronic shoulder pain
      - Adhesive capsulitis [2]
      - Arthritic [3]
      - Nonspecific [3]
   (c) Decreased range of motion associated with:
      - Adhesive capsulitis
      - Reflex sympathetic dystrophy (RSD) [aka complex regional pain syndrome (CRPS)]
   (d) Shoulder girdle pathology involving structures innervated by the suprascapular nerve (i.e., AC joint, glenohumeral joint, or shoulder capsule)
   (e) Shoulder reconstruction rehabilitation, that is, facilitation of more aggressive physical therapy
   (f) Suprascapular nerve entrapment syndrome [1]

2. Contraindications especially pertinent to this procedure:
   (a) None documented

3. Possible side effects especially pertinent to this procedure:
   (a) Pneumothorax [1], particularly if the needle is positioned too anteriorly along the suprascapular nerve and past the coracoclavicular ligament
   (b) Suprascapular artery or vein injury, particularly if the needle is within the suprascapular notch
   (c) Suprascapular nerve injury, which can be recognized due to the production of temporary numbness in the shoulder or arm [4]

4. Technical details of note for this procedure (Fig. 6.15) [5]:
   (a) Preferred needle gauge; length; type: *25-gauge; 50 mm, 2½-in.; Myo-ject™* or comparable EMG-adapted disposable hypodermic needle electrode (for use with nerve stimulator guidance)
   (b) Need for image guidance: Optional
      - Accuracy rates have been documented to be between 10 and 50%. A study by Schneider–Kolsky and colleagues reported that the safety and accuracy of suprascapular nerve blocks can be improved using CT guidance [4]. This study found that, in patients with soft tissue pathologies who did not respond to conventional treatment, CT-guided suprascapular nerve blocks can provide safe short- and long-term relief.
      - One proposed technique to reduce the need for imaging is by increasing the volume of the anesthetic to ensure both the nerve and its branches are

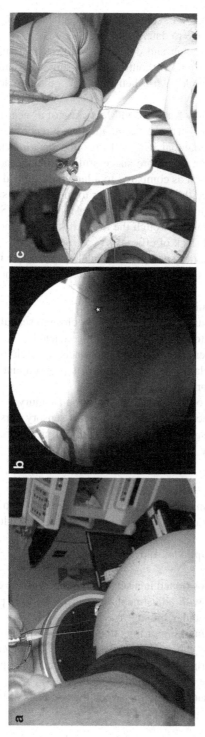

Fig. 6.15 Suprascapular nerve block (fluoroscopic-guided). (**a**) Suprascapular nerve block-human model. (**b**) Fluoroscopic image of needle placement near suprascapular nerve. (**c**) Skeletal representation of suprascapular nerve block

covered. However, clinical studies on injectate efficacy at various levels have not been done to date.

- A study by Shanahan and colleagues showed that suprascapular nerve blocks are efficacious without imaging using ultrasound or fluoroscopy. However, it is unknown whether image guidance leads to increased efficacy [2].
- In another study by Karataş and Meray, use of a "near-nerve electromyography technique" (nerve stimulation and recording of a compound muscle action potential [CMAP] pre- and post-injection) to help with nerve localization was more successful at relieving pain within 60 min following injection as compared to a landmark guided technique [3].

(c) The goal is to place the needle anterior to the scapular spine, between the suprascapular notch (SSN) and the spinoglenoid notch (SGN), without letting needle slip upward through the SSN (risk of pneumothorax) or downward into the SGN (lack of efficacy).

(d) The suprascapular artery and vein run in close proximity to the suprascapular nerve; caution should be taken to avoid injecting medication into this vascular bundle.

(e) Avoiding complications:
- Initial needle entry should be relatively close to scapular spine.
- Avoid going in too deep if bone is not contacted.
- While using nerve stimulation guidance, the relative contraction of infraspinatus relative to supraspinatus is proportional to how distal the block is, therefore:
  - Less chance of pneumothorax or vascular injury
  - Greater chance of relative blocking of sensory nerves and sparing of motor nerves. Since the usual purpose of procedure is for pain relief, it is probably better to block more distally.

5. Step-by-step procedure:
  (a) Informed consent
  (b) Preprocedural testing: Identify and record the response to a physical examination preprocedural provocative maneuver if the procedure is a diagnostic injection.
  (c) Image guidance: Optional: Fluoroscopic-guidance
  (d) Patient positioning:
  - The patient is positioned in a seated position, with the c-arm fluoroscope in an AP view with adjustments made in a lordotic plane to optimally visualize the scapular spine.
  (e) Identification and marking of injection site:
  - The position of the suprascapular notch is estimated as follows: An imaginary line runs horizontally, along the scapular spine, from the vertebral end to the acromial end.
    - A mark is made halfway between the two ends of the scapular spine.

- Another mark is made to bisect the first mark and the lateral end of the scapular spine.
- A third mark, 1.5 cm anterior to the above one, is identified as the spot for needle insertion and marked with needle cap depression or marker.
- The c-arm fluoroscope is then adjusted in the lordotic plane to optimally visualize the scapular notch region.
- The patient is connected to an EMG instrument as follows:
  - A *25-gauge, 50 mm, 2½-in. Myo-jectTM (or comparable) disposable hypodermic needle electrode* is attached to the cathode portal of the stimulator.
  - A *reference disc electrode* is then attached to the anode portal of the stimulator.
  - The reference disc electrode is taped to the anterior chest wall, directly across from the proposed needle entry site for the *Myo-ject™* electrode.
  - A *needle recording electrode* is inserted into the *infraspinatus* muscle. The infraspinatus muscle should be chosen rather the supraspinatus muscle in order to avoid the possibility of inadvertent needle placement into the trapezius muscle, which overlies the supraspinatus muscle (but not the infraspinatus muscle).
  - A *surface reference electrode* is taped to the overlying skin, besides near the infraspinatus recording electrode.
  - Proper recording needle placement into the infraspinatus is confirmed by having the patient externally rotate the shoulder from an adducted position. Note the production of voluntary motor unit potentials detected by the needle recording electrode.
  - The patient's elbow is then allowed to rest on an adjustable-height table so as to place the shoulder at 90° of adduction.
- (f) Skin preparation: Initial: Betadine® preparation using the no-touch technique
- (g) Medication preparation: 3 mL of 1% preservative-free lidocaine
- (h) Skin preparation: Final: Alcohol prep
- (i) Local anesthesia administration:
  - Anesthetize the overlying skin and soft tissue using a *small amount of 1% lidocaine contained delivered via* a 25-gauge, 1½-in. needle.
- (j) Needle placement:
  - A *25-gauge, 50 mm, 2½-in. Myo-ject™ disposable hypodermic needle electrode* is advanced, under intermittent fluoroscopic-guidance, into the region of the suprascapular nerve in the suprascapular notch area. The needle is initially inserted perpendicular to the skin surface so as to contact the posterior surface of the scapula.
  - When contact with bone is made, the needle is angled inferiorly, toward the entrance of the notch.

- Nerve stimulation is performed through the Myo-ject™ disposable hypodermic needle electrode.
- Needle position is adjusted based upon:
  - Absence of paresthesias, which would suggest that the suprascapular nerve has been inadvertently contacted
  - Reproducible CMAP from the infraspinatus muscle
  - Intermittent fluoroscopic guidance to help guide the needle into the suprascapular notch region
  - Further needle positioning should be performed so as to achieve a reproducible CMAP with the minimal amount of electrical stimulus.
(k) Contrast injection:
  - *A small amount of Omnipaque™ contained in a 1 mL non-Luer lock syringe* is then injected through the Myo-ject™ disposable hypodermic needle electrode. If vascular uptake is noted, the needle should be repositioned in such a way so as to eliminate this.
(l) Aspiration: Rule out intravascular entry and confirm entry into target structure.
(m) Injection:
  - The above-mentioned medication injectate is then slowly injected through the Myo-ject™ disposable needle.
(n) Postprocedural testing:
  - Reassess the response to the same aforementioned preprocedural provocative maneuver.
(o) Repeat injection with therapeutic injectate: Not applicable
(p) *Adhesive bandage* application over the needle entry site.
(q) Postprocedural care discussion:
  - A successful block is generally characterized by:
    - Weakness of the supraspinatus and especially the infraspinatus muscles
    - Improvement of shoulder pain (if pain is coming from the glenohumeral joint and/or acromioclavicular joint)

References

1. Waldman SD. Differential Neural Blockade for the Diagnosis of Pain. In Lampert R, Ross A, Ruzycka A, eds. Atlas of Interventional Pain Management. Philadelphia, PA: WB Saunders; 2004:163–164.
2. Shanahan EM, Ahern M, Smith M, Wetherall M, Bresnihan B, Fitzgerald O. Suprascapular nerve block (using bupivacaine and methylprednisolone acetate) in chronic shoulder pain. Ann Rheum Dis 2003;62(5):400–6.
3. Karatas GK, Meray J. Suprascapular nerve block for pain relief in adhesive capsulitis: comparison of 2 different techniques. Arch Phys Med Rehabil 2002;83(5):593–7.
4. Schneider-Kolsky ME, Pike J, Connell DA. CT-guided suprascapular nerve blocks: a pilot study. Skeletal Radiol 2004;33(5):277–82.
5. Stitik TP, Foye PM, Fossati J. Shoulder injections for osteoarthritis and other disorders. Phys Med Rehabil Clin N Am 2004; 15:407–446.

Injection Procedure: Supraspinatus Tendon Region Injection

1. Indications:
   (a) Supraspinatus tendonitis [1] diagnosis as pain generator or treatment
2. Contraindications especially pertinent to this procedure:
   (a) Previous injections. Repeat injections should be avoided due to the risk of tendon rupture [2]. The exact number of injections that increases the risk is not known with certainty.
3. Possible side effects especially pertinent to this procedure:
   (a) Iatrogenic injury to the tendon, including degeneration and rupture [3]
4. Technical details of note for this procedure (Fig. 6.16):
   (a) The tendon sheath can be injected 1 cm proximal to the insertion site on the greater tuberosity, which is the main site of pathology [1].
   (b) Preferred needle gauge; length; type: 22-gauge; *2½-in.; spinal*
   (c) Need for image guidance: Optional
      • In the authors' collective experience, ultrasound guidance should be used whenever available to better localize and inject the tendon insertion site.
   (d) A literature review found only one study (Withrington and colleagues) that compared supraspinatus tendon sheath injections with a placebo. In this population of 25 patients with supraspinatus tendonitis, there was no difference in pain or analgesic consumption at 2 or 8 weeks following the injection [4].

5. Step-by-step procedure:
   (a) Informed consent
   (b) Preprocedural testing: Identify and record the response to a physical examination pre-procedural provocative maneuver if the procedure is a diagnostic one.
   (c) Image guidance:
      • Fluoroscopy: Optional
      • Ultrasound: Recommended
   (d) Patient positioning:
      • Place the patient in a supine position on the exam table.
      • Internally rotate the arm (i.e., by placing it behind the patient's back) to expose the supraspinatus insertion site, along the anterior aspect of the humeral head. The patient's hand can also be placed on the ipsilateral hip, with the first digit pointing downward.
   (e) Identification and marking of injection site:
      • Locate a point on the skin below the anterior edge of the acromion. Have the patient activate the supraspinatus tendon and palpate this area to identify the course of the tendon as it approaches/inserts onto the greater tuberosity. Mark the skin over the site identified above with a plastic needle cap or marker, with or without image guidance.

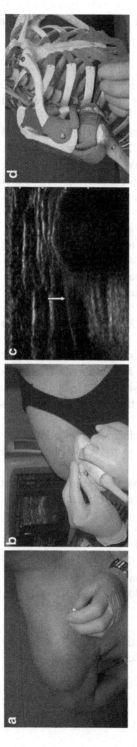

Fig. 6.16 Supraspinatus tendon injection (ultrasound-guided). (**a**) Supraspinatus tendon injection-human model. (**b**) Ultrasound showing transducer positioning for visualizing supraspinatus tendon-human model. (**c**) Ultrasound image of supraspinatus tendon injection. (**d**) Skeletal representation of supraspinatus tendon injection

(f) Skin preparation: Initial: Betadine® preparation using the no-touch technique
(g) Medication preparation:
- Diagnostic
  - Skin anesthesia: Optional: small amount of 1% lidocaine
  - Injection: 3 mL of 1% preservative-free lidocaine
- Therapeutic
  - Skin anesthesia: Optional: small amount of 1% lidocaine
  - Injection: 40 mg of Depo-Medrol® and ½ mL of 0.5% bupivacaine
(h) Local anesthesia administration:
- Optional: Anesthetize the overlying skin and soft tissue using a *small amount of 1% lidocaine* delivered via a *25-gauge, 2-½ in. needle.*
(i) Needle placement:
- Pierce the previously anesthesized skin entry site with a 22–gauge, 2½-in. needle attached to an empty 10 mL syringe.
- If ultrasound-guided: Use ultrasound to directly visualize needle placement into the supraspinatus tendon sheath.
(j) Aspirate to rule out intravascular entry.
(k) Injection:
- If ultrasound-guided: Use ultrasound guidance to directly visualize the injection.
- Advance the needle through the subcutaneous tissue until the needle impinges on bone. Withdraw the needle slightly, out of the periosteum, and inject under slight resistance. Increased resistance to flow may indicate placement of needle in the tendon itself as opposed to the peri-tendinous sheath.
(l) Postprocedural testing: If diagnostic injection:
- Reassess the response to the same aforementioned preprocedural provocative maneuver.
- If it is a positive response, repeat injection with therapeutic injectate
(m) Repeat injection with therapeutic injectate:
- Repeat steps (d) to (f).
- Medication preparation
  - Diagnostic injection
    - 1 mL of 1% preservative-free lidocaine contained in a X-mL syringe
  - Therapeutic injection:
    - Depo-Medrol® 40 mg and 0.5 mL of 0.5% preservative-free bupivacaine
- Repeat steps (h) to (l).
(n) Adhesive bandage application over the needle entry site
- Postprocedural care discussion

References

1. Stitik TP, Foye PM, Fossati J. Shoulder injections for osteoarthritis and other disorders. Phys Med Rehabil Clin N Am 2004;15(2):407–46.
2. Tallia AF, Cardone DA. Diagnostic and therapeutic injection of the shoulder region. Am Fam Physician 2003;67(6):1271–8.
3. Sofka CM, Collins AJ, Adler RS. Use of ultrasonographic guidance in interventional musculo-skeletal procedures: a review from a single institution. J Ultrasound Med 2001;20(1):21–6.
4. Withrington RH, Girgis FL, Seifert MH. A placebo-controlled trial of steroid injections in the treatment of supraspinatus tendonitis. Scand J Rheumatol 1985;14:76–78.
5. Waldman SD. Atlas of pain management injection techniques. Philadelphia, PA: WB Saunders, 2000.

Injection Procedure Templates

Injection Procedure Template: Acromioclavicular Joint Injection

---

PROCEDURE: Acromioclavicular Joint Injection

Image guidance- None unless indicated as follows: ☐- Fluoroscopy   ☐- Ultrasound

Injection Type: ☐-Diagnostic ☐-Therapeutic ☐-Diagnostic/Therapeutic

Side: ☐-Right   ☐-Left   ☐-Bilateral

- The potential benefits and side effects of the procedure were explained to the patient, an opportunity for questions was provided, then the patient signed informed consent.
- The following physical examination pre-procedural provocative maneuver was performed: ☐- N/A; ☐-
- The target was identified by appropriately positioning the patient.
- The overlying skin was prepped with Betadine® and alcohol.
- The overlying skin and soft tissue was anesthetized using a small amount of 1% lidocaine in a 3 mL syringe delivered via a 30-gauge 1" needle.

For Non-Image-Guided Procedure:

- The following needle was selected for the procedure:
  ☐-25G 1½" straight; ☐-22G 1½" straight; ☐-18G 1½" straight; ☐-Other:
- The above needle was attached to a syringe containing the following injectate:
  ☐-Diagnostic injection: 1 mL 2% preservative-free lidocaine
  ☐-Therapeutic injection: 20 mg Depo-Medrol® & 1/2 mL 1% preservative-free lidocaine
  ☐- Other injectate: _____
- Visual inspection was used to confirm entry into the target structure. The needle position was adjusted as needed such that aspiration did not reveal blood return. Then the above solution was injected into the target structure.

For Image-Guided Procedure:

- Fluoroscopic guidance was used to confirm entry of the following needle into the target: ☐-25G 2" spinal; ☐-22G 2" spinal; ☐-Other: _____
- The target structure was injected with a small amount of Omnipaque? that was contained in a 1 mL syringe and was connected to the spinal needle using extension tubing. The needle was adjusted accordingly in order to confirm proper placement without inadvertent vascular entry.
- The needle position was adjusted as needed such that aspiration did not reveal blood return. Then the syringe was unclamped, a 3 mL syringe containing the following injectate was attached and injected into the target structure:
  ☐-Diagnostic injection: 1 mL 1% preservative-free lidocaine
  ☐-Therapeutic injection: 20 mg Depo-Medrol® & 1/2 mL 1% preservative-free lidocaine
  ☐-Other injectate: _____
- An adhesive bandage was placed over the needle entry site.

If the above was a diagnostic procedure, then proceed to section immediately below.

If above was a therapeutic procedure, then proceed to Procedure Summary Section.

- The above listed pre-procedural physical examination provocative maneuver was repeated and pain relief was: ☐- N/A; ☐-significant; ☐-some ; ☐-equivocal; ☐-none; ☐-Other_____
- Based on the amount of pain relief noted above:
  ☐-a therapeutic injection will be scheduled.
  ☐-a therapeutic injection will not be scheduled. See plan in office note below.
  ☐-a therapeutic injection following the same procedure described above was done using:
       ☐- 20 mg Depo-Medrol? & 1/2 mL 1% preservative-free lidocaine
       ☐- Other injectate: _____

Procedure Summary:

For Aspiration Procedures:

- Total volume of fluid removed from the structure: _____mL
- Fluid Appearance: _____ ☐ N/A

Patient tolerance for the procedure: ☐-Excellent ☐-Good ☐-Fair ☐-Other:_____

Additional comments regarding the procedure: ☐- None; Other: _____

Post-Procedural Treatment Advice:

Avoid non-essential use of the structure until seen for follow up. Apply ice for 20-30 min. up to q2 hrs prn until seen

for follow-up, unless instructed as follows: _____

Injection Procedure Template: Bicipital Tendon Sheath Injection

---

PROCEDURE: **Bicipital Tendon Sheath Injection**
Side:　　　　☐-Right　　　　☐-Left　　　　☐-Bilateral
Procedure Type: Aspiration: ☐-Diagnostic aspiration
　　　　　Injection: ☐-Diagnostic　☐-Therapeutic　☐-Diagnostic then Therapeutic
Image guidance: None unless indicated as follows- ☐-Fluoroscopy ☐-Ultrasound

- The potential benefits and side effects of the procedure and alternative treatment options were explained to the patient, an opportunity for questions was provided, and the patient signed informed consent.
- ☐- If checked, the following physical examination pre-procedural provocative maneuver(s) was (were) performed: ☐-_____
- The patient was positioned for the procedure and the target structure was identified.
- The overlying skin was prepped with Betadine® followed by alcohol prep pad after the Betadine® dried.
- ☐- If checked, the overlying skin and soft tissue was anesthetized using a small amount of 1% lidocaine delivered via the following needle ☐-30G1"; ☐-25G1½ "; ☐-Other: _____
- The following needle was then used for the procedure:

Non-image-guided: straight needle ☐-25G1½";☐-22G1½ ";☐-21G1½";☐-18G1½ ";☐-Other:_____

Image-guided:
○　spinal needle ☐-25G2";☐-25G2½";☐-22G1½";☐-22G2½";☐-22G3½";☐-Other:_____
○　Image guidance as specified above was used to confirm needle entry into target structure.
○　☐-If checked, contrast dye contained in a syringe that was connected to the injection needle, was also used.

- The needle was adjusted accordingly to confirm proper placement without inadvertent vascular entry.
- An attempt was made to aspirate from the structure, and a syringe containing the following injectate was attached and injected into the target structure:
  ☐-Diagnostic injection: 3 mL 1% preservative-free lidocaine; ☐-Other injectate: _____
  ☐-Therapeutic injection: 40 mg Depo-Medrol® & ☐- 1 mL 1% preservative-free bupivacaine
  　　　　☐-Other injectate: _____
- The needle was removed and an adhesive bandage was placed over the needle entry site.

-**If the above was a diagnostic injection, then proceed to section immediately below.**
-**If above was a therapeutic injection procedure, aspiration only procedure, or aspiration and therapeutic injection, then proceed to Procedure Summary Section.**

For Diagnostic Injection Procedure:
- ☐-If checked, the above listed pre-procedural physical examination provocative maneuver was repeated and pain relief was: ☐-N/A; ☐-significant; ☐-some; ☐-equivocal; ☐-none; ☐-Other:_____
- Based on the amount of pain relief noted above:
  ☐-a therapeutic injection will be scheduled.
  ☐-a therapeutic injection will not be scheduled. See plan in corresponding office note.
  ☐-a therapeutic injection following the same procedure described above was done using
  　　　　☐- 40 mg Depo-Medrol® & ☐- 0.5 mL 1% preservative-free lidocaine
  　　　　☐- Other injectate: _____
- The needle was removed and an adhesive bandage was placed over the needle entry site.

Procedure Summary:
If fluid aspirated from the target structure during the procedure:
- Total volume of fluid aspirated: ___ mL; Fluid appearance: ☐- N/A; ☐-Clear yellow; ☐-Slightly cloudy; ☐-Cloudy; ☐-Purulent; ☐-Blood-tinged; ☐-Bloody; ☐-Other:_____
Patient tolerance for the procedure: ☐-Excellent; ☐-Good; ☐-Fair; ☐-Other:_____

Additional comments regarding the procedure: ☐-None; ☐Other:_____
_____

Post-Procedural Treatment Advice:
Activity modification: Avoid non-essential use of the structure until seen for follow up. ☐-Other:_____

Orthotic instructions: N/A unless indicated as follows _____

Modalities: Apply ice over the injection site prn for 20-30 min. up to q2 hrs until seen for follow-up, unless instructed as follows: ☐-Heat; ☐-Other:_____

Injection Procedure Template: Glenohumeral Joint Capsule Distention Arthrography

PROCEDURE: Glenohumeral Joint Capsule Distention Arthrography
Side: ☐-Right   ☐-Left   ☐-Bilateral
Procedure Type: Aspiration: ☐-Diagnostic aspiration
         Injection: ☐-Diagnostic   ☐-Therapeutic   ☐-Diagnostic then Therapeutic
Image guidance: None unless indicated as follows- ☐-Fluoroscopy   ☐-Ultrasound
- The potential benefits and side effects of the procedure and alternative treatment options were explained to the patient, an opportunity for questions was provided, and the patient signed informed consent.
- ☐- If checked, the following physical examination pre-procedural provocative maneuver(s) was (were) performed: ☐_____
- The patient was positioned for the procedure and the target structure was identified.
- The overlying skin was prepped with Betadine® followed by alcohol prep pad after the Betadine® dried.
- ☐- If checked, the overlying skin and soft tissue was anesthetized using a small amount of 1% lidocaine delivered via the following needle ☐-30G1"; ☐-25G1½ "; ☐-Other: _____
- The following needle was then used for the procedure:

Non-image-guided: straight needle ☐-25G1½"; ☐-22G1½ "; ☐-21G1½"; ☐-18G1½ "; ☐-Other:_____

Image-guided:
o spinal needle ☐-25G2"; ☐-25G2½"; ☐-22G1½"; ☐-22G2½"; ☐-22G3½"; ☐-Other:_____
o Image guidance as specified above was used to confirm needle entry into target structure.
o ☐-If checked, contrast dye contained in a syringe that was connected to the injection needle, was also used.

- The needle was adjusted accordingly to confirm proper placement without inadvertent vascular entry.
- An attempt was made to aspirate from the structure, and a syringe containing the following injectate was attached and injected into the target structure:
    ☐-Therapeutic injection: ☐- 40 mg Depo-Medrol® & ☐- 4 mL of Omnipaque®   &
             ☐- 5 mL of lidocaine   & ☐- 10 mL of saline
         ☐-Other injectate: _____
- The needle was removed and an adhesive bandage was placed over the needle entry site.

Procedure Summary:
If fluid aspirated from the target structure during the procedure:
- Total volume of fluid aspirated: ___ mL; Fluid appearance: ☐- N/A; ☐-Clear yellow; ☐-Slightly cloudy; ☐-Cloudy; ☐-Purulent; ☐-Blood-tinged; ☐-Bloody; ☐-Other:_____
Patient tolerance for the procedure: ☐-Excellent; ☐-Good; ☐-Fair; ☐-Other:_____

Additional comments regarding the procedure: ☐-None; ☐Other:_____

Post-Procedural Treatment Advice:
Activity modification: Avoid non-essential use of the structure until seen for follow up. ☐-Other:_____

Orthotic instructions: N/A unless indicated as follows _____
Modalities: Apply ice over the injection site prn for 20-30 min. up to q2 hrs until seen for follow-up, unless instructed as follows: ☐-Heat; ☐-Other:_____

Injection Procedure Template: Glenohumeral Joint Injection

PROCEDURE: Glenohumeral Joint Injection
Side: ☐-Right   ☐-Left   ☐-Bilateral
Procedure Type: Aspiration: ☐-Diagnostic aspiration
             Injection: ☐-Diagnostic   ☐-Therapeutic   ☐-Diagnostic then Therapeutic
Image guidance: None unless indicated as follows- ☐-Fluoroscopy   ☐-Ultrasound
- The potential benefits and side effects of the procedure and alternative treatment options were explained to the patient, an opportunity for questions was provided, and the patient signed informed consent.
- ☐- If checked, the following physical examination pre-procedural provocative maneuver(s) was (were) performed: ☐
- The patient was positioned for the procedure and the target structure was identified.
- The overlying skin was prepped with Betadine® followed by alcohol prep pad after the Betadine® dried.
- ☐- If checked, the overlying skin and soft tissue was anesthetized using a small amount of 1% lidocaine delivered via the following needle ☐-30G1"; ☐-25G1½"; ☐-Other: _____
- The following needle was then used for the procedure:

Non-image-guided: straight needle ☐-25G1½"; ☐-22G1½ "; ☐-21G1½"; ☐-18G1½ "; ☐-Other: _____

Image-guided:
o   spinal needle ☐-25G2"; ☐-25G2½"; ☐-22G1½"; ☐-22G2½"; ☐-22G3½"; ☐-Other: _____
o   Image guidance as specified above was used to confirm needle entry into target structure.
o   ☐-If checked, contrast dye contained in a syringe that was connected to the injection needle, was also used.

- The needle was adjusted accordingly to confirm proper placement without inadvertent vascular entry.
- An attempt was made to aspirate from the structure, and a syringe containing the following injectate was attached and injected into the target structure:
  ☐-Diagnostic injection: 10 mL 1% preservative-free lidocaine; ☐-Other injectate: _____
  ☐-Therapeutic injection: 80 mg Depo-Medrol® & ☐- 2 mL 1% preservative-free lidocaine
       ☐-Other injectate: _____
- The needle was removed and an adhesive bandage was placed over the needle entry site.

-If the above was a diagnostic injection, then proceed to section immediately below.
-If above was a therapeutic injection procedure, aspiration only procedure, or aspiration and therapeutic injection, then proceed to Procedure Summary Section.

For Diagnostic Injection Procedure:
- ☐-If checked, the above listed pre-procedural physical examination provocative maneuver was repeated and pain relief was: ☐-N/A; ☐-significant; ☐-some; ☐-equivocal; ☐-none; ☐-Other: _____
- Based on the amount of pain relief noted above:
  ☐-a therapeutic injection will be scheduled.
  ☐-a therapeutic injection will not be scheduled. See plan in corresponding office note.
  ☐-a therapeutic injection following the same procedure described above was done using
       ☐- 80 mg Depo-Medrol® & ☐- 0.5 mL 1% preservative-free lidocaine
       ☐- Other injectate: _____
- The needle was removed and an adhesive bandage was placed over the needle entry site.

Procedure Summary:
If fluid aspirated from the target structure during the procedure:
- Total volume of fluid aspirated: ___ mL; Fluid appearance: ☐- N/A; ☐-Clear yellow; ☐-Slightly cloudy; ☐-Cloudy; ☐-Purulent; ☐-Blood-tinged; ☐-Bloody; ☐-Other: _____
Patient tolerance for the procedure: ☐-Excellent; ☐-Good; ☐-Fair; ☐-Other: _____

Additional comments regarding the procedure: ☐-None; ☐Other: _____

Post-Procedural Treatment Advice:
Activity modification: Avoid non-essential use of the structure until seen for follow up. ☐-Other: _____

Orthotic instructions: N/A unless indicated as follows _____

Modalities: Apply ice over the injection site prn for 20-30 min. up to q2 hrs until seen for follow-up, unless instructed as follows: ☐-Heat; ☐-Other: _____

Injection Procedure Template: Infraspinatus Tendon Region

PROCEDURE: **Infraspinatus Tendon Region Injection**

Side: ☐-Right   ☐-Left   ☐-Bilateral

Procedure Type: Aspiration: ☐-Diagnostic aspiration

        Injection: ☐-Diagnostic   ☐-Therapeutic ☐-Diagnostic then Therapeutic

Image guidance: None unless indicated as follows- ☐-Fluoroscopy ☐-Ultrasound

- The potential benefits and side effects of the procedure and alternative treatment options were explained to the patient, an opportunity for questions was provided, and the patient signed informed consent.
- ☐- If checked, the following physical examination pre-procedural provocative maneuver(s) was (were) performed: ☐ _____
- The patient was positioned for the procedure and the target structure was identified.
- The overlying skin was prepped with Betadine® followed by alcohol prep pad after the Betadine® dried.
- ☐- If checked, the overlying skin and soft tissue was anesthetized using a small amount of 1% lidocaine delivered via the following needle ☐-30G1"; ☐-25G1½ "; ☐-Other: _____
- The following needle was then used for the procedure:

Non-image-guided: straight needle ☐-25G1½"; ☐-22G1½ "; ☐-21G1½"; ☐-18G1½ "; ☐-Other: _____

Image-guided:

- ○ spinal needle ☐-25G2"; ☐-25G2½"; ☐-22G1½"; ☐-22G2½"; ☐-22G3½"; ☐-Other: _____
- ○ Image guidance as specified above was used to confirm needle entry into target structure.
- ○ ☐-If checked, contrast dye contained in a syringe that was connected to the injection needle, was also used.

- The needle was adjusted accordingly to confirm proper placement without inadvertent vascular entry.
- An attempt was made to aspirate from the structure, and a syringe containing the following injectate was attached and injected into the target structure:
  - ☐-Diagnostic injection: 3 mL 1% preservative-free lidocaine; ☐-Other injectate: _____
  - ☐-Therapeutic injection: 40 mg Depo-Medrol® & ☐- 0.5 mL 0.5% preservative-free bupivacaine
    - ☐-Other injectate: _____
- The needle was removed and an adhesive bandage was placed over the needle entry site.

-If the above was a diagnostic injection, then proceed to section immediately below.

-If above was a therapeutic injection procedure, aspiration only procedure, or aspiration and therapeutic injection, then proceed to Procedure Summary Section.

For Diagnostic Injection Procedure:

- ☐-If checked, the above listed pre-procedural physical examination provocative maneuver was repeated and pain relief was: ☐-N/A; ☐-significant; ☐-some; ☐-equivocal; ☐-none; ☐-Other: _____
- Based on the amount of pain relief noted above:
  - ☐-a therapeutic injection will be scheduled.
  - ☐-a therapeutic injection will not be scheduled. See plan in corresponding office note.
  - ☐-a therapeutic injection following the same procedure described above was done using
    - ☐- 40 mg Depo-Medrol® & ☐- 0.5 mL 1% preservative-free lidocaine
    - ☐- Other injectate: _____
- The needle was removed and an adhesive bandage was placed over the needle entry site.

Procedure Summary:

If fluid aspirated from the target structure during the procedure:

- Total volume of fluid aspirated: ___ mL; Fluid appearance: ☐- N/A; ☐-Clear yellow; ☐-Slightly cloudy; ☐-Cloudy; ☐-Purulent; ☐-Blood-tinged; ☐-Bloody; ☐-Other: _____

Patient tolerance for the procedure: ☐-Excellent; ☐-Good; ☐-Fair; ☐-Other: _____

Additional comments regarding the procedure: ☐-None; ☐Other: _____

Post-Procedural Treatment Advice:

Activity modification: Avoid non-essential use of the structure until seen for follow up. ☐-Other: _____

Orthotic instructions: N/A unless indicated as follows _____

Modalities: Apply ice over the injection site prn for 20-30 min. up to q2 hrs until seen for follow-up, unless instructed as follows: ☐-Heat; ☐-Other: _____

Injection Procedure Template: Sternoclavicular Joint Injection

---

PROCEDURE: Sternoclavicular Joint Injection

Side: ☐-Right   ☐-Left   ☐-Bilateral
Procedure Type: Aspiration: ☐-Diagnostic aspiration
                Injection: ☐-Diagnostic   ☐-Therapeutic ☐-Diagnostic <u>then</u> Therapeutic
Image guidance: None unless indicated as follows- ☐-Fluoroscopy ☐-Ultrasound

- The potential benefits and side effects of the procedure and alternative treatment options were explained to the patient, an opportunity for questions was provided, and the patient signed informed consent.
- ☐- If checked, the following physical examination pre-procedural provocative maneuver(s) was (were) performed: ☐_____
- The patient was positioned for the procedure and the target structure was identified.
- The overlying skin was prepped with <u>Betadine® followed by alcohol prep pad</u> after the Betadine® dried.
- ☐- If checked, the overlying skin and soft tissue was anesthetized using a <u>small amount of 1% lidocaine</u> delivered via the following needle ☐-30G1"; ☐-25G1½ "; ☐-Other: _____
- The following needle was then used for the procedure:

Non-image-guided: straight needle ☐-25G1½";☐-22G1½ ";☐-21G1½";☐-18G1½ ";☐-Other:_____

Image-guided:
○   spinal needle ☐-25G2";☐-25G2½";☐-22G1½";☐-22G2½";☐-22G3½";☐-Other:_____
○   Image guidance as specified above was used to confirm needle entry into target structure.
○   ☐-If checked, contrast dye contained in a syringe that was connected to the injection needle, was also used.

- The needle was adjusted accordingly to confirm proper placement without inadvertent vascular entry.
- An attempt was made to aspirate from the structure, and a <u>syringe containing the following injectate</u> was attached and injected into the target structure:
  ☐-Diagnostic injection: 1 mL 2% preservative-free lidocaine; ☐-Other injectate: _____
  ☐-Therapeutic injection: 40 mg Depo-Medrol® & ☐- 1 mL 2% preservative-free lidocaine
      ☐-Other injectate: _____
- The needle was removed and an <u>adhesive bandage</u> was placed over the needle entry site.

-If the above was a <u>diagnostic injection</u>, then proceed to section immediately below.
-If above was a <u>therapeutic injection procedure, aspiration only procedure,</u> or <u>aspiration and therapeutic injection</u>, then proceed to Procedure Summary Section.

For Diagnostic Injection Procedure:
- ☐-If checked, the above listed pre-procedural physical examination provocative maneuver was repeated and pain relief was: ☐-N/A; ☐-significant; ☐-some; ☐-equivocal; ☐-none; ☐-Other:_____
- Based on the amount of pain relief noted above:
  ☐-a therapeutic injection will be scheduled.
  ☐-a therapeutic injection will <u>not</u> be scheduled. See plan in corresponding office note.
  ☐-a therapeutic injection following the same procedure described above was done using
      ☐- 40 mg Depo-Medrol® & ☐- 1 mL 1% preservative-free lidocaine
      ☐- Other injectate: _____
- The needle was removed and an <u>adhesive bandage</u> was placed over the needle entry site.

Procedure Summary:
If fluid aspirated from the target structure during the procedure:
- Total volume of fluid aspirated: ____ mL; Fluid appearance: ☐- N/A; ☐-Clear yellow; ☐-Slightly cloudy; ☐-Cloudy; ☐-Purulent; ☐-Blood-tinged; ☐-Bloody; ☐-Other:_____
Patient tolerance for the procedure: ☐-Excellent; ☐-Good; ☐-Fair; ☐-Other:_____

Additional comments regarding the procedure: ☐-None; ☐Other:_____

Post-Procedural Treatment Advice:
Activity modification: Avoid non-essential use of the structure until seen for follow up. ☐-Other:_____

Orthotic instructions: N/A unless indicated as follows _____

Modalities: Apply ice over the injection site prn for 20-30 min. up to q2 hrs until seen for follow-up, unless instructed as follows: ☐-Heat; ☐-Other:_____

Injection Procedure Template: Subacromial Injection

PROCEDURE: Subacromial Injection
Side: ☐-Right   ☐-Left   ☐-Bilateral
Procedure Type: Aspiration: ☐-Diagnostic aspiration
                    Injection: ☐-Diagnostic   ☐-Therapeutic   ☐-Diagnostic <u>then</u> Therapeutic
Image guidance: None unless indicated as follows- ☐-Fluoroscopy ☐-Ultrasound
- The potential benefits and side effects of the procedure and alternative treatment options were explained to the patient, an opportunity for questions was provided, and <u>the patient signed informed consent</u>.
- ☐- If checked, the following physical examination <u>pre-procedural provocative maneuver(s)</u> was (were) performed: ☐-_____
- The patient was positioned for the procedure and the target structure was identified.
- The overlying skin was prepped with <u>Betadine® followed by alcohol prep pad</u> after the Betadine® dried.
- ☐- If checked, the overlying skin and soft tissue was anesthetized using a <u>small amount of 1% lidocaine</u> delivered via the following needle ☐-30G1"; ☐-25G1½ "; ☐-Other: _____
- The following needle was then used for the procedure:

Non-image-guided: straight needle ☐-25G1½";☐-22G1½ ";☐-21G1½";☐-18G1½ ";☐-Other:_____

Image-guided:
- o spinal needle ☐-25G2";☐-25G2½";☐-22G1½";☐-22G2½";☐-22G3½";☐-Other:_____
- o Image guidance as specified above was used to confirm needle entry into target structure.
- o ☐-If checked, contrast dye contained in a syringe that was connected to the injection needle, was also used.

- The needle was adjusted accordingly to confirm proper placement without inadvertent vascular entry.
- An attempt was made to aspirate from the structure, and a <u>syringe containing the following injectate</u> was attached and injected into the target structure:
  ☐-Diagnostic injection: 8 mL 1% preservative-free lidocaine; ☐-Other injectate: _____
  ☐-Therapeutic injection: 80 mg Depo-Medrol® & ☐- .5 mL 0.5% preservative-free bupivacaine
            ☐-Other injectate: _____
- The needle was removed and an <u>adhesive bandage</u> was placed over the needle entry site.

-If the above was a <u>diagnostic injection</u>, then proceed to section immediately below.
-If above was a <u>therapeutic injection procedure, aspiration only procedure</u>, or <u>aspiration and therapeutic injection</u>, then proceed to Procedure Summary Section.

For Diagnostic Injection Procedure:
- ☐-If checked, the above listed pre-procedural physical examination provocative maneuver was repeated and pain relief was: ☐-N/A; ☐-significant; ☐-some; ☐-equivocal; ☐-none; ☐-Other:_____
- Based on the amount of pain relief noted above:
  ☐-a therapeutic injection will be scheduled.
  ☐-a therapeutic injection will <u>not</u> be scheduled. See plan in corresponding office note.
  ☐-a therapeutic injection following the same procedure described above was done using
        ☐- 40 mg Depo-Medrol® & ☐- 0.5 mL 1% preservative-free lidocaine
        ☐- Other injectate: _____
- The needle was removed and an <u>adhesive bandage</u> was placed over the needle entry site.

Procedure Summary:
If fluid aspirated from the target structure during the procedure:
- Total volume of fluid aspirated: ___ mL; Fluid appearance: ☐- N/A; ☐-Clear yellow; ☐-Slightly cloudy; ☐-Cloudy; ☐-Purulent; ☐-Blood-tinged; ☐-Bloody; ☐-Other:_____
Patient tolerance for the procedure: ☐-Excellent; ☐-Good; ☐-Fair; ☐-Other:_____

Additional comments regarding the procedure: ☐-None; ☐Other:_____
_____

Post-Procedural Treatment Advice:
<u>Activity modification</u>: Avoid non-essential use of the structure until seen for follow up. ☐-Other:_____
_____
<u>Orthotic instructions</u>: N/A unless indicated as follows _____
<u>Modalities:</u> Apply ice over the injection site prn for 20-30 min. up to q2 hrs until seen for follow-up, unless instructed as follows: ☐-Heat; ☐ Other:_____

Injection Procedure Template: Subscapularis Tendon Region Injection

---

PROCEDURE: Subscapularis Tendon Region Injection
Image guidance- None unless indicated as follows: ☐-Fluoroscopy   ☐- Ultrasound
Injection Type: ☐-Diagnostic   ☐-Therapeutic   ☐-Diagnostic/Therapeutic
Side: ☐-Right   ☐-Left   ☐-Bilateral
- The potential benefits and side effects of the procedure were explained to the patient, an opportunity for questions was provided, then the patient signed informed consent.
- The following physical examination pre-procedural provocative maneuver was performed: ☐- N/A; ☐-
- The target was identified by appropriately positioning the patient.
- The overlying skin was prepped with Betadine® and alcohol.

- -

For Non-Image-Guided Procedure:
- The following needle was selected for the procedure:
  ☐-22G 2½" spinal; ☐-Other: _____
- The above needle was attached to a syringe containing the following injectate:
  ☐-Diagnostic injection: 5 mL 1% preservative-free Lidocaine
  ☐-Therapeutic injection: 40 mg Depo-Medrol® & 0.5 mL 0.5% bupivicaine
  ☐- Other injectate: _____
- Visual inspection was used to confirm entry into the target structure. The needle position was adjusted as needed such that aspiration did not reveal blood return, the patient did not report paresthesias related to the needle and there was no significant resistance to injection. Then the above solution was injected into the target structure.

For Image-Guided Procedures:
- Fluoroscopic guidance was used to confirm entry of the following needle into the target: ☐-25G 1 ½ " straight; ☐-Other: _____
- The above needle was attached to a syringe containing the following injectate:
  ☐-Diagnostic injection: 5 mL 1% preservative-free lidocaine
  ☐-Therapeutic injection: 40 mg Depo-Medrol® & 0.5 mL 0.5% bupivicaine
  ☐- Other injectate: _____
- The needle position was adjusted as needed under image guidance such that aspiration did not reveal blood return. Then the above solution was injected into the target structure.

- An adhesive bandage was placed over the needle entry site.

If the above was a diagnostic procedure, then proceed to section immediately below.
If above was a therapeutic procedure, then proceed to Procedure Summary Section.

- -

- The above listed pre-procedural physical examination provocative maneuver was repeated and pain relief was: ☐-N/A; ☐-significant; ☐-some ; ☐-equivocal; ☐-none; ☐-Other_____
- Based on the amount of pain relief noted above:
  ☐-a therapeutic injection will be scheduled.
  ☐-a therapeutic injection will not be scheduled. See plan in office note below.
  ☐-a therapeutic injection following the same procedure described above was done using:
      ☐- 40 mg Depo-Medrol® & 0.5 mL 0.5% bupivicaine
      ☐- Other injectate: _____

- -

Procedure Summary:
Patient tolerance for the procedure: ☐-Excellent ☐-Good ☐-Fair ☐-Other:_____ _
_____
_____
Additional comments regarding the procedure: ☐- None; Other:_____
_____
_____

Post-Procedural Treatment Advice:
Avoid non-essential use of the structure until seen for follow up.
Splinting instructions: ☐-N/A; ☐-Other: _____
Apply ice for 20-30 min. up to q2 hrs prn until seen for follow-up, unless instructed as follows:

Injection Procedure Template: Suprascapular Nerve Block

PROCEDURE: **Suprascapular Nerve Block**
Side: □-Right   □-Left   □-Bilateral
Procedure Type: □-Diagnostic □-Therapeutic □-Diagnostic/Therapeutic
Image guidance- None unless indicated as follows: □- Fluoroscopy □- Ultrasound
- The potential benefits and side effects of the procedure were explained to the patient, an opportunity for questions was provided, then the patient signed informed consent.
- The following physical examination pre-procedural provocative maneuver was performed: □- N/A;
  □-_____
- The target was identified by landmark palpation as follows:
  - o
  - o
  - o
- The overlying skin was prepped with Betadine® and alcohol.
- The overlying skin and soft tissue was anesthetized using a small amount of 1% lidocaine in a 3 mL syringe delivered via a 25-gauge 1 ½ " needle.

For Non-Image-Guided but EMG-Guided Procedure:
- The following needle was selected for the procedure:
  □-25G 50 mm 2 ½ " Myo-ject™ disposable hypodermic needle electrode □-Other: _____
- Patient was **connected to an EMG instrument as follows:**
  - o A ground electrode was taped to the patient's thorax in the general vicinity of the scapula
  - o A surface recording electrode was placed over the infraspinatus muscle. Proper placement was confirmed by having the patient perform external rotation with the shoulder in an adducted position and observing a marked increase in EMG activity..
  - o A surface reference electrode was taped over the spine of the scapula
  - o A 2nd surface reference electrode was taped to the patients anterior chest wall
- The Myo-ject™ disposable hypodermic needle electrode was then advanced into the region of the suprascapular nerve in the suprascapular notch area. The needle was initially inserted perpendicular to the skin surface so as to contact the posterior surface of the scapula.
- Nerve stimulation was then performed through the Myo-ject™ disposable hypodermic needle electrode.
- Needle position was adjusted based upon:
  - o The absence of paresthesias that would suggest that the suprascapular nerve was inadvertently contacted.
  - o The presence of a reproducible CMAP from the infraspinatus muscle.
  - o Intermittent fluoroscopic guidance to help guide the needle into the suprascapular notch region
  - o Further needle positioning was performed so as to achieve a reproducible CMAP with the minimal amount of electrical stimulus.
- After aspiration did not reveal blood return, the syringe was unclamped, a non-Luer Lock 5 mL syringe containing the following injectate was attached and was injected into the target structure:
  □- 3 ml 1% preservative-free lidocaine □- Other: _____

For Image-Guided/EMG-guided Procedure:
- Fluoroscopic guidance was used to confirm entry of the following needle into the target:
- The following needle was selected for the procedure:
  □-25G 50 mm 2 ½ " Myo-ject™ disposable hypodermic needle electrode □-Other:_____
- Prior to needle entry, the patient was **connected to an EMG instrument as follows:**
  - o A ground electrode was taped to the patient's thorax in the general vicinity of the scapula.
  - o A surface recording electrode was placed over the infraspinatus muscle. Proper placement was confirmed by having the patient perform external rotation with the shoulder in an adducted position and observing a marked increase in EMG activity.A surface reference electrode was taped over the spine of the scapula
  - o A 2nd surface reference electrode was taped to the patients anterior chest wall
- The Myo-ject™ disposable hypodermic needle electrode was then advanced under fluoroscopic guidance into the region of the suprascapular nerve in the suprascapular notch area. The needle was initially inserted perpendicular to the skin surface so as to contact the posterior surface of the scapula.
- Nerve stimulation was then performed through the Myo-ject™ disposable hypodermic needle electrode.
- Needle position was adjusted based upon:
  - o The absence of paresthesias that would suggest that the suprascapular nerve was inadvertently contacted.
  - o The presence of a reproducible CMAP from the infraspinatus muscle·
  - o Intermittent fluoroscopic guidance to help guide the needle into the suprascapular notch region
  - o Further needle positioning was performed so as to achieve a reproducible CMAP with the minimal amount of electrical stimulus.
- Additional confirmation of successful needle entry into the target without inadvertent intravascular

Injection Procedure Template: Supraspinatus Tendon Region Injection

- injection was achieved with injection of Omnipaque® (contained in a non-Luer lock syringe) along with further adjustment of needle placement as needed.
- After aspiration did not reveal blood return, the syringe was unclamped, a non-Luer Lock 5 mL syringe containing the following injectate was attached and was injected:
  ☐- 3 ml 1% preservative-free lidocaine ☐- Other: _____
- An adhesive bandage was placed over the needle entry site.

If the above was a diagnostic procedure, then proceed to section immediately below.
If above was a therapeutic procedure, then proceed to Procedure Summary Section.

- The above listed pre-procedural physical examination provocative maneuver was repeated and pain relief was:☐-N/A; ☐-significant; ☐-some ; ☐-equivocal; ☐-none; ☐-Other_____
- Based on the amount of pain relief noted above:
  ☐-a therapeutic injection will be scheduled.
  ☐-a therapeutic injection will not be scheduled. See plan in corresponding office note.
  ☐-a therapeutic injection following the same procedure described above was done using:
    ☐- 80 mg Depo-Medrol® & 2 mL 1% preservative-free lidocaine ☐- Other_____

Procedure Summary:
Patient tolerance for the procedure: ☐-Excellent ☐-Good ☐-Fair ☐-Other:_____

Additional comments regarding the procedure: ☐- None; Other: _____

Post-Procedural Treatment Advice:
Activity modification: Avoid non-essential use of the structure until seen for follow up. ☐-Other:_____
Orthotic instructions: ☐-N/A; ☐-Other: _____
Modalities: Apply the following modality for 20-30 min. up to q2 hrs prn until seen for follow-up, unless otherwise instructed- ☐-Ice; ☐-Heat; ☐-Other:_____

Chapter 7
The Elbow

Peter P. Yonclas, Michael J. Mehnert, Todd P. Stitik,
Mohammad Hossein Dorri, Jong H. Kim, David J. Van Why,
Jose Ibarbia, Lisa Schoenherr, Naimish Baxi, Ladislav Habina,
and Jiaxin J. Tran

Introduction

Elbow region injection/aspiration procedures include those into joints, bursae, and tendon insertion sites as summarized in Table 7.1. Unlike injections into other body regions, in particular the shoulder where diagnostic injection procedures can play a major role in patient management, elbow region injections are more commonly therapeutic than diagnostic in intent. Exceptions to this, however, include aspiration in the setting of suspected crystalline arthropathy or suspected radial head fractures. Therapeutic injection procedures into the elbow region are commonly performed in conjunction with rehabilitation therapy or after conservative measures have failed.

Lateral Epicondylitis (Lateral Epicondylosis)

It has been the authors' experience during clinical practice and from a 2-year study within their practice on office-based musculoskeletal injection procedures that the lateral epicondyle is the most commonly injected elbow region structure [1]. This sentiment is supported by a survey of primary care physicians that found these injections to be the second most common office-based injection procedure after shoulder region injections [2].

Lateral epicondylitis (LE) [aka tennis elbow] are terms used to describe a syndrome of pain involving the common extensor origin of the wrist extensor forearm muscles where they arise from the lateral epicondyle. The term epicondylosis is probably a more accurate one given the likely absence of true inflammation in the non-acute setting. It can be a self-limiting condition that is often due to repetitive activities such as golf, racquet, and throwing sports as well as repetitive occupation related movements such as lifting, typing, or point and click motions from using a

T.P. Stitik (✉)
Department of Physical Medicine and Rehabilitation, New Jersey Medical School,
Newark, NJ, USA
e-mail: todd.stitik@gmail.com

Table 7.1 Summary of elbow region injection procedures

Injection type	Specific structure	Meta-analysis(es)	Prospective study (studies)	Case series/report(s) retrospective study	Described in review article(s) and/or injection textbook(s)
Bursa	Cubital				16
	Olecranon			13	17
Joint	Elbow		12	14	18
	Radiocapitellar			15	
Nerve block procedure	Cubital tunnel			19	20, 21
	Lateral antebrachial cutaneous nerve				22
	Radial tunnel				21, 23
Tendon: musculotendinous junction	Lateral epicondyle	5	3, 4, 6, 8	7	24
	Medial epicondyle		9–11	25	26

Listed within each injection type in order of descending amount of current evidence supporting its use. Except in the case of randomized clinical trials for lateral epicondylitis where there is a large amount of literature, references are provided for all meta-analyses, prospective studies, and case series/case reports along with at least one reference to descriptions in review articles or injection textbooks. For those procedures that are only described in review articles and/or textbooks, representative references are provided

mouse. Patients typically present with a history of an insidious onset of pain and tenderness in the region of the lateral epicondyle and pain-limited weakness with grip strength. Physical examination typically reveals point tenderness in the region of the lateral epicondyle as well as pain and weakness with resisted wrist extension or supination and passive stretching of the extensor muscles.

There is no current consensus within the literature about the timing, dose, and ideal patient for corticosteroid injection. The long-term potential benefit has recently come under scrutiny, as it appears that in certain patients who receive corticosteroid injections, there may be a paradoxical worsening of symptoms after initial relief [3]. A general rule is that indications for a corticosteroid injection for LE include severe acute pain with functional impairment or chronic pain and/or disability not relieved by conservative treatment [4]. A meta-analysis found that corticosteroid injections appear to be most effective in the short term (2–6 weeks) [5]. It also appears that, to be most effective, they should be given early in the course of the disease (4 weeks or less). This timing is in keeping with the belief that the disorder evolves from one of a traumatic inflammatory tendonitis to an ongoing tendinosis involving deep tissue formation.

Because recalcitrant or chronic LE is thought to be due to an incomplete healing response characterized by tendinosis, percutaneous needle tenotomy (PNT) injection of autologous blood or botulism toxin A have recently been advocated for patients with chronic LE. Theoretically, an injection of autologous blood might provide the necessary cellular and humoral mediators to induce a healing cascade. To date, there have been several prospective studies that have shown some short-term to intermediate duration relief, but no studies to date have looked at the long-term benefits of autologous blood injections [6, 7]. Similarly, botulism toxin A is thought to provide temporary paralysis of the common extensor muscles, allowing a healing response to occur. However, to date, no studies have demonstrated a beneficial effect when compared to placebo [8].

Medial Epicondylitis (Medial Epicondylosis)

Medial epicondylitis (ME) (aka golfer's elbow) involves the pathologic alteration in the musculotendinous origins of the pronator flexor bundle at the medial epicondyle. As was stated for the lateral epicondyle region, the medial epicondyle region pathology is also likely to involve chronic tendinopathy rather than an acute inflammatory process. Thus the term medial epicondylosis is probably more accurate. ME is characterized by pain along the medial elbow that is worsened by resisted forearm pronation and/or wrist flexion. It is estimated that occurrence of the disease is ten times less likely than LE, and, as a result, the literature regarding ME has been scant in comparison [9].

Like LE injections. ME corticosteroid injections are likely most beneficial in the short-term. Several prospective, randomized studies have documented short-term efficacy of corticosteroid injections. Stahl and Kaufman noted significantly less pain at 6 weeks but no significant difference from placebo at 3 months and 1 year [10].

A study on autologous blood injections was also performed on patients with medial epicondylitis. This study found that the combined action of dry needling and autologous blood injection under ultrasound guidance appeared to be an effective treatment for refractory medial epicondylitis [11].

Olecranon Bursitis

Olecranon bursitis commonly occurs after repetitive trauma to the elbow, in patients with rheumatoid or crystalloid arthritis, or in patients with an underlying bursal infection. On exam, the patient generally presents with a swollen, painless fluid-filled bursal sac. The sac can be aspirated and, if symptoms are recurrent, can be injected with corticosteroid. The only blinded, prospective study to evaluate injections for olecranon bursitis found that injection with a corticosteroid led to the quickest decrease in fluid content and had the least amount of fluid recurrence [12]. When performed, care should be taken to utilize a zigzag pattern of needle entry through the skin and subcutaneous tissue, if possible, to reduce the chances of creating a communicating fistula with the skin. While image guidance should not be necessary in the majority of cases as the distended bursa is usually easily palpable, ultrasound guidance has been reported as being used to assist with two such injections [13] and could prove to be particularly helpful in cases of a loculated bursitis.

Elbow Joint Arthropathy

The major indications for injection into the elbow joint are symptomatic osteoarthritis, rheumatoid arthritis, and crystal arthropathies. Occasionally, an aspiration may be performed from the elbow to assist with diagnosis of suspected elbow fractures as well as to provide relief from pain and swelling in the setting of an elbow fracture. Specifically, the presence of blood or fat globules in conjunction with a history of trauma raises the possibility of fracture. Although there is no consensus in the literature regarding the need for image guidance, case reports has been published regarding the use of MR imaging as well as ultrasound to help guide an elbow joint injection [14].

Another approach into the elbow joint per se is via the radiocapitellar articulation, as it is contiguous with the elbow joint proper. The radiocapitellar joint can also be injected with local anesthetic in cases of recalcitrant lateral epicondylitis where the diagnosis is unclear. In this setting, pain relief would be more suggestive of the radiocapitellar joint as the primary pain generator. The radiocapitellar approach to the elbow joint may be used in cases of osteochondritis dessicans of the capitellum (Panner's Disease), where local anesthetic may be used to confirm the capitellum as the primary pain generator and better help guide treatment [15].

Miscellaneous Procedures

In addition to the more commonly performed injections at the elbow, several other nerve blocks procedures of potentially entrapped nerves at the elbow as well as therapeutic injections in smaller bursa around the elbow have been described. Although not well-studied or commonly performed in the authors' practices (and therefore templates for these procedures have not been provided), they deserve mention and are included in Table 7.1. The use of ultrasound guidance makes possible the injection of large volumes of saline and anesthetic mixtures in an attempt to hydrodissect fibrous adhesions off of entrapped peripheral nerves.

References

1. Stitik TP, Foye PM, Nadler SF, Chen B, Schoenherr L, Von Hagen S. Injections in patients with osteoarthritis and other musculoskeletal disorders: use of synthetic injection models for teaching physiatry residents. Am J Phys Med Rehabil 2005;84:550–9.
2. Gormley GJ, Corrigan M, Steele WK, Stevenson M, Taggart AJ. Joint and soft tissue injections in the community: questionnaire survey of general practitioners' experiences and attitudes. Ann Rheum Dis 2003;62(1):61–4.
3. Bisset L, Beller E, Jull G, Brooks P, Darnell R, Vicenzino B. Mobilisation with movement and exercise, corticosteroid injection, or wait and see for tennis elbow: randomised trial. BMJ 2006;333(7575):939. Epub.
4. Field LD, Savoie FH. Common elbow injuries in sport. Sports Med 1998;26:193–205. Hay EM, Patterson SM, Lewis M, Hosie G, Croft P. Pragmatic randomized controlled trial of local corticosteroid injection and naproxen for treatment of lateral epicondylitis of elbow in primary care. BMJ 1999;319:964–8.
5. Assendelft WJ, Hay EM, Adshead R, Bouter LM. Corticosteroid injections for lateral epicondylitis: a systematic overview. Br J Gen Pract 1996;46:209–16.
6. Zeebregts CJ, Tielliu IF, Hulsebos RG, de Bruin C, Verhoeven EL, Huisman RM et al. Ultrasound-guided autologous blood injection for tennis elbow. Skeletal Radiol 2006;35(6):371–7. Epub 2006 Mar 22.
7. Edwards SG, Calandruccio JH. Autologous blood injections for refractory lateral epicondylitis. J Hand Surg [Am] 2003;28(2):272–8.
8. Hayton MJ, Sanitin AJ, Hughes J, Frostick SP, Trail IA, Stanley JK. Botulinum toxin injection in the treatment of tennis elbow. A double-blind, randomized, controlled pilot study. J Bone Joint Surg Am 2005;87(3):503–7.
9. Ciccotti MG, Ramani MH. Medial epicondylitis. Sports Med Arthrosc Rev 2003;11(1):57–62.
10. Stahl S, Kaufman T. The efficacy of an injection of steroids for medial epicondylitis: a prospective study of sixty elbows. J Bone Joint Surg Am 1997;79:1648–1652.
11. Suresh SP, Ali KE, Jones H, Connell DA. Medial Epicondylitis: is ultrasound guided autologous blood transfer an effective treatment? Br J Sports Med 2006;40(11):935–9.
12. Smith DL, McAfee JH, Lucas LM, Kumar KL, Romney DM. Treatment of nonseptic olecranon bursitis. A controlled, blinded prospective trial. Arch Intern Med 1989;149(11):2527–30.
13. Sofka CM, Collins AJ, Adler RS. Use of ultrasonographic guidance in interventional musculoskeletal procedures: a review from a single institution. J Ultrasound Med 2001;20(1):21–6.
14. Genant JW, Vandevenne JE, Bergman AG, Beaulieu CF, Kee ST, Norbash AM et al. Interventional musculoskeletal procedures performed by using MR imaging guidance with a vertically open MR unit: assessment of techniques and applicability. Radiology 2002;223(1):127–36.

15. Poddar SK, Hill J, Loeffler R. Elbow pain in a twenty year old football player. Med Sci Sports Exerc 2001;33(5):S8.
16. Sofka CM, Adler RS. Sonography of Cubital Bursitis. AJR Am J Roentgenol 2004;183(1):51–3.
17. Waldman SD. Olecranon Bursitis Pain. Atlas of Pain Management Injection Techniques. Philadelphia, PA: WB Saunders; 2000:90–92.
18. Waldman SD. Intra-articular Injection of the Elbow Joint. Atlas of Pain Management Injection Techniques. Philadelphia, PA: WB Saunders; 2000:77–79.
19. Elhassan B. Steinmann SP. Entrapment neuropathy of the ulnar nerve. J Am Acad Orthop Surg 2007; 15(11):672–81.
20. Waldman SD. Cubital Tunnel. Atlas of Pain Management Injection Techniques. Philadelphia, PA: WB Saunders; 2000:103–6.
21. Bracker MD, Ralph LO. The numb arm and hand. Am Fam Physician 1995;51(1):103–16.
22. Waldman SD. Lateral Antebrachial Cutancous Nerve Entrapment Syndrome. Atlas of Pain Management Injection Techniques. Philadelphia, PA: WB Saunders; 2000:107–9.
23. Waldman SD. Radial Nerve Block at the Elbow. Atlas of Pain Management Injection Techniques. Philadelphia, PA: WB Saunders; 2000:175–77.
24. Waldman SD. Tennis Elbow Syndrome. Atlas of Pain Management Injection Techniques. Philadelphia, PA: WB Saunders; 2000:80–83
25. Marmor L. Medial epicondylitis. Calif Med 1959;91(1):23.
26. Waldman SD. Golfer's Elbow Syndrome. Atlas of Pain Management Injection Techniques. Philadelphia, PA: WB Saunders; 2000:87–89.

Procedure Instructions

Injection Procedure: Lateral Epicondylitis Injection

1. Indications:
   (a) Lateral epicondylitis: diagnosis as pain generator or treatment [1]
2. Contraindications especially pertinent to this procedure:
   (a) None documented
3. Possible side effects especially pertinent to this procedure:
   (a) Iatrogenic injury to the common extensor tendon, including degeneration and rupture.
   (b) Iatrogenic injury to the radial nerve
4. Technical details of note for this procedure (Fig. 7.1):
   (a) Preferred needle gauge: 25-gauge [2]
   (b) Need for image guidance: Optional
      • Ultrasound has been used to guide injections and monitor tendon healing following autologous blood injections [3].
      • Although fluoroscopic guidance has not been formally described for this procedure, the authors have provided an example to illustrate how this injection would appear if fluoroscopic guidance was used.
   (c) Need for image guidance: Optional; generally not required
5. Step-by-step procedure:
   (a) Informed consent
   (b) Pre-procedural testing: Identify and record the response to a physical examination preprocedural provocative maneuver if the procedure is a diagnostic one.
   (c) Image guidance: Optional: ultrasound guidance
   (d) Patient positioning: With the patient in a seated position, the elbow resting on a flat surface, the hand is in full pronation, and the elbow is flexed to 60–90°.
   (e) Identification and marking of injection site:
      • If nonimage-guided:
        – Identify the lateral epicondyles by direct palpation and with palpation of the origin of the common extensor tendon as the patient extends and relaxes the wrist on the affected side.
      • If image-guided:
        – Image the underlying target structure. If ultrasound-guided, the target structure is the common extensor tendon insertion onto the lateral epicondyle. If fluoroscopic-guided, the target structure is the distal aspect of the lateral epicondyle.
      • Mark the target using a marker or by depressing the skin with a plastic needle cap.
   (f) Skin preparation: Initial: Betadine® preparation using the no-touch technique
   (g) Medication preparation:

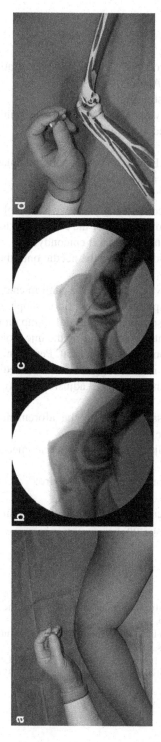

Fig. 7.1 Lateral epicondylar region injection (fluoroscopic-guided). (**a**) Lateral epicondylar region injection-human model. (**b**) Fluoroscopic image of needle entry into lateral epicondylar region. (**c**) Fluoroscopic image of lateral epicondylar region dye pattern. (**d**) Skeletal representation of lateral epicondylar region injection

- Diagnostic injection:
  - 1 mL of 2% preservative-free lidocaine
- Therapeutic injection:
  - 40-mg Depo-Medrol® and 1 mL of 1% preservative-free lidocaine
(h) Skin preparation: Final: Alcohol prep
(i) Local anesthesia administration: Optional
  - Anesthetize the overlying skin and soft tissue using a *small amount of 1% lidocaine* delivered via a *30-gauge*.
(j) Needle placement:
  - If non-image-guided: Direct the needle perpendicular to the skin towards the lateral epicondyle and tendon attachment.
  - If image-guided:
    - If ultrasound-guided: Directly visualize needle placement between the tendon and the tendon sheath of the common extensor tendon close to the insertion site onto the lateral epicondyle.
    - If fluoroscopic-guided: Direct the needle onto the distal aspect of the lateral epicondyle.
(k) Aspiration: Rule out intravascular entry and confirm entry into target structure.
(l) Contrast injection: Not applicable unless fluoroscopic guidance
(m) Injection: Unclamp the aspiration syringe and clamp on the injection syringe.
  - If resistance is encountered early during the injection, rotate the needle to dislodge the bevel from sides of the joint. Persistent very high resistance despite bevel rotation instead suggests that the needle may be embedded in the tendon and further positional adjustment may be necessary.
(n) Postprocedural testing:
  - If applicable, reassess response to the aforementioned preprocedural provocative maneuver.
(o) If (+) response, repeat injection with therapeutic injectate:
  - Repeat steps (d)–(f).
  - Medication preparation: 40-mg Depo-Medrol®
  - Repeat steps (h)–(m).
(p) *Adhesive bandage* application over the needle entry site
(q) Postprocedural care discussion

References

1. Cardone DA, Tallia AF. Diagnostic and therapeutic injection of the elbow region. Am Fam Physician 2002;66(11):2097–100.
2. Saunders S. Elbow treatments. In Law M, ed. Injection Techniques in Orthopaedic and Sports Medicine. London: WB Saunders; 2002:50.
3. Connell DA, Ali KE, Ahmad M, Lambert S, Corbett S, Curtis M. Ultrasound-guided autologous blood injection for tennis elbow. Skeletal Radiol 2006;35(6):371–7.

Injection Procedure: Medial Epicondylitis Injection

1. Indications:
   (a) Medial epicondylitis: diagnosis as pain generator or treatment [1]

2. Contraindications especially pertinent to this procedure:
   (a) None documented

3. Possible side effects especially pertinent to this procedure:
   (a) Iatrogenic injury to the common extensor tendon, including degeneration and rupture.

4. Technical details of note for this procedure (Fig. 7.2):
   (a) Preferred needle gauge: 25-gauge [2]
   (b) Need for image guidance: Optional; generally not required
       • Ultrasound has been used for diagnosis to guide injections and monitor tendon healing following autologous blood injections [3].
       • Although fluoroscopic guidance has not been formally described for this procedure, the authors have provided an example to illustrate how this injection would appear if fluoroscopic guidance was used.

5. Step-by-step procedure:
   (a) Informed consent
   (b) Preprocedural testing: Identify and record the response to a physical examination preprocedural provocative maneuver if the procedure is a diagnostic one.
   (c) Image guidance: Optional: Fluoroscopic and/or ultrasound guidance
   (d) Patient positioning: With the patient in a seated position, the elbow resting on a flat surface, the hand is in full pronation, and the elbow is flexed to 60–90°.
   (e) Identification and marking of injection site:
       • If nonimage-guided:
           – Identify the medial epicondyle by direct palpation and with palpation of the origin of the common extensor tendon as the patient extends and relaxes the wrist on the affected side.
       • If image-guided:
           – Image the underlying target structure. If fluoroscopic-guided, the target structure is the distal aspect of the medial epicondyle. If ultrasound-guided, the target structure is the common extensor tendon insertion onto the medial epicondyle.
       • Mark the target using a marker or by depressing the skin with a plastic needle cap.
   (f) Skin preparation: Initial: Betadine® preparation using the no-touch technique

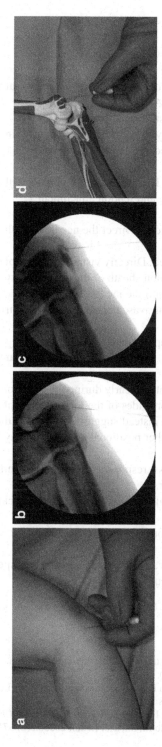

Fig. 7.2 Medial epicondylar region injection (fluoroscopic-guided). (**a**) Medial epicondylar region injection-human model. (**b**) Fluoroscopic image of needle entry into medial epicondylar region. (**c**) Fluoroscopic image of medial epicondylar region dye pattern. (**d**) Skeletal representation of medial epicondylar region injection

(g) Medication preparation:
- Diagnostic injection:
  - 1 mL of 2% preservative-free lidocaine
- Therapeutic injection:
  - 40-mg Depo-Medrol® and 1 mL of 1% preservative-free lidocaine

(h) Skin preparation: Final: Alcohol prep

(i) Local anesthesia administration: Optional
- Anesthetize the overlying skin and soft tissue using a *small amount of 1% lidocaine* delivered via a *30-gauge needle.*

(j) Needle placement:
- If non-image-guided: Direct the needle perpendicular to the skin toward the medial epicondyle and tendon attachment.
- If image-guided:
  - If fluoroscopic-guided: Direct the needle onto the distal aspect of the medial epicondyle.
  - If ultrasound-guided: Directly visualize needle placement between the tendon and the tendon sheath of the common extensor tendon close to the insertion site onto the medial epicondyle.

(k) Aspiration: Rule out intravascular entry and confirm entry into target structure.

(l) Contrast injection: Not applicable

(m) Injection: Unclamp the aspiration syringe and clamp on the injection syringe.
- If resistance is encountered early during the injection, rotate the needle to dislodge the bevel from sides of the joint. Persistent very high resistance despite bevel rotation instead suggests that the needle may be embedded in the tendon and further positional adjustment may be necessary.

(n) Postprocedural testing:
- If applicable, reassess response to the aforementioned preprocedural provocative maneuver.

(o) If (+) response, repeat injection with therapeutic injectate:
- Repeat steps (d)–(f).
- Medication preparation: 40-mg Depo-Medrol®
- Repeat steps (h)–(m).

(p) Adhesive bandage application over the needle entry site

(q) Postprocedural care discussion

References

1. Cardone DA, Tallia AF. Diagnostic and therapeutic injection of the elbow region. Am Fam Physician 2002;66(11):2097–100.
2. Saunders S. Elbow treatments . In Law M, ed. Injection Techniques in Orthopaedic and Sports Medicine. London: WB Saunders; 2002:50.
3. Connell DA, Ali KE, Ahmad M, Lambert S, Corbett S, Curtis M. Ultrasound-guided autologous blood injection for tennis elbow. Skeletal Radiol 2006;35(6):371–7.

Injection Procedure: Olecranon Bursa Aspiration/Injection

1. Indications:
   (a) Diagnosis of Olecranon bursa as a pain generator and/or treatment [1]

2. Contraindications especially pertinent to this procedure:
   (a) None documented

3. Possible side effects especially pertinent to this procedure:
   (a) There is a theoretical risk of injury to the ulnar nerve with this injection, as the ulnar nerve courses around the epicondyle groove. This risk is decreased by aiming the needle toward the lateral aspect of the bursa.

4. Technical details of note for this procedure (Fig. 7.3):
   (a) Preferred needle gauge: 18-gauge
       • A 25-gauge needle has been suggested if the goal is to just inject the olecranon bursa without aspirating it [2].
   (b) Need for image guidance: No
       • This procedure is generally performed for bursal swelling, and image guidance is unnecessary in the authors' opinion.

5. Step-by-step procedure:
   (a) Informed consent
   (b) Preprocedural testing: Not applicable
   (c) Image guidance: Optional: Ultrasound-guided procedure
       • In the vast majority of cases, the swelling is so apparent to inspection that image guidance to ensure successful needle entry into the bursa is not necessary. In cases of very subtle swelling, ultrasound guidance could be of help in guiding needle placement.
   (d) Patient positioning:
       • Place the patient in a seated position with the elbow resting on a flat surface, the hand in full pronation, and the elbow flexed to 90°. Approaching the bursa from a posterolateral angle is preferred to avoid potential injury to the ulnar nerve.
   (e) Identification and marking of injection site:
       • Identify the center of the distended, painful bursa, or the olecranon process if the bursa is not significantly distended. Care should be taken to select an injection site slightly lateral to the area described earlier to avoid the ulnar nerve.
       • Mark the target using a marker or by depressing the skin with a plastic needle cap.
   (f) Skin preparation: Initial: Betadine® preparation using the no-touch technique
   (g) Medication preparation
       • Therapeutic injection:
         – 80-mg Depo-Medrol® ½ ml preservative-free lidocaine
   (h) Skin preparation: Final: Alcohol prep

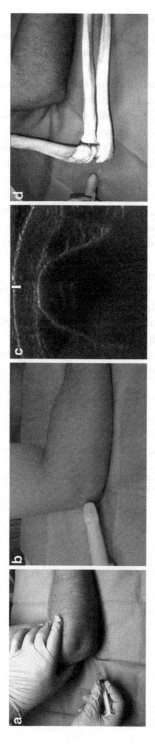

Fig. 7.3 Olecranon bursa aspiration and/or injection (ultrasound-guided). (**a**) Olecranon bursa injection-human model. (**b**) Ultrasound transducer positioning for visualizing olecranon bursa-human model. (**c**) Ultrasonogram corresponding to previous image. (**d**) Skeletal representation of Olecranon bursa aspiration/injection

(i) Local anesthesia administration: Optional
  - Anesthetize the overlying skin and soft tissue using a *small amount of 1% lidocaine* delivered via a *30-gauge needle*.
(j) Needle placement:
  - Pierce the previously anesthetized skin and subcutaneous tissue site with the needle attached to a 10 or 20-mL syringe.
  - After needle insertion, the needle should be directed in a zig-zag direction to prevent leakage of the reaccumulated fluid through a needle tract that can develop if the needle is directed straight through the tissue.
(k) Aspiration: Rule out intravascular entry and confirm entry into bursa (if enough bursal fluid is present to allow aspiration).
  - Maintain continuous aspiration during needle advancement.
  - Aspirate fluid from the bursa. Bursal fluid may be bloody or blood-tinged depending on the pathology. A purely hemorrhagic aspirate may indicate placement of the needle tip in a blood vessel and require needle adjustment.
(l) Contrast injection: Not applicable
(m) Injection (if applicable): Unclamp the aspiration syringe and clamp on the injection syringe containing the injectate.
  - If resistance is encountered early during the injection, rotate the needle to dislodge the bevel from the side of the joint.
(n) *Adhesive bandage* application over the needle entry site
(o) Postprocedural care discussion

References

1. Cardone DA, Tallia AF. Diagnostic and therapeutic injection of the elbow region. Am Fam Physician 2002;66(11):2097–100.
2. Saunders S. Elbow treatments. In Law M, ed. Injection Techniques in Orthopaedic and Sports Medicine, second edition. London: WB Saunders; 2002:48.

Injection Procedure: Radiocapitellar Injection
Approach to Elbow Joint

1. Indications:
   (a) Diagnosis of radiocapitellar joint as a pain generator
   (b) Radiocapitellar joint pain

2. Contraindications especially pertinent to this procedure:
   (a) None documented

3. Possible side effects especially pertinent to this procedure:
   (a) None documented

4. Technical details of note for this procedure (Fig. 7.4):
   (a) Preferred needle gauge:
      • Aspiration +/- injection: *18–21 gauge*
      • Injection only: *25 gauge*
   (b) Need for image guidance: Optional

5. Step-by-step procedure:
   (a) Informed consent
   (b) Preprocedural testing: Identify and record the response to a physical exami-
       nation preprocedural provocative maneuver if the procedure is a diagnostic
       injection.
   (c) Image guidance: Optional: Fluoroscopic-guided procedure
   (d) Patient positioning:
      • Place the patient in a seated position on the side and positioned in the
        X-ray beam.
      • The elbow is placed on a flat surface and positioned in 50–90° of elbow
        flexion, with the palm facing downward (pronated).
   (e) Identification and marking of injection site:
      • If nonimage-guided:
        – The capitellum and radial head are palpated and identified. The space
          between the capitellum and radial head is identified by palpation.
      • If image-guided:
        – Use image guidance in order to identify the underlying radiocapitellar
          joint.
      • Mark the target using a marker or by depressing the skin with a plastic
        needle cap.
   (f) Skin preparation: Initial: Betadine® preparation using the no-touch
       technique
   (g) Medication preparation: 3 mL of 2% preservative-free lidocaine
   (h) Skin preparation: Final: Alcohol prep
   (i) Local anesthesia administration: Optional
      • Anesthetize the overlying skin and soft tissue using a *small amount of
        1% lidocaine* delivered via a *30-gauge, 1-in. needle.*

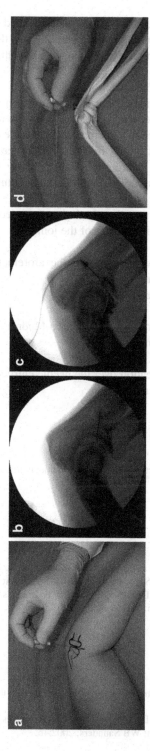

Fig. 7.4 Radiocapitellar joint injection (fluoroscopic-guided). (**a**) Radiocapitellar joint injection-human model. (**b**) Fluoroscopic image of needle entry into radiocapitellar joint. (**c**) Fluoroscopic image of radiocapitellar arthrogram. (**d**) Skeletal representation of radiocapitellar joint injection

(j) Needle placement: Pierce the previously anesthetized skin and subcutaneous tissue site with the appropriate needle and direct to the target.

(k) Aspiration: Rule out intravascular entry and confirm entry into target structure.

(l) Contrast injection: If applicable.

- Inject the joint with enough contrast to confirm entry into the target structure. Connecting the contrast dye syringe to the needle using extension tubing is recommended to prevent a shift in needle position during attachment and detachment to and from the spinal needle. Adjust the needle position, if necessary, in order to obtain a clearly defined arthrogram.

(m) Injection: Unclamp the syringe from the extension tubing and clamp on the injection syringe.

- If resistance is encountered early during the injection, rotate the needle to dislodge the bevel from sides of the joint.

(n) Postprocedural testing:

- If applicable, reassess response to the aforementioned preprocedural provocative maneuver.

(o) Repeat injection with therapeutic injectate:

- Ρεπεατ στεπσ (δ)–(φ).
- Medication preparation: 40 mg of Depo-Medrol® and 2 mL of 1% preservative-free lidocaine
- Repeat steps (h)–(m).

(p) *Adhesive bandage* application over the needle entry site

(q) Postprocedural care discussion

Bibliography

These textbook entries describe injections into the radiohumeral articulation, but not specifically into the radiocapitellar joint

References

1. Waldman SD. Radial nerve block at the elbow. In Andjelkovic N, Chappelle A, eds. Atlas of Interventional Pain Management, Second edition. Philadelphia, PA; 2004:175–177.
2. Saunders S. Elbow treatments. In Law M, ed. Injection Techniques in Orthopaedic and Sports Medicine, Second edition. London: WB Saunders; 2002:50–52.

References

1. Cardone DA, Tallia AF. Diagnostic and therapeutic injection of the elbow region. Am Fam Physician 2002;66(11):2097–100.
2. Saunders S. Elbow treatments. In Law M, ed. Injection Techniques in Orthopaedic and Sports Medicine, Second edition. London: WB Saunders; 2002:46.

Injection Procedure: Elbow Joint Aspiration and/or Injection

1. *Indications*:
   (a) Crystal arthropathy [1]
   (b) Osteoarthritis
   (c) Relief from swelling/pain due to trauma
   (d) Rheumatoid arthritis
   (e) Trauma: Diagnosis of fracture and/or relief of pain due to effusion

2. Contraindications especially pertinent to this procedure:
   (a) None documented

3. Possible side effects especially pertinent to this procedure:
   (a) None documented

4. Technical details of note for this procedure (Fig. 7.5):
   (a) Preferred needle gauge:
      • Aspiration +/- injection: *18–21 gauge*
      • Injection only: Use of a *25-gauge* needle has been suggested [2]
   (b) Need for image guidance: Optional
      • A review of the literature did not yield any decisive studies to strongly recommend doing the injection with or without imaging guidance

5. Step-by-step procedure:
   (a) Informed consent
   (b) Pre-procedural testing: Identify and record the response to a physical examination preprocedural provocative maneuver if the procedure is a diagnostic injection.
   (c) Image guidance: Optional: Fluoroscopic- or ultrasound-guided procedure
   (d) Patient positioning:
      • The elbow is placed on a flat surface and positioned in 50–90° of elbow flexion, with the palm facing downward (pronated).
   (e) Identification and marking of injection site:
      • The lateral epicondyle, radial head, and posterior aspect of the olecranon are palpated and identified.
      • If non-image-guided:
        – Identify the groove between the lateral epicondyle and posterior olecranon; it is palpated lateral to the radial head.
      • If fluoroscopic-guided:
        – Obtain a fluoroscopic picture in order to identify the needle entry site in the center of the triangle formed by the lateral epicondyle, radial head, and posterior aspect of the olecranon.
        – Make adjustments in the metallic marker location and/or relative position of the c-arm–c-arm fluoroscope as needed.

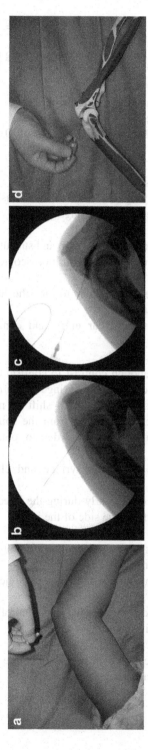

Fig. 7.5 Elbow joint injection (fluoroscopic-guided). (**a**) Elbow joint injection-human model. (**b**) Fluoroscopic image of needle entry into elbow joint. (**c**) Fluoroscopic image of elbow joint arthrogram. (**d**) Skeletal representation of elbow joint injection

- Mark the target using a marker or by depressing the skin with a plastic needle cap.
(f) Skin preparation: Initial: Betadine® preparation using the no-touch technique
(g) Medication preparation:
    - Diagnostic injection:
        - 3 mL of 2% preservative-free lidocaine
    - Therapeutic injection:
        - 80 mg of Depo-Medrol® and 2 mL of 0.25% preservative-free bupivacaine
(h) Skin preparation: Final: Alcohol prep
(i) Local anesthesia administration: Optional
    - Anesthetize the overlying skin and soft tissue using a *small amount of 1% lidocaine* delivered via a *30-gauge needle*.
(j) Needle placement:
    - Pierce the previously anesthetized skin and subcutaneous tissue site with the spinal needle and use intermittent fluoroscopic guidance to direct the spinal needle into the elbow joint.
    - The needle is directed proximally toward the head of the radius and medially into the joint.
(k) Aspiration: Rule out intravascular entry and confirm entry into target structure.
(l) Contrast injection:
    - Inject the joint with enough contrast to confirm entry into target structure. Connecting the contrast dye syringe to the needle using extension tubing is recommended to prevent a shift in needle position during attachment and detachment to and from the spinal needle. Adjust the needle position, if necessary, in order to obtain a clearly defined arthrogram.
(m) Injection: Unclamp the aspiration syringe and clamp on the injection syringe.
    - If resistance is encountered early during the injection, rotate the needle to dislodge the bevel from the side of the joint.
(n) Postprocedural testing:
    - If applicable, reassess the response to the aforementioned pre-procedural provocative maneuver.
(o) If (+) response, repeat injection with therapeutic injectate:
    - Repeat steps (d)–(f).
    - Medication preparation: 80 mg of Depo-Medrol® and 1 mL of 0.25% preservative-free bupivacaine
    - Repeat steps (h)–(m).
(p) *Adhesive bandage* application over needle entry site
(q) Postprocedural care discussion

Injection Procedure Templates

Injection Procedure Template: Lateral Epicondylitis Injection

---

PROCEDURE: Lateral Epicondylitis Injection
Side: ☐-Right   ☐-Left   ☐-Bilateral
Procedure Type: Aspiration: ☐-Diagnostic aspiration
        Injection: ☐-Diagnostic   ☐-Therapeutic   ☐-Diagnostic then Therapeutic
Image guidance: None unless indicated as follows- ☐-Fluoroscopy ☐-Ultrasound

- The potential benefits and side effects of the procedure and alternative treatment options were explained to the patient, an opportunity for questions was provided, and the patient signed informed consent.
- ☐- If checked, the following physical examination pre-procedural provocative maneuver(s) was (were) performed: ☐-_____
- The patient was positioned for the procedure and the target structure was identified.
- The overlying skin was prepped with Betadine® followed by alcohol prep pad after the Betadine® dried.
- ☐- If checked, the overlying skin and soft tissue was anesthetized using a small amount of 1% lidocaine delivered via the following needle ☐-30G1"; ☐-25G1½ "; ☐-Other: _____
- The following needle was then used for the procedure:
  - Type: Straight needle unless indicated as follows: ☐-Spinal needle; ☐-Other:_____
  - Gauge: ☐-30; ☐-27; ☐-25; ☐-22; ☐-21; -18; -Other:_____
  - Length: ☐-5/8"; ☐- 1"; ☐- 1 ½"; ☐- 2"; ☐- 2 ½"; ☐- 3";☐- 3½"; ☐-Other:_____

○ Image guidance if indicated above was used to confirm needle entry into target structure.
○ ☐-If checked, contrast dye was then injected and the needle position was adjusted accordingly to confirm proper placement without inadvertent intravascular entry.

- Needle was adjusted accordingly to confirm proper placement without inadvertent vascular entry.
- An attempt was made to aspirate from the structure and then the following injectate was delivered into the target structure:
  - ☐-Diagnostic injection: 1 mL 2% preservative-free lidocaine; ☐-Other injectate: _____
  - ☐-Therapeutic injection: 40 mg Depo-Medrol® & ☐- 1 mL 1% preservative-free lidocaine
    ☐-Other injectate: _____
- The needle was removed and an adhesive bandage was placed over the needle entry site.

-If the above was a diagnostic injection, then proceed to section immediately below.
-If above was a therapeutic injection procedure, aspiration only procedure, or aspiration and therapeutic injection, then proceed to Procedure Summary Section.

For Diagnostic Injection Procedure:

- ☐-If checked, the above listed pre-procedural physical examination provocative maneuver was repeated and pain relief was: ☐-N/A; ☐-significant; ☐-some; ☐-equivocal; ☐-none; ☐-Other:_____
  Based on the amount of pain relief noted above:
  - ☐-a therapeutic injection will be scheduled.
  - ☐-a therapeutic injection will not be scheduled. See plan in corresponding office note.
  - ☐-a therapeutic injection following the same procedure described above was done using
    - ☐- 40 mg Depo-Medrol® & ☐- 1 mL 1% preservative-free lidocaine
    - ☐- Other injectate:_____
- The needle was removed and an adhesive bandage was placed over the needle entry site.

Procedure Summary:
If fluid aspirated from the target structure during the procedure:

- Total volume of fluid aspirated: ___ mL; Fluid appearance: ☐- N/A; ☐-Clear yellow; ☐-Slightly cloudy; ☐-Cloudy; ☐-Purulent; ☐-Blood-tinged; ☐-Bloody; ☐-Other:_____

Patient tolerance for the procedure: ☐-Excellent; ☐-Good; ☐-Fair; ☐-Other:_____
Additional comments regarding the procedure: ☐-None; ☐-Other:_____
_____

Post-Procedural Treatment Advice:
Activity modification: Avoid non-essential use of the structure until seen for follow up. ☐-Other:_____
Orthotic instructions: N/A unless indicated as follows _____
Modalities: Apply ice over the injection site prn for 20-30 min. up to q2 hrs until seen for follow-up, unless instructed as follows: ☐-Heat;
☐-Other:_____

Injection Procedure Template: Medial Epicondylitis Injection

PROCEDURE: Medial Epicondylitis Injection
Side: ☐-Right   ☐-Left   ☐-Bilateral
Procedure Type: Aspiration: ☐-Diagnostic aspiration
            Injection: ☐-Diagnostic   ☐-Therapeutic   ☐-Diagnostic <u>then</u> Therapeutic
Image guidance: None unless indicated as follows- ☐-Fluoroscopy   ☐-Ultrasound

- The potential benefits and side effects of the procedure and alternative treatment options were explained to the patient, an opportunity for questions was provided, and <u>the patient signed informed consent</u>.
- ☐- If checked, the following physical examination <u>pre-procedural provocative maneuver(s)</u> was (were) performed: ☐-_____
- The patient was positioned for the procedure and the target structure was identified.
- The overlying skin was prepped with <u>Betadine® followed by alcohol prep pad</u> after the Betadine® dried.
- ☐- If checked, the overlying skin and soft tissue was anesthetized using a <u>small amount of 1% lidocaine</u> delivered via the following needle ☐-30G1"; ☐-25G1½ "; ☐-Other: _____
- The following needle was then used for the procedure:
  - <u>Type</u>: Straight needle unless indicated as follows: ☐-Spinal needle; ☐-Other:_____
  - <u>Gauge</u>: ☐-30; ☐-27; ☐-25; ☐-22; ☐-21; -18; -Other:_____
  - <u>Length</u>: ☐-5/8"; ☐- 1"; ☐- 1 ½"; ☐- 2"; ☐- 2 ½"; ☐- 3"; ☐- 3½"; ☐-Other:_____
- ○ Image guidance if indicated above was used to confirm needle entry into target structure.
- ○ ☐-If checked, contrast dye was then injected and the needle position was adjusted accordingly to confirm proper placement without inadvertent intravascular entry.
- Needle was adjusted accordingly to confirm proper placement without inadvertent vascular entry.
- An attempt was made to aspirate from the structure and then the following injectate was delivered into the target structure:
  - ☐-Diagnostic injection: <mark>1 mL 2% preservative-free lidocaine</mark>; ☐-Other injectate: _____
  - ☐-Therapeutic injection: <mark>40 mg Depo-Medrol®</mark> & ☐- <mark>1 mL 1% preservative-free lidocaine</mark>
    - ☐-Other injectate: _____
- The needle was removed and an <u>adhesive bandage</u> was placed over the needle entry site.

-If the above was a <u>diagnostic injection</u>, then proceed to section immediately below.
-If above was a <u>therapeutic injection procedure</u>, <u>aspiration only procedure</u>, or <u>aspiration and therapeutic injection</u>, then proceed to Procedure Summary Section.

For Diagnostic Injection Procedure:
- ☐-If checked, the above listed pre-procedural physical examination provocative maneuver was repeated and pain relief was : ☐-N/A; ☐-significant; ☐-some; ☐-equivocal; ☐-none; ☐-Other:_____
- Based on the amount of pain relief noted above:
  - ☐-a therapeutic injection will be scheduled.
  - ☐-a therapeutic injection will <u>not</u> be scheduled. See plan in corresponding office note.
  - ☐-a therapeutic injection following the same procedure described above was done using
    - ☐- <mark>40 mg Depo-Medrol®</mark> & ☐- <mark>1 mL 1% preservative-free lidocaine</mark>
    - ☐- Other injectate:_____
- The needle was removed and an <u>adhesive bandage</u> was placed over the needle entry site.

Procedure Summary:
If fluid aspirated from the target structure during the procedure:
- Total volume of fluid aspirated: ___ mL; Fluid appearance: ☐- N/A; ☐-Clear yellow; ☐-Slightly cloudy; ☐-Cloudy; ☐-Purulent; ☐-Blood-tinged; ☐-Bloody; ☐-Other:_____
Patient tolerance for the procedure: ☐-Excellent; ☐-Good; ☐-Fair; ☐-Other:_____
Additional comments regarding the procedure: ☐-None; ☐Other:_____
_____

Post-Procedural Treatment Advice:
Activity modification: Avoid non-essential use of the structure until seen for follow up. ☐-Other:_____
Orthotic instructions: N/A unless indicated as follows _____
Modalities: Apply ice over the injection site prn for 20-30 min. up to q2 hrs until seen for follow-up, unless instructed as follows: ☐-Heat;
☐-Other:_____

Injection Procedure Template: Olecranon Bursa Injection/Aspiration

PROCEDURE: Olecranon Bursa Injection/Aspiration
Side: ☐-Right   ☐-Left   ☐-Bilateral
Procedure Type: Aspiration: ☐-Diagnostic aspiration
                Injection: ☐-Diagnostic   ☐-Therapeutic   ☐-Diagnostic then Therapeutic
Image guidance: None unless indicated as follows- ☐-Fluoroscopy   ☐-Ultrasound
- The potential benefits and side effects of the procedure and alternative treatment options were explained to the patient, an opportunity for questions was provided, and the patient signed informed consent.
- ☐- If checked, the following physical examination pre-procedural provocative maneuver(s) was (were) performed: ☐-_____
- The patient was positioned for the procedure and the target structure was identified.
- The overlying skin was prepped with Betadine® followed by alcohol prep pad after the Betadine® dried.
- ☐- If checked, the overlying skin and soft tissue was anesthetized using a small amount of 1% lidocaine delivered via the following needle ☐-30G1"; ☐-25G1½ "; ☐-Other: _____
- The following needle was then used for the procedure:
    Type: Straight needle unless indicated as follows: ☐-Spinal needle; ☐-Other:_____
    Gauge: ☐-30; ☐-27; ☐-25; ☐-22; ☐-21; -18; -Other:_____
    Length: ☐-5/8"; ☐- 1"; ☐- 1 ½"; ☐- 2"; ☐- 2 ½"; ☐- 3";☐- 3½"; ☐-Other:_____
○ Image guidance if indicated above was used to confirm needle entry into target structure.
○ ☐-If checked, contrast dye was then injected and the needle position was adjusted accordingly to confirm proper placement without inadvertent intravascular entry.
- Needle was adjusted accordingly to confirm proper placement without inadvertent vascular entry.
- An attempt was made to aspirate from the structure and then the following injectate was delivered into the target structure:
    ☐-Diagnostic injection: 3 mL 2% preservative-free lidocaine; ☐-Other injectate: _____
    ☐-Therapeutic injection: 80 mg Depo-Medrol® & ☐- 0.5 mL 1% preservative-free lidocaine
        ☐-Other injectate: _____
- The needle was removed and an adhesive bandage was placed over the needle entry site.

-If the above was a diagnostic injection, then proceed to section immediately below.
-If above was a therapeutic injection procedure, aspiration only procedure, or aspiration and therapeutic injection, then proceed to Procedure Summary Section.

For Diagnostic Injection Procedure:
- ☐- If checked, the above listed pre-procedural physical examination provocative maneuver was repeated and pain relief was: ☐-N/A; ☐-significant; ☐-some; ☐-equivocal; ☐-none; ☐-Other:_____
- Based on the amount of pain relief noted above:
    ☐-a therapeutic injection will be scheduled.
    ☐-a therapeutic injection will not be scheduled. See plan in corresponding office note.
    ☐-a therapeutic injection following the same procedure described above was done using
        ☐- 80 mg Depo-Medrol® & ☐- 0.5 mL 1% preservative-free lidocaine
        ☐- Other injectate: _____
- The needle was removed and an adhesive bandage was placed over the needle entry site.

Procedure Summary:
If fluid aspirated from the target structure during the procedure:
- Total volume of fluid aspirated: ___ mL; Fluid appearance: ☐- N/A; ☐-Clear yellow; ☐-Slightly cloudy;
    ☐-Cloudy; ☐-Purulent; ☐-Blood-tinged; ☐-Bloody; ☐-Other:_____
Patient tolerance for the procedure: ☐-Excellent; ☐-Good; ☐-Fair; ☐-Other:_____
Additional comments regarding the procedure: ☐-None; ☐Other:_____
_____
_____

Post-Procedural Treatment Advice:
Activity modification: Avoid non-essential use of the structure until seen for follow up. ☐-Other:_____
Orthotic instructions: N/A unless indicated as follows _____
Modalities: Apply ice over the injection site prn for 20-30 min. up to q2 hrs until seen for follow-up, unless instructed as follows: ☐-Heat;
☐-Other:_____

Injection Procedure Template

Radiocapitellar Injection Approach to Elbow Joint

PROCEDURE: Radiocapitellar Injection Approach to Elbow Joint
Side: ☐-Right   ☐-Left   ☐-Bilateral
Procedure Type: Aspiration: ☐-Diagnostic aspiration
            Injection: ☐-Diagnostic   ☐-Therapeutic   ☐-Diagnostic <u>then</u> Therapeutic
Image guidance: None unless indicated as follows- ☐-Fluoroscopy   ☐-Ultrasound

- The potential benefits and side effects of the procedure and alternative treatment options were explained to the patient, an opportunity for questions was provided, and the patient signed informed consent.
- ☐- If checked, the following physical examination pre-procedural provocative maneuver(s) was (were) performed: ☐- _____
- The patient was positioned for the procedure and the target structure was identified.
- The overlying skin was prepped with <u>Betadine® followed by alcohol prep pad</u> after the Betadine® dried.
- ☐- If checked, the overlying skin and soft tissue was anesthetized using a <u>small amount of 1% lidocaine</u> delivered via the following needle ☐-30G1"; ☐-25G1½ "; ☐-Other: _____
- The following needle was then used for the procedure:
  - <u>Type:</u> Straight needle unless indicated as follows: ☐-Spinal needle; ☐-Other:_____
  - <u>Gauge:</u> ☐-30; ☐-27; ☐-25; ☐-22; ☐-21; -18; -Other: _____
  - <u>Length:</u> ☐-5/8"; ☐- 1"; ☐- 1 ½"; ☐- 2"; ☐- 2 ½"; ☐- 3";☐- 3½"; ☐-Other:_____
- o Image guidance if indicated above was used to confirm needle entry into target structure.
- o ☐-If checked, contrast dye was then injected and the needle position was adjusted accordingly to confirm proper placement without inadvertent intravascular entry.
- Needle was adjusted accordingly to confirm proper placement without inadvertent vascular entry.
- An attempt was made to aspirate from the structure and then the following injectate was delivered into the target structure:
  - ☐-Diagnostic injection: 3 mL 1% preservative-free lidocaine   ☐-Other injectate: _____
  - ☐-Therapeutic injection: 40 mg Depo-Medrol® & ☐- 2 mL 1% preservative-free lidocaine
    - ☐-Other injectate: _____
- The needle was removed and an <u>adhesive bandage</u> was placed over the needle entry site.

-If the above was a <u>diagnostic injection</u>, then proceed to section immediately below.
-If above was a <u>therapeutic injection procedure</u>, <u>aspiration only procedure</u>, or <u>aspiration and therapeutic injection</u>, then proceed to Procedure Summary Section.

For Diagnostic Injection Procedure:
- ☐-If checked, the above listed pre-procedural physical examination provocative maneuver was repeated and pain relief was: ☐-N/A; ☐-significant; ☐-some; ☐-equivocal; ☐-none; ☐-Other:_____
- Based on the amount of pain relief noted above:
  - ☐-a therapeutic injection will be scheduled.
  - ☐-a therapeutic injection will <u>not</u> be scheduled. See plan in corresponding office note.
  - ☐-a therapeutic injection following the same procedure described above was done using
    - ☐- 40 mg Depo-Medrol® & ☐- 2 mL 1% preservative-free lidocaine
    - ☐- Other injectate: _____
- The needle was removed and an <u>adhesive bandage</u> was placed over the needle entry site.

Procedure Summary:
If fluid aspirated from the target structure during the procedure:
- Total volume of fluid aspirated: ___ mL; Fluid appearance: ☐- N/A; ☐-Clear yellow; ☐-Slightly cloudy; ☐-Cloudy; ☐-Purulent; ☐-Blood-tinged; ☐-Bloody; ☐-Other:_____
Patient tolerance for the procedure: ☐-Excellent; ☐-Good; ☐-Fair; ☐-Other:_____

Additional comments regarding the procedure: ☐-None; ☐Other:_____

Post-Procedural Treatment Advice:
Activity modification: Avoid non-essential use of the structure until seen for follow up. ☐-Other:_____

Orthotic instructions: N/A unless indicated as follows _____
Modalities: Apply ice over the injection site prn for 20-30 min. up to q2 hrs until seen for follow-up, unless instructed as follows: ☐-Heat; ☐-Other:_____

Injection Procedure Template: Elbow Joint Aspiration and/or Injection

---

PROCEDURE: Elbow Joint Aspiration and/or Injection
Side:　　　　　☐-Right　　　　　☐-Left　　　　　☐-Bilateral
Procedure Type: Aspiration:　　☐-Diagnostic aspiration
　　　　　　　　　Injection:　　☐-Diagnostic　　☐-Therapeutic　☐-Diagnostic then Therapeutic
Image guidance: None unless indicated as follows- ☐-Fluoroscopy ☐-Ultrasound

- The potential benefits and side effects of the procedure and alternative treatment options were explained to the patient, an opportunity for questions was provided, and the patient signed informed consent.
- ☐- If checked, the following physical examination pre-procedural provocative maneuver(s) was (were) performed: ☐-_____
- The patient was positioned for the procedure and the target structure was identified.
- The overlying skin was prepped with Betadine® followed by alcohol prep pad after the Betadine® dried.
- ☐- If checked, the overlying skin and soft tissue was anesthetized using a small amount of 1% lidocaine delivered via the following needle ☐-30G1"; ☐-25G1½ "; ☐-Other:_____
- The following needle was then used for the procedure:
  　　Type: Straight needle unless indicated as follows: ☐-Spinal needle; ☐-Other:_____
  　　Gauge: ☐-30; ☐-27; ☐-25; ☐-22; ☐-21; -18; -Other:_____
  　　Length: ☐-5/8"; ☐- 1"; ☐- 1 ½"; ☐- 2"; ☐- 2 ½"; ☐- 3";☐- 3½"; ☐-Other:_____
- ○ Image guidance if indicated above was used to confirm needle entry into target structure.
- ○ ☐-If checked, contrast dye was then injected and the needle position was adjusted accordingly to confirm proper placement without inadvertent intravascular entry.
- Needle was adjusted accordingly to confirm proper placement without inadvertent vascular entry.
- An attempt was made to aspirate from the structure and then the following injectate was delivered into the target structure:
  　　☐-Diagnostic injection: 3 mL 2% preservative-free lidocaine; ☐-Other injectate:_____
  　　☐-Therapeutic injection: 80 mg Depo-Medrol® & ☐- 1 mL 0.25% preservative-free bupivacaine
  　　　　　　　☐-Other injectate:_____
- The needle was removed and an adhesive bandage was placed over the needle entry site.

-If the above was a diagnostic injection, then proceed to section immediately below.
-If above was a therapeutic injection procedure, aspiration only procedure, or aspiration and therapeutic injection, then proceed to Procedure Summary Section.

For Diagnostic Injection Procedure:
- ☐-If checked, the above listed pre-procedural physical examination provocative maneuver was repeated and pain relief was: ☐-N/A; ☐-significant; ☐-some; ☐-equivocal; ☐-none; ☐-Other:_____
- Based on the amount of pain relief noted above:
  　☐-a therapeutic injection will be scheduled.
  　☐-a therapeutic injection will not be scheduled. See plan in corresponding office note.
  　☐-a therapeutic injection following the same procedure described above was done using
  　　　　☐- 80 mg Depo-Medrol® & ☐- 1 mL 0.25% preservative-free lidocaine
  　　　　☐- Other injectate:_____
- The needle was removed and an adhesive bandage was placed over the needle entry site.

Procedure Summary:
If fluid aspirated from the target structure during the procedure:
- Total volume of fluid aspirated: ____ mL; Fluid appearance: ☐- N/A; ☐-Clear yellow; ☐-Slightly cloudy; ☐-Cloudy; ☐-Purulent; ☐-Blood-tinged; ☐-Bloody; ☐-Other:

Patient tolerance for the procedure: ☐-Excellent; ☐-Good; ☐-Fair; ☐-Other:_____

Additional comments regarding the procedure: ☐-None; ☐Other:_____

Post-Procedural Treatment Advice:
Activity modification: Avoid non-essential use of the structure until seen for follow up. ☐-Other:_____

Orthotic instructions: N/A unless indicated as follows _____
Modalities: Apply ice over the injection site prn for 20-30 min. up to q2 hrs until seen for follow-up, unless instructed as follows: ☐-Heat; ☐-Other:_____

Chapter 8
The Wrist

Patrick M. Foye, Debra S. Ibrahim, Michael J. Mehnert, Todd P. Stitik, Jong H. Kim, Mohammad Hossein Dorri, David J. Van Why, Jose Ibarbia, Lisa Schoenherr, Naimish Baxi, Ladislav Habina, and Jiaxin J. Tran

Introduction

Injections at the wrist region are frequently performed in musculoskeletal practice. Prior to injection at the wrist or any site, the physician should perform a careful history and a physical exam to hone in on the source of the patient's presenting symptoms. The literature provides a variety of descriptions regarding how to perform various injections for various procedures, and variable degrees of evidence regarding their effectiveness (Table 8.1).

Carpal tunnel injection (CTI) with corticosteroid is a common procedure, largely due to the high incidence of carpal tunnel syndrome (CTS). CTI can be performed via various techniques. Perhaps the most notable potential complication from CTI is median nerve injury [1–4]. This, however, is usually transient [4]. Most CTI techniques involve insertion of a thin (e.g., 25 gauge) needle along the wrist crease and angle the injection posteriorly-distally into the carpal tunnel, beneath the transverse carpal ligament. Authors often suggest that needle placement medial (ulnar) to the palmaris longus tendon can minimize the risk of inadvertent median nerve injury [4]. However, another study suggests that the median nerve often travels on the ulnar side of the palmaris longus tendon, thus those authors suggest that injection through the flexor carpi radialis (FCR) tendon may be least likely to pierce the median nerve [5]. Another approach uses a very thin (29 gauge) half inch needle inserted 2–3 cm distal to the middle of the wrist crease [6]. This approach was found to be less time-consuming and less painful. Transient ulnar nerve irritation is also possible [1]. Proper technique should minimize the risk of median or ulnar nerve irritation. Ultrasound guidance offers major advantages with respect to minimizing the risk of inadvertent median nerve injury.

Although some studies have found that CTI was not effective for CTS [7, 8], most studies have found these injections to be effective when provided, at least as a short-term relief for CTS (e.g., while postponing surgical treatment) [9, 10]. CTI

T.P. Stitik (✉)
Department of Physical Medicine and Rehabilitation, New Jersey Medical School,
Newark, NJ, USA
e-mail: todd.stitik@gmail.com

P.M. Foye et al.

Table 8.1 Summary of wrist region injection procedures

Injection type	Specific structure	Meta-analysis (es)	Prospective study (studies)	Case series/report(s)	Described in review article(s) and/or injection textbook(s)
Articulation/joint	Distal radioulnar joint		23	22	27–29
	TFCC (triangular fibrocartilage complex)				30
	Wrist joint		23, 26, 24	31	32–34
Other:	Carpal tunnel	8	14, 5, 10, 11, 7, 12, 13, 6	2, 1, 3, 4	35–38, 8
Bursa/cyst	Ganglion cyst		45, 46	39, 21	40, 38
Tendons	de Quervain's tenosynovitis		15, 18	17, 41, 16	42–44, 38

The content of this table is listed within each injection type in order of descending amount of current evidence supporting its use. References are provided for all meta-analyses, prospective studies, and case series/case reports along with at least one reference to descriptions in review articles or injection textbooks. For those procedures that are only described in review articles and/or textbooks, representative references are provided

can be particularly effective at providing good long-term results for mild CTS [11] and also in helping to identify which patients will not require surgery[12]. About half of CTS patients obtain long-lasting improvement via a single injection.[13] Higher doses of injected steroids tend to produce more favorable results, and repeat injections are often beneficial [13]. In fact, a prospective, randomized trial of 163 wrists with electrodiagnostically-confirmed CTS showed that in patients without thenar atrophy, CTI was as effective as surgical decompression at producing symptomatic relief at 3 months and 12 months after intervention [14]. A key to management along with the injection is to try and identify, if possible, the underlying risk factors for CTS and to correct these. Ultrasound guidance now offers an alternative type of injection procedure known as nerve hydrodissection as was described in the introductory chapter of this text.

Corticosteroid injections for de Quervain's tenosynovitis are also quite commonly performed. Indeed, a prospective study found that the injections rapidly relieved signs/symptoms, without significant adverse reactions, and recommended injection as the preferred treatment for this condition [15]. In addition, one prospective study has shown tendon sheath corticosteroid injection to be more effective than splinting [16]. These injections can provide complete relief [17]. Suprafibrous injections may be easier than intrasynovial injections, with the same benefits [18]. A review article calculated that de Quervain's injections have complication rates of, at most, 5% for skin color changes (none of which were reported to be permanent), 1.4% for flare, 0.6% for nontender nodules, and 0.3% for superficial thrombophlebitis [19]. The literature contains only 1 case report of resultant persistent cheiralgia paresthetica (radial nerve dysesthesias) [20].

Ganglion cysts at the wrists are sometimes treated by aspiration/injection to obtain temporary symptomatic relief, but, due to the high recurrence rates, surgical excision is often considered the definitive treatment [21].

Corticosteroid injections into the wrist joints can help relieve inflammatory conditions such as rheumatoid arthritis. Isolated injection to the distal radial ulnar joint (DRUJ) can be performed fairly simply and without complications [22]. However, patients with more diffuse wrist involvement seem to benefit more from injection not only into the DRUJ but also into the mid carpal joint [23]. Both of these joint spaces can be injected via a single puncture site, without reinsertion [24]. In addition to injections of steroids, arthritic wrist joints can alternatively be injected with hyaluronic acid in osteoarthritis [25] or with a inhibitor of TNF-alpha for rheumatoid arthritis [26].

References

1. Tavares SP, Giddins GE. Nerve injury following steroid injection for carpal tunnel syndrome. A report of two cases. J Hand Surg [Br] 1996;21(2):208–9.
2. Kasten SJ, Louis DS. Carpal tunnel syndrome: a case of median nerve injection injury and a safe and effective method for injecting the carpal tunnel. J Fam Pract 1996;43(1):79–82.
3. Linskey ME, Segal R. Median nerve injury from local steroid injection in carpal tunnel syndrome. Neurosurgery 1990;26(3):512–5.

4. McConnell JR, Bush DC. Intraneural steroid injection as a complication in the management of carpal tunnel syndrome. A report of three cases. Clin Orthop Relat Res 1990;(250):181–4.
5. Racasan O, Dupert T. J Hand Surg: J Br Soc Surg Hand 2005;30(4):412–4.
6. Habib GS, Badarny S, Rawashdeh H. A novel approach of local corticosteroid injection for the treatment of carpal tunnel syndrome. Clin Rheumatol 2006;25(3):338–40.
7. Sevim S, Dogu O, Camdeviren H, Kaleagasi H, Aral M, Arslan E, Milcan A. Long-term effectiveness of steroid injections and splinting in mild and moderate carpal tunnel syndrome. Neurol Sci 2004;25(2):48–52.
8. Marshall S, Tardif G, Ashworth N. Local corticosteroid injection for carpal tunnel syndrome. Cochrane Database Syst Rev 2002;(4):CD001554.
9. Wood MR. Hydrocortisone injections for carpal tunnel syndrome. Hand 1980;12(1):62–4.
10. Armstrong T, Devor W, Borschel L, Contreras R. Intracarpal steroid injection is safe and effective for short-term management of carpal tunnel syndrome. Muscle Nerve 2004;29(1):82–8.
11. Agarwal V, Singh R, Sachdev A, Wiclaff, Shekhar S, Goel D. A prospective study of the long-term efficacy of local methyl prednisolone acetate injection in the management of mild carpal tunnel syndrome. Rheumatology (Oxford) 2005;44(5):647–50.
12. Graham RG, Hudson DA, Solomons M, Singer M. A prospective study to assess the outcome of steroid injections and wrist splinting for the treatment of carpal tunnel syndrome. Plast Reconstr Surg 2004;113(2):550–6.
13. Dammers JW, Roos Y, Veering MM, Vermeulen M. Injection with methylprednisolone in patients with the carpal tunnel syndrome: a randomised double blind trial testing three different doses. J Neurol 2006;253(5):574–7.
14. Ly-Pen D, Andreu JL, de Blas G, Sánchez-Olaso A, Millán I. Surgical decompression versus local steroid injection in carpal tunnel syndrome: a one-year, prospective, randomized, open, controlled clinical trial. Arthritis Rheum 2005;52: 612–9.
15. Anderson BC, Manthey R, Brouns MC. Treatment of De Quervain's tenosynovitis with corticosteroids. A prospective study of the response to local injection. Arthritis Rheum 1991;34(7):793–8.
16. Avci S, Yilmaz C, Sayli U. Comparison of nonsurgical treatment measures for de Quervain's disease of pregnancy and lactation. J Hand Surg [Am] 2002;27(2):322–4.
17. Rankin ME, Rankin EA. Injection therapy for management of stenosing tenosynovitis (de Quervain's disease) of the wrist. J Natl Med Assoc 1998;90(8):474–6.
18. Apimonbutr P, Budhraja N. Suprafibrous injection with corticosteroid in de Quervain's disease. J Med Assoc Thai 2003;86(3):232–7.
19. Foye PM, Sullivan WJ, Panagos A, Zuhosky JP, Sable AW, Irwin RW. Industrial medicine and acute musculoskeletal rehabilitation. 6. Upper- and lower-limb injections for acute musculoskeletal injuries and injured workers. Arch Phys Med Rehabil 2007;88(3 Suppl 1):S29–33.
20. Chodoroff G, Honet JC. Cheiralgia paresthetica and linear atrophy as a complication of local steroid injection. Arch Phys Med Rehabil 1985;66(9):637–9.
21. Wright TW, Cooney WP, Ilstrup DM. Anterior wrist ganglion. J Hand Surg [Am]. 1994;19(6):954–8.
22. Lomasney LM, Cooper RA. Distal radioulnar joint arthrography: simplified technique. Radiology 1996;199(1):278–9.
23. Koski JM, Hermunen H. Intra-articular glucocorticoid treatment of the rheumatoid wrist. An ultrasonographic study. Scand J Rheumatol 2001;30(5):268–70.
24. Pesquer L, Glon Y, Scepi M, Hardit C, Hannequin J, Tasu JP. A new method for radio-carpal joint injection. J Radiol. 2005;86(12 Pt 1):1795–7.
25. Fuchs S, Mönikes R, Wohlmeiner A, Heyse T. Intra-articular hyaluronic acid compared with corticoid injections for the treatment of rhizarthrosis. Osteoarthritis Cartilage 2006; 14(1):82–8.
26. Bliddal H, Terslev L, Qvistgaard E, Recke P, Holm CC, Danneskiold-Samsoe B et al. Safety of intra-articular injection of etanercept in small-joint arthritis: an uncontrolled, pilot-study with independent imaging assessment. Joint Bone Spine 2006;73(6):714–7.

27. Saunders S. Wrist treatments. In Saunders S, ed. Injection Techniques in Orthopaedic and Sports Medicine. Second edition. London: WB Saunders; 2002:70–81; 58–59.

28. Kesson M, Atkins E, Davies I. Wrist and hand. In Kesson M, Atkins E, Davies I, eds. Musculoskeletal Injection Skills. New York: Butterworth Heinemann; 2002:80–82.

29. Waldman SD. Intra-articular Injection of the Inferior Radio-ulnar Joint. Atlas of Pain Management Injection Techniques. Philadelphia, PA: WB Saunders; 2000:116–118.

30. Levinsohn EM, Rosen ID, Palmer AK. Wrist arthrography: value of the three-compartment injection method. Radiology 1991;179(1):231–9.

31. Mondal LK, Sarkar K, Datta H, Chatterjee PR. Acute bilateral central serous chorioretinopathy following intra-articular injection of corticosteroid. Indian J Ophthalmol 2005;53(2):132–4.

32. Waldman SD. Intra-articular Injection of the Wrist Joint. Atlas of Pain Management Injection Techniques. Philadelphia, PA: WB Saunders; 2000:113–5.

33. Saunders S. Wrist treatments. In Saunders S, ed. Injection Techniques in Orthopaedic and Sports Medicine. Second edition. London: WB Saunders; 2002:70–81; 56–57.

34. Kesson M, Atkins E, Davies I. Wrist and hand. In Kesson M, Atkins E, Davies I, eds. Musculoskeletal Injection Skills. New York: Butterworth Heinemann; 2002:83–5.

35. Saunders S. Wrist treatments. In Saunders S, ed. Injection Techniques in Orthopaedic and Sports Medicine. Second edition. London: WB Saunders; 2002:70–81;66–7.

36. Kesson M, Atkins E, Davies I. Wrist and hand. In Kesson M, Atkins E, Davies I, eds. Musculoskeletal Injection Skills. New York: Butterworth Heinemann; 2002:95–8.

37. Waldman SD. Carpal Tunnel Syndrome. Atlas of Pain Management Injection Techniques. Philadelphia, PA: WB Saunders; 2000:144–7.

38. Tallia AF, Cardone DA. Diagnostic and therapeutic injection of the wrist and hand region. Am Fam Physician 2003;67(4):745–50.

39. Stapczynski JS. Localized depigmentation after steroid injection of a ganglion cyst on the hand. Ann Emerg Med 1991;20(7):807–9.

40. Waldman SD. Ganglion Cysts of the Wrist. Atlas of Pain Management Injection Techniques. Philadelphia, PA: WB Saunders; 2000:153–5.

41. Yuen A, Coombs CJ. Abductor pollicis longus tendon rupture in De Quervain's disease. J Hand Surg [Br] 2006;31(1):72–5.

42. Waldman SD. De Quervain's Tenosynovitis. Atlas of Pain Management Injection Techniques. Philadelphia, PA: WB Saunders; 2000:122–4.

43. Saunders S. Wrist treatments. In Saunders S, ed. Injection Techniques in Orthopaedic and Sports Medicine. Second edition. London: WB Saunders; 2002:70–81; 62–63.

44. Kesson M, Atkins E, Davies I. Wrist and hand. In Kesson M, Atkins E, Davies I, eds. Musculoskeletal Injection Skills. New York: Butterworth Heinemann; 2002:102–104.

45. Dias J, Buch K. Palmar wrist ganglion: does intervention improve outcome? A prospective study of the natural history and patient-reported treatment outcomes. J Hand Surg [Br] 2003;28(2):172–6.

46. Stephen AB, Lyons AR, Davis TR. A prospective study of two conservative treatments for ganglia of the wrist.J Hand Surg [Br] 1999;24(1):104–5.

Procedure Instructions

Injection Procedure: Carpal Tunnel Injection

1. Indications:
   (a) Carpal Tunnel Syndrome diagnosis as pain generator or treatment
2. Contraindications especially pertinent to this procedure:
   (b) None documented
3. Possible side effects especially pertinent to this procedure [1–3]:
   (c) Damage to flexor tendons
   (d) Damage to the median or ulnar nerve causing increased symptoms or permanent neurological deficit.
4. Technical details of note for this procedure (Fig. 8.1):
   (e) Preferred needle gauge; length; type:
   • Aspiration ± injection: 25 gauge;1 ½ in.; straight
   (f) Need for image guidance: Optional
   • Grassi and colleagues [4] has suggested use of imaging, particularly ultra-sound, to help avoid iatrogenic lesions to tendons and nerves caused by needle insertion to these structures. This could improve clinical efficacy by allowing corticosteroid placement into the most appropriate target area.
   • The location of the median nerve in the carpal tunnel is radial 43% of the time, middle 22% of the time, and ulnar 12% of the time [3]. This varia-tion in location makes guidance a useful tool, since it will allow direct localization of the nerve.
   • If ultrasound-guided: In a study by Grassi and colleagues [4], the follow-ing procedure was used:
     – A fine metal clip was placed between the skin and the transducer.
     – The best injection site could be selected when the clip crossed the carpal tunnel at a safe distance from blood vessels, tendons, and the median nerve.
     – The median nerve is determined by position and the typical isolated echoic dots against an anechoic background surrounded by a sharply echoic contour corresponding to the perineurium. This contrasts with the appearance of tendons, which are multiple, tight packed echoic dots.
     – This point was marked with a skin marker.
     – Needle insertion into the target area was performed under sonographic guidance. The needle is a distinct, hyperechoic, small round spot generating a "comet-tail" artifact.
     – The optimal entrance point was located between the median nerve and the flexor carpi radialis tendon.
     – The aspiration and injection of steroid was performed under sono-graphic control.

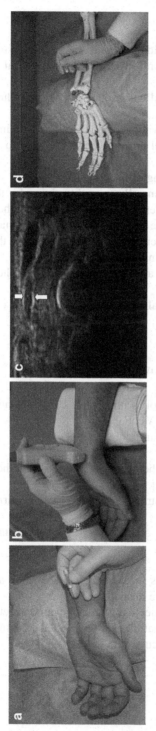

Fig. 8.1 Injection into carpal tunnel (ultrasound-guided). (**a**) Injection into carpal tunnel- human model. (**b**) Ultrasound transducer positioning for visualizing median nerve- human model. (**c**) Ultrasonogram corresponding to previous picture. (**d**) Skeletal representation of injection into carpal tunnel

5. Step-by-step procedure:
   (a) Informed consent
   (b) Pre-procedural testing: Identify and record the response to a physical examination pre-procedural provocative maneuver if the procedure is a diagnostic injection.
   (c) Image guidance: Optional: Ultrasound-guided procedure
   (d) Patient positioning:
       • The patient is seated with the hand resting in a supinated position on the exam table and a towel rolled up under the wrist so as to slightly extend the wrist.
   (e) Identification and marking of injection site:
       • The median nerve generally runs directly under the palmaris longus tendon, which can often be identified by having the patient oppose the thumb to the tip of the fifth finger. Once the palmaris longus has been identified, the needle entry site can be marked on the skin between the palmaris longus tendon and the FCR tendon.
       • Mark the target using a marker or by depressing the skin with a plastic needle cap.
   (f) Skin preparation: Initial: Betadine® preparation using the no-touch technique
   (g) Medication preparation:
       • Diagnostic injection:
         – 1 mL 1% preservative-free lidocaine

       • Therapeutic injection:
         – 40 mg Depo-Medrol® with 0.5 mL 1% preservative-free lidocaine
   (h) Skin preparation: Final: Alcohol prep
   (i) Local anesthesia administration: Not applicable
   (j) Needle placement:
       • Pierce the skin and subcutaneous tissue site with the appropriate needle and direct to the target.
   (k) Aspiration: Rule out intravascular entry and confirm entry into target structure.
   (l) Injection: Unclamp the aspiration syringe and clamp on the injection syringe.
   (m) Post-procedural testing:
       • If applicable, reassess the response to the same aforementioned pre-procedural provocative maneuver.
   (n) If (+) response, repeat injection with therapeutic injectate: Not applicable
   (o) *Adhesive bandage* application over the needle entry site
   (p) Post-procedural care discussion

References

1. Habib GS, Badarny S, Rawashdeh H. A novel approach of local corticosteroid injection for the treatment of carpal tunnel syndrome. Clin Rheumatol 2006;25(3):338–40.
2. Kasten SJ, Louis DS. Carpal tunnel syndrome: a case of median nerve injection injury and a safe and effective method for injecting the carpal tunnel. J Fam Pract 1996;43(1):79–82.
3. Racasan O, Dubert T. The safest location for steroid injection in the treatment of carpal tunnel syndrome. J Hand Surg [Br] 2005;30(4):412–4.
4. Grassi W, Farina A, FilippumLi E, Cervini C. Intralesional therapy in carpal tunnel syndrome: a sonographic-guided approach. Clin Exp Rheumatol 2002;20(1):73–6.

Injection Procedure: de Quervain's Tenosynovitis Injection

1. Indications:
   (a) Clinical diagnosis of de Quervain's tenosynovitis (inflammation of the abductor pollicis longus and/or extensor pollicis brevis tendons) as pain generator or treatment [1]

2. Contraindications especially pertinent to this procedure:
   (b) None documented

3. Possible side effects especially pertinent to this procedure:
   (c) Increased risk of skin depigmentation

4. Technical details of note for this procedure (Fig. 8.2):
   (d) Preferred needle gauge; length; type:
     • Injection: 25 gauge; 1½ in.; straight
   (e) Need for image guidance: Optional
   (f) In a study by Zingas and colleagues [2], injections into the first dorsal compartment were confirmed by dye visualization in 16/19 cases. Pain relief of symptoms occurred in 11/19 patients. Although the sample size was small, 4/5 patients who had injections into the abductor pollicis longus and extensor pollicis brevis had pain relief. In contrast, none of the three patients who did not have dye in either compartment had pain relief. The authors concluded from this that the accurate injection of steroid and lidocaine solutions is required for pain relief of de Quervain's tendonitis. The extensor pollicis brevis compartment was missed in 13/19 patients, possibly due to the small size and deep location. The compartment is separate in 41–47% of patients, and failed injection of this region has been suggested to be the cause of persistent pain following corticosteroid injections of the region in 30% of those injected. Accurate injection of both compartments is suggested in order to maximize the number of effective injections.
   (g) The use of ultrasound as a diagnostic tool, a guide to therapeutic injections, and an objective way to monitor the efficacy of therapy has been documented for wrist and other small joint injections. Ultrasound guidance of needle positions has been documented as a simple procedure, easy to perform, not time consuming, and a nondamaging method for the metacarpophalangeal joints and carpal joints [3, 4].

5. Step-by-step procedure:
   (h) Informed consent
   (i) Pre-procedural testing: Identify and record the response to a physical examination pre-procedural provocative maneuver (e.g., Finkelstein test: painful passive combined thumb opposition/passive wrist ulnar deviation) if the procedure is a diagnostic injection.
   (j) Image guidance: Optional: Ultrasound-guided procedure

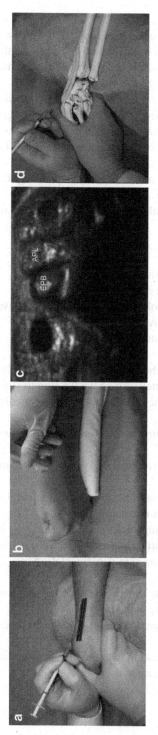

Fig. 8.2 Injection for de Quervain's disease: (ultrasound-guided). (**a**) Injection for de Quervain's disease- human model. (**b**) Ultrasound transducer positioning for visualizing extensor pollicis brevis (EPB) and abductor pollicis longus (APL) tendons- human model. (**c**) Ultrasonogram corresponding to previous image. (**d**) Skeletal representation of injection for de Quervain's disease

(k) Patient positioning:
  • Place the patient in a seated position with the elbow and forearm resting on a flat surface. The forearm should be resting on the ulnar surface with the thumb pointed upwards and the hand in a "vertical" position.

(l) Identification and marking of injection site:
  • Have the patient actively extend the thumb to identify the two tendons noted previously. Passively flex the thumb, and again note the location of these tendons by palpation over the base of the first metacarpal. If possible, palpate a space between the tendons and mark this as the ideal injection site.
  • Mark the target using a marker or by depressing the skin with a plastic needle cap.

(m) Skin preparation: Initial: Betadine® preparation using the no-touch technique

(n) Medication preparation:
  • Diagnostic injection:
    – 1 mL 1% preservative-free lidocaine
  • Therapeutic injection:
    – 20 mg Depo-Medrol® with 1 mL 1% preservative-free lidocaine

(o) Skin preparation: Final: Alcohol prep

(p) Local anesthesia administration: Not applicable

(q) Needle placement:
  • Pierce the skin and subcutaneous tissue site with the appropriate needle at an angle approximately 20° above the skin to slide the needle into the first dorsal compartment/tendon sheath proximally (between the tendons if able).

(r) Aspiration: Rule out intravascular entry and confirm entry into target structure.

(s) Injection: Unclamp the aspiration syringe and clamp on the injection syringe.
  • Inject the tendon sheath/first dorsal compartment with the previously mentioned medication injectate.
  • Increased resistance suggests that the needle may be embedded in one of the tendons, and further positional adjustment may be necessary.
  • Flush the site to prevent skin depigmentation.

(t) Post-procedural testing:
  • If applicable, reassess the response to the same aforementioned pre-procedural provocative maneuver.

(u) If (+ve) response, repeat injection with therapeutic injectate: Not applicable

(v) *Adhesive bandage* application over the needle entry site.

(w) Post-procedural care discussion

References

1. Tallia AF, Cardone DA. Diagnostic and therapeutic injection of the wrist and hand region. Am Fam Physician 2003;67(4):745–50.
2. Zingas C, Failla JM, Van Holsbeeck M. Injection accuracy and clinical relief of de Quervain's tendinitis. J Hand Surg [Am] 1998;23(1):89–96.
3. Koski JM, Hermunen H. Intra-articular glucocorticoid treatment of the rheumatoid wrist. An ultrasonographic study. Scand J Rheumatol 2001;30(5):268–70.
4. Grassi W, Lamanna G, Farina A, Cervini C. Synovitis of small joints: sonographic guided diagnostic and therapeutic approach. Ann Rheum Dis 1999;58(10):595–7.

Injection Procedure: Distal Radio-Ulnar Joint Injection

1. Indications:
   (a) Distal radio-ulnar joint diagnosis as pain generator [1] or treatment
2. Contraindications especially pertinent to this procedure:
   (b) None documented
3. Possible side effects especially pertinent to this procedure:
   (c) None documented
4. Technical details of note for this procedure (Fig. 8.3):
   (a) Preferred needle gauge; length; type:
       • Aspiration ± injection: 25 gauge; 1½ in.; straight
   (b) Need for image guidance: Recommended
       • Lomasney and Cooper [1] reportedly described an injection technique using fluoroscopy that was less painful than nonimage-guided injections presumably due to more accurate localization and less needle repositioning to get the needle into the small space.
       • In a study by Beaulieu and Ladd [2], a technique described contrast administration into the distal radio-ulnar joint. No fluoroscopic guidance was used for the injection of the contrast, and no statistical data were provided as part of this study from which injection accuracy could be inferred.
5. Step-by-step procedure:
   (a) Informed consent
   (b) Pre-procedural testing: Identify and record the response to a physical examination pre-procedural provocative maneuver if the procedure is a diagnostic injection.
   (c) Image guidance: Recommended: Fluoroscopic-guided or Ultrasound-guided
       • If fluoroscopic guidance is used, the technique described by Lomansey and Cooper[1] can be explained as follows:
         – Patient is placed in a supine positon or seated with are in table with palm of hand placed flat on the table.
         – The distal radioulnar joint was visualized with fluoroscopy and roughly profiled.
         – Although visualizing the joint in profile is not required, supination should be avoided because the radial bone margin may be superimposed over the ulnar head.
         – A point was localized on the skin over the ulnar head, approximately 3 mm proximal to the distal horizontal ulnar margin and 1–2 mm ulnar to the cortical margin of the articular aspect of the ulnar head.
         – After sterile preparation and use of local anesthesia with 1% lidocaine, either a 25 gauge, 1 in. straight needle, or a 23-gauge butterfly

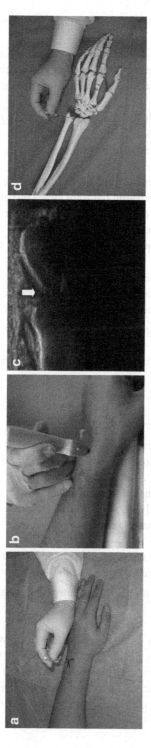

Fig. 8.3 Distal radioulnar joint injection (ultrasound-guided). (**a**) Distal radioulnar joint injection- human model. (**b**) Ultrasound transducer positioning for visualizing distal radioulnar joint- human model. (**c**) Ultrasonogram corresponding to previous image. (**d**) Skeletal representation of distal radioulnar joint injection

needle was advanced perpendicular to the skin until the bone margin was reached.

  - After a test injection showed a flow of contrast material away from the needle tip, confirming intra-articular placement, 1–2 mL of contrast was injected to visualize the joint after full distension of the joint.

(d) Patient positioning:
  • Place the patient with the arm and hand resting on the procedure table and the palm facing downwards.

(e) Identification and marking of injection site:
  • If nonimage-guided:
    - Palpate the radio-ulnar joint by feeling for the mobility of the radius and ulnar and identifying the joint space in-between. After localizing the separation of the radius and ulna, the distal end of the ulna is identified by palpating the prominent distal tip. The joint space is generally located just medial and proximal to this most distal tip.
  • If image-guided:
    - Identify the radio-ulnar joint using imaging by localizing the distal tip of the ulna and noting the joint space, generally located just medial and proximal to this most distal tip of the ulna.

  • Mark the target using a marker or by depressing the skin with a plastic needle cap.

(f) Skin preparation: Initial: Betadine® preparation using the no-touch technique

(g) Medication preparation:
  • Diagnostic injection:
    - 2 mL of 2% preservative-free lidocaine

  • Therapeutic injection:
    - 40 mg Depo-Medrol® and 0.5 mL of 1% preservative-free lidocaine

(h) Skin preparation: Final: Alcohol prep pad wipe

(i) Local anesthesia administration: Optional
  • Anesthetize the overlying skin and soft tissue using a *small amount of 1% lidocaine* delivered via a 25-guage needle.

(j) Needle placement:
  • Pierce the previously anesthetized skin and subcutaneous tissue site with the appropriate needle and direct to the target.

(k) Aspiration: Rule out intravascular entry and confirm entry into target structure.

(l) Contrast injection:
  • Inject the joint with enough contrast to confirm entry into the target structure. Connecting the contrast dye syringe to the needle using extension tubing is recommended to prevent a shift in needle position during attachment and detachment to and from the spinal needle. Adjust the needle position, if necessary, in order to obtain a clearly defined arthrogram.

(m) Injection: Unclamp the aspiration syringe and clamp on the injection syringe.
   • If resistance is encountered during the injection, rotate the needle to dislodge the bevel from the side of the joint.
(n) Post-procedural testing
   • If applicable, reassess the response to the same aforementioned pre-procedural provocative maneuver.
(o) If (+ve) response, repeat injection with therapeutic injectate:
   • Repeat steps #4–6.
   • Medication preparation: 40 mg Depo-Medrol®
   • Repeat steps # 8–13.
(p) *Adhesive bandage* application over the needle entry site
(q) Post-procedural care discussion

References

1. Lomasney LM, Cooper RA. Distal radioulnar joint arthrography: simplified technique. Radiology 1996;199(1):278–9.
2. Beaulieu CF, Ladd AL. MR arthrography of the wrist: scanning-room injection of the radio-carpal joint based on clinical landmarks. AJR Am J Roentgenol 1998;170(3):606–8.

Injection Procedure: Ganglion Cyst Aspiration/Injection

1. Indications:
   (a) Ganglion cyst diagnosis: Under those circumstances when it is unclear on physical examination if a mass represents a ganglion cyst, attempted aspiration of the mass can clarify the diagnosis.
   (b) Symptomatic ganglion cyst [1] treatment

2. Contraindications especially pertinent to this procedure:
   (c) None documented

3. Possible side effects especially pertinent to this procedure:
   (d) None documented, though recurrence rate of ganglion cyst formation/fluid accumulation is relatively high.

4. Technical details of note for this procedure (Fig. 8.4):
   (e) Preferred needle gauge; length; type:
      • Aspiration ± injection: 18 gauge; 1½ in.; straight
   (f) Need for ultrasound guidance: Optional

5. Step-by-step procedure:
   (a) Informed consent
   (b) Pre-procedural testing: Identify and record the response to a physical examination pre-procedural provocative maneuver if the procedure is a diagnostic injection.
   (c) Image-guidance: Optional: Ultrasound-guided
   (d) Patient positioning:
      • Position the patient with the affected joint resting on a table and the most superficial aspect of the ganglion cyst easily accessible.
   (e) Identification and marking of injection site:
      • If nonimage-guided:
         – Palpate the ganglion cyst and attempt to identify an approach that will allow entrance into the structure without passing the needle in close proximity to neurovascular structures.

      • If ultrasound-guided: Use ultrasound guidance, to identify the cystic structure, ascertain the fluid volume present within the cyst, and identify any adjacent neurovascular structures.
      • Mark the target using a marker or by depressing the skin with a plastic needle cap.
   (f) Skin preparation: Initial: Betadine® preparation using the no-touch technique
   (g) Medication preparation:
      • Therapeutic injection:
         – 40 mg Depo-Medrol® and 1 mL 1% preservative-free lidocaine
   (h) Skin preparation: Final: Alcohol prep pad wipe

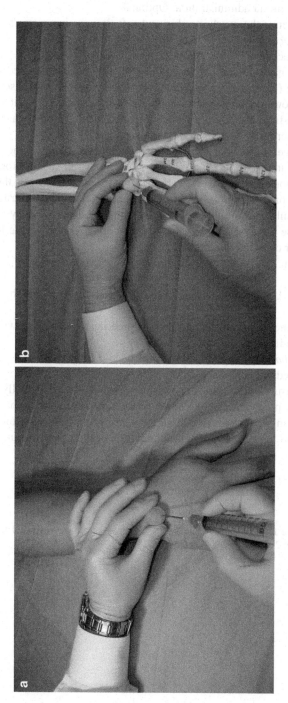

Fig. 8.4 Ganglion cyst aspiration/injection. (**a**) Ganglion cyst aspiration/injection- human model. (**b**) Skeletal representation of ganglion cyst aspiration/injection.

(i) Local anesthesia administration: Optional
  • Anesthetize the overlying skin and soft tissue using a *small amount of 1% lidocaine* delivered via a 25- or 30-guage needle.
(j) Needle placement:
  • If nonimage-guided: Advance the 18-gauge needle attached to a 20cc syringe (for increased vacuum force during aspiration of viscous cystic fluid) towards the target site with the syringe under constant aspiration. Successful entry into the cystic structure usually results in aspiration of thick, serosanguinous ganglion cyst contents.
  • If image-guided: Using ultrasound guidance, advance the 18-gauge needle attached to a 20 mL syringe (for increased vacuum force during aspiration of viscous cystic fluid) into the ganglion with the syringe under constant aspiration. Successful entry into the cystic structure usually results in aspiration of thick, serosanguinous ganglion cyst contents. Because the cyst may be loculated, this may require needle manipulation for complete drainage.
(k) Aspiration: Rule out intravascular entry and confirm entry into target structure.
(l) Injection: Unclamp the aspiration syringe and clamp on the injection syringe.
  • Inject the cyst with the previously-noted injectate prior to withdrawing the needle from the skin.
(m) *Adhesive bandage* application over the needle entry site
(n) Post-procedural care discussion:
  • Emphasis on the following considerations that are especially pertinent to this procedure: avoid unnecessary repetitive motion of the body region in order to prevent rapid clearance of the corticosteroid from the cyst and to prevent rapid reaccumulation of the ganglion fluid.

References

1. Tallia AF, Cardone DA. Diagnostic and therapeutic injection of the wrist and hand region. Am Fam Physician 2003;67(4):745–50.

Injection Procedure: Triangular Fibrocartilage (TFCC) Complex Injection

1. Indications:
   (a) TFCC diagnosis as a pain generator
   (b) Symptomatic TFCC Injury/Arthritis [1] treatment

2. Contraindications especially pertinent to this procedure:
   (c) None documented

3. Possible side effects especially pertinent to this procedure:
   (d) None documented

4. Technical details of note for this procedure (Fig. 8.5):
   (e) Preferred needle gauge; length; type:
   - Aspiration ± injection: 25 gauge; 1½ in.; straight
   (d) Need for image guidance: Optional
   - The use of ultrasound as a diagnostic tool, a guide to therapeutic injections, and an objective way to monitor the efficacy of therapy has been documented for wrist and other small joint injections. Ultrasound guidance of needle positions has been documented as a simple procedure, easy to perform, not time consuming, and a nondamaging method for the metacarpophalangeal joints and carpal joints [1, 2].
   - In the opinion of the authors of this chapter, fluoroscopy is highly useful as a means of verifying placement into the true triangular fibrocartilage complex if ultrasound guidance is not available

5. Step-by-step procedure:
   (a) Informed consent
   (b) Pre-procedural testing: Identify and record the response to a physical examination pre-procedural provocative maneuver if the procedure is a diagnostic injection
   (c) Image-guidance: Recommended: Fluoroscopic-guided or Ultrasound-guided
   (d) Patient positioning:
   - Place the patient in a seated position with the hand placed flat on a table (palm down) in a resting position.
   (e) Identification and marking of injection site:
   - If nonimage-guided:
     - Palpate the junction of the ulna and the most proximal carpal bones in an attempt to identify the distal end of the ulna with the TFCC present in-between the carpal bones and the distal end of the ulna.
   - If image-guided:
     - Locate the distal end of the ulnar and the space between the ulna and the most proximal articulating carpal bones. The TFCC will lie in-between.

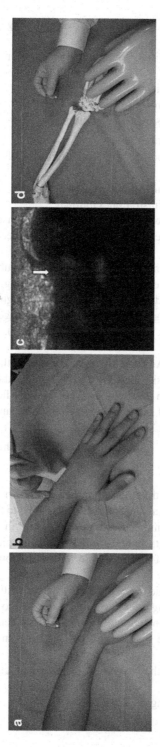

Fig. 8.5 Triangular fibrocartilage complex (TFCC) injection. (**a**) TFCC injection. (**a**) TFCC injection- human model. (**b**) Ultrasound transducer positioning for visualizing TFCC- human model. (**c**) Ultrasonogram corresponding to previous image. (**d**) Skeletal representation of TFCC injection

- Mark the target using a marker or by depressing the skin with a plastic needle cap.
(f) Skin preparation: Initial: Betadine® preparation using the no-touch technique
(g) Medication preparation:
  - Diagnostic injection:
    - 1 mL of 1% preservative-free lidocaine
  - Therapeutic injection:
    - 20 mg of Depo-Medrol® and 0.5 mL of 1% preservative-free lidocaine
(h) Skin preparation: Final: Alcohol prep pad wipe
(i) Local anesthesia administration: Optional
  - Anesthetize the overlying skin and soft tissue using a *small amount of 1% lidocaine* delivered via a 25- or 30-guage needle.
(j) Needle placement:
  - Pierce the previously anesthetized skin and subcutaneous tissue site with the appropriate needle and direct to the target.
  - If nonimage-guided: Advance the needle through the subcutaneous tissue towards the target site until the needle engages the triangular fibrocartilage complex (with a gelatinous feel). Inject under slight resistance.
  - If image-guided: Advance the needle through the subcutaneous tissue towards the target site until the needle engages the triangular fibrocartilage complex (with a gelatinous feel). The needle should be visualized at the distal end of the ulna between the ulna and the proximal carpal bones. Inject under slight resistance.
(k) Aspiration: Rule out intravascular entry and confirm entry into target structure.
(l) Contrast injection:
  - Inject the joint with enough contrast to confirm entry into the target structure. Connecting the contrast dye syringe to the needle using extension tubing is recommended to prevent a shift in needle position during attachment and detachment to and from the spinal needle. Adjust the needle position, if necessary, in order to obtain a clearly defined arthrogram.
  - If fluoroscopic-guidance: Inject the target with *several milliliter of Omnipaque™ using a 5 mL syringe* connected to the straight needle via extension tubing. Injection of contrast should demonstrate filling of the space between the distal aspect of the ulna and the proximal carpal bones.
(m) Injection: Unclamp the aspiration syringe and clamp on the injection syringe
(n) Post-procedural testing:

- If applicable, reassess the response to the aforementioned pre-procedural provocative maneuver.

(e) If (+ve) response, repeat injection with therapeutic injectate:
- Repeat steps #4–6.
- Medication preparation: 20 mg Depo-Medrol®
- Repeat steps # 8–13.

(f) *Adhesive bandage* application over the needle entry site

(g) Post-procedural care discussion

References

1. Koski JM, Hermunen H. Intra-articular glucocorticoid treatment of the rheumatoid wrist. An ultrasonographic study. Scand J Rheumatol 2001;30(5):268–70.
2. Grassi W, Lamanna G, Farina A, Cervini C. Synovitis of small joints: sonographic guided diagnostic and therapeutic approach. Ann Rheum Dis 1999;58(10):595–7.

Injection Procedure: Wrist Joint Injection: Intercarpal Approach

1. Indications:
   (a) Wrist joint diagnosis as a pain generator or aspiration of joint fluid for diagnosis of inflammatory arthropathy, crystal arthropathy or infection
   (b) Wrist joint arthropathy treatment

2. Contraindications especially pertinent to this procedure:
   (a) None documented

3. Possible side effects especially pertinent to this procedure:
   (d) None documented

4. Technical details of note for this procedure (Fig. 8.6):
   (e) Preferred needle gauge; length; type:
      • Aspiration ± injection: 25 gauge; 1½ in.; straight
   (f) Need for fluoroscopic guidance: Recommended
   (g) One text notes that the wrist joint capsule encompassing the carpal bones is not continuous but rather is septated with multiple isolated divisions. Thus, the joint as a whole cannot be injected with one site of needle entry but requires multiple needle insertions [1].

5. Step-by-step procedure:
   (a) Informed consent
   (b) Pre-procedural testing: Identify and record the response to a physical examination pre-procedural provocative maneuver if the procedure is a diagnostic injection.
   (c) Image-guidance: Recommended: Fluoroscopic-guided
   (d) Patient positioning:
      • Patient is positioned with the arm and hand resting on the procedure table and the palm facing downwards. The affected wrist may be better accessed by resting the wrist over a rolled-up towel.
   (e) Identification and marking of injection site:
      • If nonimage-guided:
        – Palpate the carpal bones and locate a spot half-way between the distal end of the radius and ulna and the proximal aspect of the metacarpals. Continue to palpate and identify locations between the carpal bones as potential injection sites. The joint can be accessed through anyone of several sites. Choose the site that appears to provide the easiest access.
      • If image-guided:
        – Identify the wrist joint articulations using imaging by localizing the carpal bones using image guidance.
      • Mark the target using a marker or by depressing the skin with a plastic needle cap.

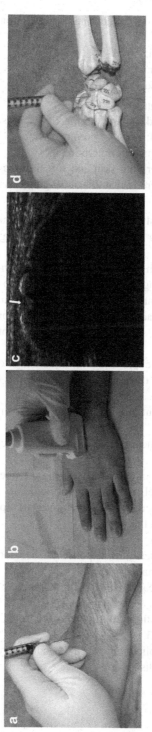

Fig. 8.6 Wrist joint injection (ultrasound-guided). (**a**) Wrist joint injection- human model. (**b**) Ultrasound transducer positioning for visualizing wrist joint- human model. (**c**) Ultrasonogram corresponding to previous image. (**d**) Skeletal representation of wrist joint injection

(f) Skin preparation: Initial: Betadine® preparation using the no-touch technique

(g) Medication preparation:
  - Diagnostic injection:
    – 1 mL of 2% preservative-free lidocaine

  - Therapeutic injection:
    – 40 mg Depo-Medrol® and 0.5 mL of 1% preservative-free lidocaine

(h) Skin preparation: Final: Alcohol prep pad wipe

(i) Local anesthesia administration: Optional
  - Anesthetize the overlying skin and soft tissue using a *small amount of 1% lidocaine* delivered via a 25- or 30-guage needle.

(j) Needle placement:
  - Pierce the previously anesthetized skin and subcutaneous tissue site with the appropriate needle and direct to the target.

(k) Contrast injection:
  - Inject the joint with enough contrast to confirm entry into the target structure. Connecting the contrast dye syringe to the needle using extension tubing is recommended to prevent a shift in needle position during attachment and detachment to and from the spinal needle. Adjust the needle position, if necessary, in order to obtain a clearly defined arthrogram.
  - With use of fluoroscopic imaging, injection of contrast should demonstrate migration of dye away from the needle tip, illustrating a well-defined arthrogram.

(l) Aspiration: Rule out intravascular entry and confirm entry into the target structure.

(m) Injection: Unclamp the aspiration syringe and clamp on the injection syringe.
  - If resistance is encountered early during the injection, rotate the needle to dislodge the bevel from the side of the joint.
  - The injectate is generally distributed over multiple injection sites across the dorsal aspect of the wrist [1].

(n) Post-procedural testing:
  - If applicable, reassess the response to the aforementioned pre-procedural provocative maneuver.

(o) If (+ve) response, repeat injection with therapeutic injectate:
  - Repeat steps #4–6.
  - Medication preparation: 20 mg Depo-Medrol®
  - Repeat steps # 8–13.

(p) *Adhesive bandage* application over the needle entry site

(q) Post-procedural care discussion

References

1. Saunders S. Wrist treatments. In Law M, ed. Injection Techniques in Orthopaedic and Sports Medicine. Second edition. London: WB Saunders;2002:56–57.

Injection Procedure Templates

Injection Procedure Template: Carpal Tunnel Injection

PROCEDURE: Carpal Tunnel Injection
Side: ☐-Right   ☐-Left   ☐-Bilateral
Procedure Type: Aspiration: ☐-Diagnostic aspiration
 Injection: ☐-Diagnostic   ☐-Therapeutic   ☐-Diagnostic then Therapeutic
Image guidance: None unless indicated as follows- ☐-Fluoroscopy   ☐-Ultrasound
- The potential benefits and side effects of the procedure and alternative treatment options were explained to the patient, an opportunity for questions was provided, and the patient signed informed consent.
- ☐- If checked, the following physical examination pre-procedural provocative maneuver(s) was (were) performed: ☐-
 _____
- The patient was positioned for the procedure and the target structure was identified.
- The overlying skin was prepped with Betadine® followed by alcohol prep pad after the Betadine® dried.
- ☐- If checked, the overlying skin and soft tissue was anesthetized using a small amount of 1% lidocaine delivered via the following needle ☐-30G1"; ☐-25G1½ "; ☐-Other: _____
- The following needle was then used for the procedure:
  Type: Straight needle unless indicated as follows: ☐-Spinal needle; ☐-Other:_____
  Gauge: ☐-30; ☐-27; ☐-25; ☐-22; ☐-21; -18; Other:_____
  Length: ☐-5/8"; ☐- 1"; ☐- 1 ½"; ☐- 2"; ☐- 2 ½"; ☐- 3";☐- 3½"; ☐-Other:_____
- o   Image guidance if indicated above was used to confirm needle entry into target structure.
- o   -If checked, contrast dye was then injected and the needle position was adjusted accordingly to confirm proper placement without inadvertent intravascular entry.
- Needle was adjusted accordingly to confirm proper placement without inadvertent vascular entry.
- An attempt was made to aspirate from the structure and then the following injectate was delivered into the target structure:
  ☐-Diagnostic injection: 1 mL 1% preservative-free lidocaine; ☐-Other injectate: _____
  ☐-Therapeutic injection: 40 mg Depo-Medrol® & ☐- 0.5 mL 1% preservative-free lidocaine
      ☐-Other injectate: _____
- The needle was removed and an adhesive bandage was placed over the needle entry site.

-If the above was a diagnostic injection, then proceed to section immediately below.
-If above was a therapeutic injection procedure, aspiration only procedure, or aspiration and therapeutic injection, then proceed to Procedure Summary Section.

For Diagnostic Injection Procedure:
- ☐-If checked, the above listed pre-procedural physical examination provocative maneuver was repeated and pain relief was: ☐-N/A; ☐-significant; ☐-some; ☐-equivocal; ☐-none; ☐-Other:_____
- Based on the amount of pain relief noted above:
  ☐-a therapeutic injection will be scheduled.
  ☐-a therapeutic injection will not be scheduled. See plan in corresponding office note.
  ☐-a therapeutic injection following the same procedure described above was done using
      ☐- 40 mg Depo-Medrol® & ☐- 0.5 mL 1% preservative-free lidocaine
      ☐- Other injectate:_____
- The needle was removed and an adhesive bandage was placed over the needle entry site.

Procedure Summary:
If fluid aspirated from the target structure during the procedure:
- Total volume of fluid aspirated: ___ mL; Fluid appearance: ☐- N/A; ☐-Clear yellow; ☐-Slightly cloudy; ☐-Cloudy; ☐-Purulent; ☐-Blood-tinged; ☐-Bloody; ☐-Other:_____
Patient tolerance for the procedure: ☐-Excellent; ☐-Good; ☐-Fair; ☐-Other:_____

Additional comments regarding the procedure: ☐-None; ☐Other:_____
_____

Post-Procedural Treatment Advice:
Activity modification: Avoid non-essential use of the structure until seen for follow up. ☐-Other:_____
_____

Orthotic instructions: N/A unless indicated as follows _____
Modalities: Apply ice over the injection site prn for 20-30 min. up to q2 hrs until seen for follow-up, unless instructed as follows: ☐-Heat; ☐-Other:_____

Injection Procedure Template: de Quervain's Tenosynovitis Injection

PROCEDURE: de Quervain's Tenosynovitis Injection

Side: ☐-Right   ☐-Left   ☐-Bilateral

Procedure Type: Aspiration: ☐-Diagnostic aspiration

        Injection: ☐-Diagnostic   ☐-Therapeutic ☐-Diagnostic then Therapeutic

Image guidance: None unless indicated as follows- ☐-Fluoroscopy ☐-Ultrasound

- The potential benefits and side effects of the procedure and alternative treatment options were explained to the patient, an opportunity for questions was provided, and the patient signed informed consent.
- ☐- If checked, the following physical examination pre-procedural provocative maneuver(s) was (were) performed: ☐-
  _____
- The patient was positioned for the procedure and the target structure was identified.
- The overlying skin was prepped with Betadine® followed by alcohol prep pad after the Betadine® dried.
- ☐- If checked, the overlying skin and soft tissue was anesthetized using a small amount of 1% lidocaine delivered via the following needle ☐-30G1"; ☐-25G1½ "; ☐-Other:_____
- The following needle was then used for the procedure:
      Type: Straight needle unless indicated as follows: ☐-Spinal needle; ☐-Other:_____
      Gauge: ☐-30; ☐-27; ☐-25; ☐-22; ☐-21; -18; Other:_____
      Length: ☐-5/8"; ☐- 1"; ☐- 1 ½"; ☐- 2"; ☐- 2 ½"; ☐- 3";☐- 3½"; ☐-Other:_____
- ○ Image guidance if indicated above was used to confirm needle entry into target structure.
- ○ ☐-If checked, contrast dye was then injected and the needle position was adjusted accordingly to confirm proper placement without inadvertent intravascular entry.
- Needle was adjusted accordingly to confirm proper placement without inadvertent vascular entry.
- An attempt was made to aspirate from the structure and then the following injectate was delivered into the target structure:
  ☐-Diagnostic injection: 1 mL 1% preservative-free lidocaine _____
  ☐-Therapeutic injection: 20 mg Depo-Medrol® & ☐- 1 mL 1% preservative-free lidocaine
      ☐-Other injectate: _____
- The needle was removed and an adhesive bandage was placed over the needle entry site.

-If the above was a diagnostic injection, then proceed to section immediately below.

-If above was a therapeutic injection procedure, aspiration only procedure, or aspiration and therapeutic injection, then proceed to Procedure Summary Section.

For Diagnostic Injection Procedure:

- ☐-If checked, the above listed pre-procedural physical examination provocative maneuver was repeated and pain relief was: ☐- N/A; ☐-significant; ☐-some; ☐-equivocal; ☐-none; ☐-Other:_____
- Based on the amount of pain relief noted above:
  ☐-a therapeutic injection will be scheduled.
  ☐-a therapeutic injection will not be scheduled. See plan in corresponding office note.
  ☐-a therapeutic injection following the same procedure described above was done using
      ☐- 20 mg Depo-Medrol® & ☐- 1 mL 1% preservative-free lidocaine
      ☐- Other injectate:_____
- The needle was removed and an adhesive bandage was placed over the needle entry site.

Procedure Summary:

If fluid aspirated from the target structure during the procedure:
- Total volume of fluid aspirated: ___ mL; Fluid appearance: ☐- N/A; ☐-Clear yellow; ☐-Slightly cloudy; ☐-Cloudy; ☐-Purulent; ☐-Blood-tinged; ☐-Bloody; ☐-Other:_____

Patient tolerance for the procedure: ☐-Excellent; ☐-Good; ☐-Fair; ☐-Other:_____

Additional comments regarding the procedure: ☐-None; ☐Other:_____
_____

Post-Procedural Treatment Advice:

Activity modification: Avoid non-essential use of the structure until seen for follow up. ☐-Other:_____

Orthotic instructions: N/A unless indicated as follows _____

Modalities: Apply ice over the injection site prn for 20-30 min. up to q2 hrs until seen for follow-up, unless instructed as follows: ☐-Heat; ☐-Other:_____

Injection Procedure Template: Distal Radio-Ulnar Injection

PROCEDURE: Distal Radio-Ulnar Injection
Side:　　□-Right　　　　□-Left　　　　□-Bilateral
Procedure Type: Aspiration:　□-Diagnostic aspiration
　　　　　　Injection:　□-Diagnostic　　□-Therapeutic　□-Diagnostic then Therapeutic
Image guidance: None unless indicated as follows- □-Fluoroscopy　□-Ultrasound
- The potential benefits and side effects of the procedure and alternative treatment options were explained to the patient, an opportunity for questions was provided, and the patient signed informed consent.
- □- If checked, the following physical examination pre-procedural provocative maneuver(s) was (were) performed: □-
_____
- The patient was positioned for the procedure and the target structure was identified.
- The overlying skin was prepped with Betadine® followed by alcohol prep pad after the Betadine® dried.
- □- If checked, the overlying skin and soft tissue was anesthetized using a small amount of 1% lidocaine delivered via the following needle □-30G1"; □-25G1½ "; □-Other: _____
- The following needle was then used for the procedure:
  - Type: Straight needle unless indicated as follows: □-Spinal needle; □-Other:_____
  - Gauge: □-30; □-27; □-25; □-22; □-21; -18; Other:_____
  - Length: □-5/8"; □- 1"; □- 1 ½"; □- 2"; □- 2 ½"; □- 3";□- 3½"; □-Other:_____
- ○ Image guidance if indicated above was used to confirm needle entry into target structure.
- ○ □-If checked, contrast dye was then injected and the needle position was adjusted accordingly to confirm proper placement without inadvertent intravascular entry.
- Needle was adjusted accordingly to confirm proper placement without inadvertent vascular entry.
- An attempt was made to aspirate from the structure and then the following injectate was delivered into the target structure:
  □-Diagnostic injection: 2 mL 2% preservative-free lidocaine; □-Other injectate: _____
  □-Therapeutic injection: 40 mg Depo-Medrol® & □- 0.5 mL 1% preservative-free bupivacaine
  　　　　　□-Other injectate: _____
- The needle was removed and an adhesive bandage was placed over the needle entry site.

-If the above was a **diagnostic injection**, then proceed to section immediately below.
-If above was a **therapeutic injection procedure, aspiration only procedure,** or **aspiration and therapeutic injection,** then proceed to Procedure Summary Section.

For Diagnostic Injection Procedure:
- □-If checked, the above listed pre-procedural physical examination provocative maneuver was repeated and pain relief was: □-N/A; □-significant; □-some; □-equivocal; □-none; □-Other:_____
- Based on the amount of pain relief noted above:
  □-a therapeutic injection will be scheduled.
  □-a therapeutic injection will not be scheduled. See plan in corresponding office note.
  □-a therapeutic injection following the same procedure described above was done using
  　　　□- 40 mg Depo-Medrol® & □- 0.5 mL 1% preservative-free lidocaine
  　　　□- Other injectate:_____
- The needle was removed and an adhesive bandage was placed over the needle entry site.

Procedure Summary:
If fluid aspirated from the target structure during the procedure:
- Total volume of fluid aspirated: ___ mL; Fluid appearance: □- N/A; □-Clear yellow; □-Slightly cloudy;
  □-Cloudy; □-Purulent; □-Blood-tinged; □-Bloody; □-Other:_____
Patient tolerance for the procedure: □-Excellent; □-Good; □-Fair; □-Other:_____

Additional comments regarding the procedure: □-None; □Other:_____
_____

Post-Procedural Treatment Advice:
Activity modification: Avoid non-essential use of the structure until seen for follow up. □-Other:_____
_____
Orthotic instructions: N/A unless indicated as follows _____
Modalities: Apply ice over the injection site prn for 20-30 min. up to q2 hrs until seen for follow-up, unless instructed as follows: □-Heat; □-Other:_____

Injection Procedure Template: Ganglion Cyst Aspiration/Injection

PROCEDURE: Ganglion Cyst Aspiration/Injection
Side: ☐-Right   ☐-Left   ☐-Bilateral
Procedure Type: Aspiration: ☐-Diagnostic aspiration
         Injection: ☐-Diagnostic   ☐-Therapeutic   ☐-Diagnostic then Therapeutic
Image guidance: None unless indicated as follows- ☐-Fluoroscopy   ☐-Ultrasound
- The potential benefits and side effects of the procedure and alternative treatment options were explained to the patient, an opportunity for questions was provided, and the patient signed informed consent.
- ☐- If checked, the following physical examination pre-procedural provocative maneuver(s) was (were) performed: ☐-
- The patient was positioned for the procedure and the target structure was identified.
- The overlying skin was prepped with Betadine® followed by alcohol prep pad after the Betadine® dried.
- ☐- If checked, the overlying skin and soft tissue was anesthetized using a small amount of 1% lidocaine delivered via the following needle ☐-30G1"; ☐-25G1½ "; ☐-Other: _____
- The following needle was then used for the procedure:
  - Type: Straight needle unless indicated as follows: ☐-Spinal needle; ☐-Other:_____
  - Gauge: ☐-30; ☐-27; ☐-25; ☐-22; ☐-21; -18; Other:_____
  - Length: ☐-5/8"; ☐- 1"; ☐- 1 ½"; ☐- 2"; ☐- 2 ½"; ☐- 3";☐- 3½"; ☐-Other:_____
- ○ Image guidance if indicated above was used to confirm needle entry into target structure.
- ○ ☐-If checked, contrast dye was then injected and the needle position was adjusted accordingly to confirm proper placement without inadvertent intravascular entry.
- Needle was adjusted accordingly to confirm proper placement without inadvertent vascular entry.
- An attempt was made to aspirate from the structure and then the following injectate was delivered into the target structure:
  - ☐-Diagnostic injection: 1 mL 1% preservative-free lidocaine; ☐-Other injectate:_____
  - ☐-Therapeutic injection: 40 mg Depo-Medrol® & ☐- 1 mL 1% preservative-free lidocaine
  - ☐-Other injectate:_____
- The needle was removed and an adhesive bandage was placed over the needle entry site.

-If the above was a **diagnostic injection,** then proceed to section immediately below.
-If above was a **therapeutic injection procedure, aspiration only procedure,** or **aspiration and therapeutic injection,** then proceed to Procedure Summary Section.

For Diagnostic Injection Procedure:
- ☐-If checked, the above listed pre-procedural physical examination provocative maneuver was repeated and pain relief was: ☐-N/A; ☐-significant; ☐-some; ☐-equivocal; ☐-none; ☐-Other:_____
- Based on the amount of pain relief noted above:
  - ☐-a therapeutic injection will be scheduled.
  - ☐-a therapeutic injection will not be scheduled. See plan in corresponding office note.
  - ☐-a therapeutic injection following the same procedure described above was done using
    ☐- 40 mg Depo-Medrol® & ☐- 1 mL 1% preservative-free lidocaine
    ☐- Other injectate:_____
- The needle was removed and an adhesive bandage was placed over the needle entry site.

Procedure Summary:
If fluid aspirated from the target structure during the procedure:
- Total volume of fluid aspirated: ___ mL; Fluid appearance: ☐- N/A; ☐-Clear yellow; ☐-Slightly cloudy; ☐-Cloudy; ☐-Purulent; ☐-Blood-tinged; ☐-Bloody; ☐-Other:_____
Patient tolerance for the procedure: ☐-Excellent; ☐-Good; ☐-Fair; ☐-Other:_____

Additional comments regarding the procedure: ☐-None; ☐-Other:_____
_____
_____

Post-Procedural Treatment Advice:
Activity modification: Avoid non-essential use of the structure until seen for follow up. ☐-Other:_____

Orthotic instructions: N/A unless indicated as follows _____
Modalities: Apply ice over the injection site prn for 20-30 min. up to q2 hrs until seen for follow-up, unless instructed as follows: ☐-Heat; ☐-Other:_____

Injection Procedure Template: Triangular Fibrocartilage Complex Injection

PROCEDURE: Triangular Fibrocartilage Complex Injection
Side: ☐-Right   ☐-Left   ☐-Bilateral
Procedure Type: Aspiration: ☐-Diagnostic aspiration
                Injection: ☐-Diagnostic   ☐-Therapeutic ☐-Diagnostic then Therapeutic
Image guidance: None unless indicated as follows- ☐-Fluoroscopy ☐-Ultrasound
- The potential benefits and side effects of the procedure and alternative treatment options were explained to the patient, an opportunity for questions was provided, and the patient signed informed consent.
- ☐- If checked, the following physical examination pre-procedural provocative maneuver(s) was (were) performed: ☐-
  _____
- The patient was positioned for the procedure and the target structure was identified.
- The overlying skin was prepped with Betadine® followed by alcohol prep pad after the Betadine® dried.
- ☐- If checked, the overlying skin and soft tissue was anesthetized using a small amount of 1% lidocaine delivered via the following needle ☐-30G1"; ☐-25G1½ "; ☐-Other: _____
- The following needle was then used for the procedure:
    Type: Straight needle unless indicated as follows: ☐-Spinal needle; ☐-Other:_____
    Gauge: ☐-30; ☐-27; ☐-25; ☐-22; ☐-21; -18; Other:_____
    Length: ☐-5/8"; ☐- 1"; ☐- 1 ½"; ☐- 2"; ☐- 2 ½"; ☐- 3";☐- 3½"; ☐-Other:_____
- o Image guidance if indicated above was used to confirm needle entry into target structure.
- o ☐-If checked, contrast dye was then injected and the needle position was adjusted accordingly to confirm proper placement without inadvertent intravascular entry.
- Needle was adjusted accordingly to confirm proper placement without inadvertent vascular entry.
- An attempt was made to aspirate from the structure and then the following injectate was delivered into the target structure:
    ☐-Diagnostic injection: 1 mL 1% preservative-free lidocaine; ☐-Other injectate: _____
    ☐-Therapeutic injection: 20 mg Depo-Medrol® & ☐- 0.5 mL 1% preservative-free lidocaine
                    ☐-Other injectate: _____
- The needle was removed and an adhesive bandage was placed over the needle entry site.

-If the above was a **diagnostic injection**, then proceed to section immediately below.
-If above was a **therapeutic injection procedure, aspiration only procedure, or aspiration and therapeutic injection,** then proceed
to Procedure Summary Section.

For Diagnostic Injection Procedure:
- ☐-If checked, the above listed pre-procedural physical examination provocative maneuver was repeated and pain relief was: ☐-
  N/A; ☐-significant; ☐-some; ☐-equivocal; ☐-none; ☐-Other:_____
- Based on the amount of pain relief noted above:
    ☐-a therapeutic injection will be scheduled.
    ☐-a therapeutic injection will not be scheduled. See plan in corresponding office note.
    ☐-a therapeutic injection following the same procedure described above was done using
        ☐- 20 mg Depo-Medrol® & ☐- 0.5 mL 1% preservative-free lidocaine
        ☐- Other injectate: _____
- The needle was removed and an adhesive bandage was placed over the needle entry site.

Procedure Summary:
If fluid aspirated from the target structure during the procedure:
- Total volume of fluid aspirated: ___ mL; Fluid appearance: ☐- N/A; ☐-Clear yellow; ☐-Slightly cloudy;
  ☐-Cloudy; ☐-Purulent; ☐-Blood-tinged; ☐-Bloody; ☐-Other:_____
Patient tolerance for the procedure: ☐-Excellent; ☐-Good; ☐-Fair; ☐-Other:_____

Additional comments regarding the procedure: ☐-None; ☐Other:_____
_____

Post-Procedural Treatment Advice:
Activity modification: Avoid non-essential use of the structure until seen for follow up. ☐-Other:_____
_____

Orthotic instructions: N/A unless indicated as follows _____
Modalities: Apply ice over the injection site prn for 20-30 min. up to q2 hrs until seen for follow-up, unless instructed as follows: ☐-
Heat; ☐-Other:_____

Injection Procedure Template: Wrist Joint Injection: Intercarpal Approach

---

PROCEDURE: Wrist Joint Injection: Intercarpal Approach
Side: ☐-Right   ☐-Left   ☐-Bilateral
Procedure Type: Aspiration: ☐-Diagnostic aspiration
          Injection: ☐-Diagnostic   ☐-Therapeutic   ☐-Diagnostic then Therapeutic
Image guidance: None unless indicated as follows- ☐-Fluoroscopy ☐-Ultrasound
- The potential benefits and side effects of the procedure and alternative treatment options were explained to the patient, an opportunity for questions was provided, and the patient signed informed consent.
- ☐- If checked, the following physical examination pre-procedural provocative maneuver(s) was (were) performed: ☐-
- The patient was positioned for the procedure and the target structure was identified.
- The overlying skin was prepped with Betadine® followed by alcohol prep pad after the Betadine® dried.
- ☐- If checked, the overlying skin and soft tissue was anesthetized using a small amount of 1% lidocaine delivered via the following needle ☐-30G1"; ☐-25G1½"; ☐-Other:_____
- The following needle was then used for the procedure:
  Type: Straight needle unless indicated as follows: ☐-Spinal needle; ☐-Other:_____
  Gauge: ☐-30; ☐-27; ☐-25; ☐-22; ☐-21; -18; Other:_____
  Length: ☐-5/8"; ☐- 1"; ☐- 1 ½"; ☐- 2"; ☐- 2 ½"; ☐- 3";☐- 3½"; ☐-Other:_____
  - Image guidance if indicated above was used to confirm needle entry into target structure.
  - ☐-If checked, contrast dye was then injected and the needle position was adjusted accordingly to confirm proper placement without inadvertent intravascular entry.
- Needle was adjusted accordingly to confirm proper placement without inadvertent vascular entry.
- An attempt was made to aspirate from the structure and then the following injectate was delivered into the target structure:
  ☐-Diagnostic injection: 1 mL 2% preservative-free lidocaine; ☐-Other injectate:_____
  ☐-Therapeutic injection: 40 mg Depo-Medrol® & ☐- .5 mL 1% preservative-free lidocaine
       ☐-Other injectate:_____
- The needle was removed and an adhesive bandage was placed over the needle entry site.

-If the above was a **diagnostic injection**, then proceed to section immediately below.
-If above was a **therapeutic injection procedure, aspiration only procedure, or aspiration and therapeutic injection**, then proceed to Procedure Summary Section.

For Diagnostic Injection Procedure:
- ☐-If checked, the above listed pre-procedural physical examination provocative maneuver was repeated and pain relief was: ☐-
  N/A; ☐-significant; ☐-some; ☐-equivocal; ☐-none; ☐-Other:_____
- Based on the amount of pain relief noted above:
  ☐-a therapeutic injection will be scheduled.
  ☐-a therapeutic injection will not be scheduled. See plan in corresponding office note.
  ☐-a therapeutic injection following the same procedure described above was done using
       ☐- 40 mg Depo-Medrol® & ☐- 0.5 mL 1% preservative-free lidocaine
       ☐- Other injectate:_____
- The needle was removed and an adhesive bandage was placed over the needle entry site.

Procedure Summary:
If fluid aspirated from the target structure during the procedure:
- Total volume of fluid aspirated: ___ mL; Fluid appearance: ☐- N/A; ☐-Clear yellow; ☐-Slightly cloudy;
  ☐-Cloudy; ☐-Purulent; ☐-Blood-tinged; ☐-Bloody; ☐-Other:_____
Patient tolerance for the procedure: ☐-Excellent; ☐-Good; ☐-Fair; ☐-Other:_____

Additional comments regarding the procedure: ☐-None; ☐Other:_____

Post-Procedural Treatment Advice:
Activity modification: Avoid non-essential use of the structure until seen for follow up. ☐-Other:_____

Orthotic instructions: N/A unless indicated as follows _____
Modalities: Apply ice over the injection site prn for 20-30 min. up to q2 hrs until seen for follow-up, unless instructed as follows: ☐-
Heat; ☐-Other:_____

Chapter 9
The Hand

Patrick M. Foye, Debra S. Ibrahim, Michael J. Mehnert, Todd P. Stitik,
Jong H. Kim, Mohammad Hossein Dorri, David J. Van Why, Jose Ibarbia,
Lisa Schoenherr, Naimish Baxi, Ladislav Habina, and Jiaxin J. Tran

Introduction

Injections at the hand region are relatively common in musculoskeletal practice.
Some of the more commonly performed injections are listed in Table 9.1, along
with relevant references from the medical literature. These hand region injections
encompass a spectrum of intra-articular joint injections for osteoarthritis and other
arthritic conditions, tendon sheath injections, nerve blocks, etc.

Perhaps the most frequently performed of these procedures is a corticosteroid
injection for trigger finger. Many clinicians consider such injections to be the first line
treatment for trigger finger, based on the known effectiveness and the low incidence
of complications. Trigger finger occurs because a hypertrophic nodule prevents
the smooth passage of the flexor tendon beneath the first annular (A1) pulley, just
anterior to the metacarpophalangeal (MCP) joint. It was classically taught that the
corticosteroid should be injected into the tendon sheath but not into the substance of
the tendon itself (to minimize the risk of tendon disruption and weakening). With the
use of ultrasound guidance, it is even possible to inject into the A-1 pulley mechanism
itself. Interestingly, recent prospective studies found that even subcutaneous (extrasynovial) corticosteroid injections outside of a tendon sheath were as effective as
intrasheath injections [1, 2]. Surgical consultation should be considered for debride-
ment of the hypertrophic nodule at the flexor tendon and/or its sheath if the patient
fails to adequately respond to corticosteroid injections. Of note, an excessive number
of steroid injections at a given flexor tendon may potentially cause weakening and
subsequent tendon rupture, thus resulting in a "jersey finger" requiring surgical
reattachment. The exact number of such injections is not known with certainty.

Osteoarthritis (OA) of the hand is extremely common, and it is becoming more
so as the population ages. The most visible signs of hand OA on physical exam are
Heberden's nodes at the distal interphalangeal (IP) joints and Bouchard's nodes at

T.P. Stitik (✉)
Department of Physical Medicine and Rehabilitation, New Jersey Medical School,
Newark, NJ, USA
e-mail: todd.stitik@gmail.com

T.P. Stitik (ed.), *Injection Procedures: Osteoarthritis and Related Conditions*,
DOI 10.1007/978-0-387-76595-2_9, © Springer Science+Business Media, LLC 2011

Table 9.1 Summary of hand region injection procedures

Injection type	Specific structure	Meta-analysis (es)	Prospective study (studies)	Case series/report(s)	Described in review article(s) and/or injection textbook(s)
Articulation/Joint	1st CMC joint		[3, 9]	[19]	[20–23]
	Metacarpo-phalangngeal joint		[5, 24]	[6, 7]	[25, 26]
	Interphalangeal (IP) joints		[5, 8–10]	[27]	[28, 29]
Nerve	Digital nerve block	[12]	[11, 13, 14, 30]	[15, 31]	[32]
Tendons	Trigger finger		[1, 2]	[33]	[34–37]
Other	Subungual hematoma		[16, 18]	[38]	[17, 39–41]

Listed within each injection type in order of descending amount of current evidence supporting its use. References are provided for all meta-analyses, prospective studies, and case series/case reports along with at least one reference to descriptions in review articles or injection textbooks. For those procedures that are only described in review articles and/or textbooks, representative references are provided

the proximal interphalangeal joints. While OA at the first carpometacarpal joint (first CMC joint, i.e., at the base of the thumb) is not usually as readily visible early on in the disease process, this is actually the earliest and most common site for hand OA. Physical exam involves differentiating first CMC joint OA from nearby pain generators such as the first dorsal compartment (de Quervain's tenosynovitis, extending up into the distal forearm), scaphoid injuries (localized over the base of the anatomic snuffbox), and trigger thumb (episodic, painful catching volar to the MCP joint, rather than at the CMC joint). Before any injections are administered, the physician should strive to determine the precise pain generator so that the optimal target can be chosen. It is important to remember that small joints such as the first CMC joint should be entered using a thin needle and that the total volume of injectate should be kept low, so as to minimize postinjection pain exacerbation. If fluoroscopic guidance is used for precise intra-articular needle placement, contrast volume should be kept to a minimum (to allow space for injection of the therapeutic medication) or avoided altogether. Ultrasound guidance offers another alternative. While not yet FDA-approved for injection into the first CMC joint, initial prospective studies have shown that viscosupplementation (e.g., hyaluronic acid) injections relieve first CMC OA [3, 4] and provide longer benefit than corticosteroid injections [3].

Metacarpophalangngeal joints can be especially affected by rheumatoid arthritis, but not generally by OA. As such, literature on MCP injections is largely limited to rheumatoid arthritis patients. Furtado and colleagues demonstrated in a prospective study that in patients with rheumatoid arthritis and symptomatic polyarticular involvement, injections into MCP joints were particularly efficacious [24]. Intra-articular 169Erbium-citrate (aka 169Er-citrate) as a method of causing radiosynoviorthesis (radiosynovectomy) was found to be effective in symptomatic MCP and PIP joints of rheumatoid arthritis patients who had failed to respond to corticosteroid injections [5]. Accuracy of intra-articular needle placement was found to be superior with ultrasound guidance compared to palpation-guided procedures for MCP (4/5 vs. 27/27) and PIP joints (6/12 vs. 24/26) [6]. A case series of ten patients with "locked" MCP joints due to either MCP joint degeneration or of spontaneous etiology whose management included MCP joint capsule distension by local anesthetic injection was published [7].

Painful and stiff interphalangeal joints, e.g., in rheumatoid arthritis patients, can be relieved via injections with corticosteroids [8, 9], 10% dextrose, [10] or radioactive 169 erbium citrate [5]. Among corticosteroids, triamcinolone seems more likely to cause skin and soft tissue atrophy, as compared with methylprednisolone [9].

Digital nerve blocks are useful prior to performing suturing or other procedures on the thumb or fingers. Local anesthetic blockade is often required at both the medial and lateral digital nerves of a given digit, to attain adequate anesthesia of the digit. Classic teaching is that one should avoid injecting local anesthetic containing epinephrine, since the vasoconstriction could result in finger ischemia. Various approaches include subcutaneous, metacarpal, and transthecal, with many authors finding that the subcutaneous digital block is equally effective [11, 12], or more effective than the other approaches [13], and that the less invasive nature of the subcutaneous approach possibly makes this the best choice [14, 15].

Subungual hematoma (blood beneath the fingernail) can be treated with fingernail trephination (bur hole). Trephination does not appear to be associated with
possible infection, osteomyelitis, or major nail deformity regardless of hematoma
size [16]. It gives good functional and cosmetic outcomes [17], while making nail
removal unnecessary [16, 18].

References

1. Taras JS, Raphael JS, Pan WT, Movagharnia F, Sotereanos DG. Corticosteroid injections for trigger digits: is intrasheath injection necessary? J Hand Surg [Am] 1998;23(4):717–22.
2. Kazuki K, Egi T, Okada M, Takaoka K. Clinical outcome of extrasynovial steroid injection for trigger finger. Hand Surg 2006;11(1–2):1–4.
3. Fuchs S, Mönikes R, Wohlmeiner A, Heyse T. Intra-articular hyaluronic acid compared with corticoid injections for the treatment of rhizarthrosis. Osteoarthritis Cartilage 2006;14(1):82–8.
4. Coaccioli S, Pinoca F, Puxeddu A. Short term efficacy of intra-articular injection of hyaluronic acid in osteoarthritis of the first carpometacarpal joint in a preliminary open pilot study. Clin Ter 2006;157(4):321–5.
5. Kahan A, Mödder G, Menkes CJ, Verrier P, Devaux JY, Bonmartin A. 169Erbium-citrate synoviorthesis after failure of local corticosteroid injections to treat rheumatoid arthritis-affected finger joints. Clin Exp Rheumatol 2004;22(6):722–6.
6. Raza K, Lee CY, Pilling D, Heaton S, Situnayake RD, Carruthers DM et al. Ultrasound guidance allows accurate needle placement and aspiration from small joints in patients with early inflammatory arthritis. Rheumatology (Oxford) 2003;42(8):976–9.
7. Posner MA, Langa V, Green SM. The locked metacarpophalangeal joint: diagnosis and treatment. J Hand Surg [Am] 1986;11(2):249–53.
8. Menkes CJ, Gô AL, Verrier P, Aignan M, Delbarre F. Double-blind study of erbium 169 injection (synoviorthesis) in rheumatoid digital joints. Ann Rheum Dis 1977;36:254–6.
9. Jalava S, Saario R. Treatment of finger joints with local steroids. A double-blind study. Scand J Rheumatol 1983;12(1):12–4.
10. Reeves KD, Hassanein K. Randomized, prospective, placebo-controlled double-blind study of dextrose prolotherapy for osteoarthritic thumb and finger (DIP, PIP, and trapeziometacarpal) joints: evidence of clinical efficacy. J Altern Complement Med 2000;6(4):311–20.
11. Low CK, Wong HP, Low YP. Comparison between single injection transthecal and subcutaneous digital blocks. J Hand Surg [Br] 1997;22(5):582–4.
12. Yin ZG, Zhang JB, Kan SL, Wang P. A comparison of traditional digital blocks and single subcutaneous palmar injection blocks at the base of the finger and a meta-analysis of the digital block trials. J Hand Surg [Br] 2006;31(5):547–55.
13. Hung VS, Bodavula VK, Dubin NH. Digital anaesthesia: comparison of the efficacy and pain associated with three digital nerve block techniques. J Hand Surg [Br] 2005;30(6):581–4.
14. Brutus JP, Baeten Y, Chahidi N, Kinnen L, Ledoux P, Moermans JP. Single injection digital block: comparison between three techniques. Chir Main 2002;21(3):182–7.
15. Kollersbeck C, Walcher T, Gradl G, Genelin F. Clinical experiences and dosage pattern in subcutaneous single-injection digital block technique. Handchir Mikrochir Plast Chir 2004;36(1):64–6.
16. Seaberg DC, Angelos WJ, Paris PM. Treatment of subungual hematomas with nail trephination: a prospective study. Am J Emerg Med 1991;9(3):209–10.
17. Batrick N, Hashemi K, Freij R. Treatment of uncomplicated subungual haematoma. Emerg Med J 2003;20(1):65.

18. Meek S, White M. Subungual haematomas: is simple trephining enough? J Accid Emerg Med 1998;15(4):269–71.
19. Joshi R. Intraarticular corticosteroid injection for first carpometacarpal osteoarthritis. J Rheumatol 2005;32(7):1305–6.
20. Saunders S. Wrist treatments. In Saunders S, ed. Injection Techniques in Orthopaedic and Sports Medicine. Second edition. London: WB Saunders; 2002:70–81, 60–61.
21. Waldman SD. Intra-articular Injection of the Carpometacarpal Joint of the Thumb. Atlas of Pain Management Injection Techniques. Philadelphia, PA: WB Saunders; 2000: 125–7.
22. Kesson M, Atkins E, Davies I. Wrist and hand. In Kesson M, Atkins E, Davies I, eds. Musculoskeletal Injection Skills. New York: Butterworth Heinemann; 2002:86–88.
23. Tallia AF, Cardone DA. Diagnostic and therapeutic injection of the wrist and hand region. Am Fam Physician. 2003;67(4):745–50.
24. Furtado RN, Oliveira LM, Natour J. Polyarticular corticosteroid injection versus systemic administration in treatment of rheumatoid arthritis patients: a randomized controlled study. J Rheumatol 2005;32(9):1691–8.
25. Kesson M, Atkins E, Davies I. Wrist and hand. In Kesson M, Atkins E, Davies I, eds. Musculoskeletal Injection Skills. New York: Butterworth Heinemann; 2002:89–90.
26. Waldman SD. Intra-articular Injection of the Metacarpophalangeal Joints. Atlas of Pain Management Injection Techniques. Second edition. Philadelphia, PA: WB Saunders; 2007: 248–51.
27. Kumar S, Singh RJ, Reed AM, Lteif AN. Cushing's syndrome after intra-articular and intradermal administration of triamcinolone acetonide in three pediatric patients. Pediatrics 2004;113(6):1820–4.
28. Waldman SD. Intra-articular Injection of the Interphalangeal Joints. Atlas of Pain Management Injection Techniques. Philadelphia, PA: WB Saunders; 2000:141–3.
29. Kesson M, Atkins E, Davies I. Wrist and hand. In Kesson M, Atkins E, Davies I, eds. Musculoskeletal Injection Skills. New York: Butterworth Heinemann; 2002:89–91.
30. Williams JG, Lalonde DH. Randomized comparison of the single-injection volar subcutaneous block and the two-injection dorsal block for digital anesthesia. Plast Reconstr Surg 2006;118(5):1195–200.
31. Castellanos J, Ramírez C, De Sena L, Bertrán C. Transthecal digital block: digital anaesthesia through the sheath of the flexor tendon. J Bone Joint Surg Br 2000;82(6):889.
32. Scarff CE, Scarff CW. Digital nerve blocks: More gain with less pain. Australas J Dermatol 2007;48(1):60–1.
33. Fitzgerald BT, Hofmeister EP, Fan RA, Thompson MA. Delayed flexor digitorum superficialis and profundus ruptures in a trigger finger after a steroid injection: a case report. J Hand Surg [Am] 2005;30(3):479–82.
34. Saunders S. Wrist treatments. In Saunders S, ed. Injection Techniques in Orthopaedic and Sports Medicine. Second edition. London: WB Saunders; 2002:70–81, 64–5.
35. Kesson M, Atkins E, Davies I. Wrist and hand. In Kesson M, Atkins E, Davies I, eds. Musculoskeletal Injection Skills. New York: Butterworth Heinemann; 2002:99–101.
36. Waldman SD. Trigger Finger Syndrome. Atlas of Pain Management Injection Techniques. Philadelphia, PA: WB Saunders; 2000:134–7.
37. Akhtar S, Burke FD. Study to outline the efficacy and illustrate techniques for steroid injection for trigger finger and thumb. Postgrad Med J 2006;82(973):763–6.
38. Salter SA, Ciocon DH, Gowrishankar TR, Kimball AB. Controlled nail trephination for subungual hematoma. Am J Emerg Med 2006;24(7):875–7.
39. Skinner PB Jr. Management of traumatic subungual hematoma. Am Fam Physician 2005; 71(5):856.
40. Kaya TI, Tursen U, Baz K, Ikizoglu G. Extra-fine insulin syringe needle: an excellent instrument for the evacuation of subungual hematoma. Dermatol Surg 2003; 29(11):1141–3.
41. Palamarchuk HJ, Kerzner M. An improved approach to evacuation of subungual hematoma. J Am Podiatr Med Assoc 1989;79(11):566–8.

Procedure Instructions

Injection Procedure: First Carpometacarpal Joint Injection

1. Indications:
   (a) Diagnosis: Pain due to first CMC arthritis
   (b) Treatment
       • Overuse pain
       • Arthritis pain [1]

2. Contraindications especially pertinent to this procedure:
   (a) None documented

3. Possible side effects especially pertinent to this procedure:
   (a) None documented

4. Technical details of note for this procedure (Fig. 9.1):
   (a) Preferred needle gauge; length; type:
       • Nonimage-guided 25-gauge
       • Image-guided 25-gauge
   (b) Need for image guidance: Recommended
       • A study by Helm and colleagues [2] was conducted to determine the accuracy of intra-articular injections of the trapeziometacarpal joint for osteoarthritis. Of 60 injections that were completed, 58% were placed correctly. Although it is not universal practice to use imaging for this injection, the author has always used imaging when available to confirm placement and states that imaging greatly enhances the correct needle placement
       • The use of ultrasound as a diagnostic tool, a guide to therapeutic injections, and an objective way to monitor the efficacy of therapy has been documented for wrist and other small joint injections. Ultrasound guidance of needle positions has been documented as a simple procedure, easy to perform, not time consuming, and a nondamaging method for the metacarpalphalangeal joints and carpal joints [3, 4]

5. Step-by-step procedure:
   (a) Informed consent
   (b) Preprocedural testing: Identify and record the response to a physical examination preprocedural provocative maneuver if the procedure is a diagnostic one
   (c) Image guidance: Optional: Fluoroscopic-guided
   (d) Patient positioning:
       • If nonimage-guided: Place the patient in a seated position with the affected hand laying flat (palm-down) on the table
       • If image-guided: Place the patient in a seated position with the affected hand laying flat (palm-down) on the fluoroscopy table with an A-P view used to visualize the joint space

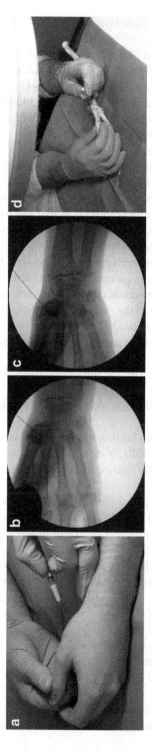

Fig. 9.1 First carpometacarpal (CMC) joint injection (fluoroscopic-guided). (**a**) First CMC joint injection–human model. (**b**) Fluoroscopic image of needle entry into first CMC joint. (**c**) Fluoroscopic image of first CMC arthrogram. (**d**) Skeletal representation of first CMC joint injection

(e) Identification and marking of injection site:
- If nonimage-guided:
  - Palpate the location of the first CMC joint by feeling for the distal end of the trapezium where it articulates with the first metacarpal in the anatomical snuff box. Entry through the skin overlying the anatomical snuff box is generally preferred. Active and passive movement of the first digit in flexion and extension while feeling for the trapezium-first metacarpal articulation is also helpful
- If fluoroscopic-guided:
  - Palpate the location of the first CMC joint by feeling for the distal end of the trapezium where it articulates with the first metacarpal in the anatomical snuff box. Entry through the skin overlying the anatomical snuff box is generally preferred. Active and passive movement of the first digit in flexion and extension while feeling for the trapezium-first metacarpal articulation is also helpful
  - Place a metallic marker such as a clamp over this site
  - Shoot a fluoroscopic picture in order to determine how well the proposed injection site correlates with the underlying joint
  - Make adjustments in the metallic marker location and/or relative position of the c-arm as needed
  - Mark the target using a marker or by depressing the skin with a plastic needle cap
- If ultrasound-guided: Use the ultrasound transducer to image the underlying target structure
  - Mark the target using a marker or by depressing the skin with a plastic needle cap
- Some common factors leading to inaccurate placement include [2]:
  - Aiming too proximally, at a "soft spot" at the apex of the anatomical snuffbox, frequently causing entrance of the scapho-trapezio-trapezoid joint
  - Difficulty entering the narrow trapeziometacarpal joint, especially when arthritis and osteophytes alter that space
  - Variability in the size and overhang of the abductor tubercle significantly constrains the angle of insertion
  - The joint line itself is not planar, which is underappreciated by many
(f) Skin preparation: Initial: Betadine® preparation using the no-touch technique
(g) Medication preparation:
- Diagnostic injection:
  - 0.5 mL of 2% preservative-free lidocaine
- Therapeutic injection:
  - 20 mg of Depo-Medrol® and 0.5 mL of 1% preservative-free lidocaine
(h) Skin preparation: Final: Alcohol prep pad wipe
(i) Local anesthesia administration: Optional, generally not needed

(j) Needle placement:
  - Pierce the previously anesthetized skin and subcutaneous tissue site with the appropriate needle and direct to the target

(k) Aspiration: Rule out intravascular entry and confirm entry into target structure

(l) Contrast injection:
  - Attempt to aspirate any synovial fluid that might be present in the joint
  - Inject the joint with enough contrast to confirm entry into the target structure. Connecting the contrast dye syringe to the needle using extension tubing is recommended to prevent a shift in needle position during attachment and detachment to and from the spinal needle. Adjust the needle position, if necessary, in order to obtain a clearly defined arthrogram
  - Aspirate back in order to remove some of the *Omnipaque*™ in order to allow for a greater volume of subsequent injectate and to confirm that blood return is not present
  - If fluoroscopic guidance: Inject the knee joint with *several cc of Omnipaque*™ *using a 5 cc syringe* connected to the straight needle via extension tubing. Adjust needle position, if necessary in order to clearly define an arthrogram

(m) Injection: Unclamp the aspiration syringe and clamp on the injection syringe

(n) Postprocedural testing:
  - If applicable, reassess response to the aforementioned preprocedural provocative maneuver

(o) If (+) response, repeat injection with therapeutic injectate:
  - Repeat steps d–f
  - Medication preparation 20 mg of Depo-Medrol®
  - Repeat steps h–m

(p) *Adhesive bandage* application over the needle entry site

(q) Postprocedural care discussion

References

1. Tallia AF, Cardone DA. Diagnostic and therapeutic injection of the wrist and hand region. Am Fam Physician 2003;67(4):745–50.
2. Helm AT, Higgins G, Rajkumar P, Redfern DR. Accuracy of intra-articular injections for osteoarthritis of the trapeziometacarpal joint. Int J Clin Pract 2003;57(4):265–6.
3. Koski JM, Hermunen H. Intra-articular glucocorticoid treatment of the rheumatoid wrist. An ultrasonographic study. Scand J Rheumatol 2001;30(5):268–70.
4. Grassi W, Lamanna G, Farina A, Cervini C. Synovitis of small joints: sonographic guided diagnostic and therapeutic approach. Ann Rheum Dis 1999;58(10):595–7.

Injection Procedure

Injection Procedure:Hand Metacarpophalangeal or Interphalangeal Joint Injection

1. Indications [1]:
   (a) Joint aspiration for fluid analysis
   (b) Crystal arthritis
   (c) Rheumatoid arthritis
   (d) Septic arthritis
   (e) Pain relief, osteoarthritis

2. Contraindications especially pertinent to this procedure:
   (a) None documented

3. Possible side effects especially pertinent to this procedure:
   (a) None documented

4. Technical details of note for this procedure (Figs. 9.2 and 9.3):
   (a) Preferred needle gauge; length; type:
      • 25-gauge
   (b) Need for ultrasound guidance: Optional
      • In a study by Raza and colleagues [2], the intra-articular accuracy of injections was 80% (4/5) with palpation. Many of the successful ones did not provide aspiration of cells with lavage. With ultrasound guidance, 100% (27/27) were intra-articular and yielded cell aspiration in 52% (14/27) of injections
      • The use of ultrasound as a diagnostic tool, a guide to therapeutic injections, and an objective way to monitor the efficacy of therapy has been documented for wrist and other small joint injections. Ultrasound guidance of needle positions has been documented as a simple procedure, easy to perform, not time consuming, and a nondamaging method for the MCP joints and carpal joints [3, 4]

5. Step-by-step procedure:
   (a) Informed consent
   (b) Preprocedural testing: Identify and record the response to a physical examination preprocedural provocative maneuver if the procedure is a diagnostic injection
   (c) Image-guidance: Optional: Ultrasound-guided
   (d) Patient positioning:
      • If nonimage guided: For MCP joint injections, the hand can be positioned resting on the procedure table with the palm down, to be accessed from the dorsal aspect of the hand. For IP joint injections, the joints can be accessed from either the medial or lateral side of the joint

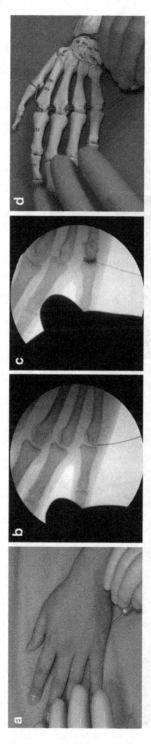

Fig. 9.2 Fifth metacarpophalangeal (MCP) joint injection (fluoroscopic-guided). (**a**) Fifth MCP joint injection–human model. (**b**) Fluoroscopic image of needle entry into fifth MCP joint. (**c**) Fluoroscopic image of fifth MCP arthrogram. (**d**) Skeletal representation of fifth MCP joint injection

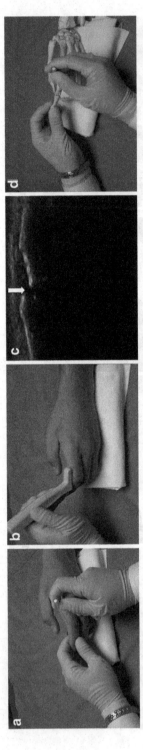

Fig. 9.3 Interphalangeal (IP) joint injection (ultrasound-guided). (**a**) IP joint injection-human model. (**b**) Ultrasound transducer positioning for visualizing IP joint – human model. (**c**) Ultrasonogram corresponding to previous image. (**d**) Skeletal representation of IP joint injection

- If image-guided: For MCP joint injections, the hand can be positioned resting on the procedure table with the palm down, to be accessed from the dorsal aspect of the hand. For IP joint injections, the joints can be accessed from either the medial or lateral side of the joint

(e) Identification and marking of injection site:
  - If nonimage-guided:
    - The target joint space can be identified by passively flexing and extending the digit across the target joint to identify the space between the two bones
  - If image-guided:
    - The target joint space is identified using imaging guidance
  - Mark the target using a marker or by depressing the skin with a plastic needle cap

(f) Skin preparation: Initial: Betadine® preparation using the no-touch technique

(g) Medication preparation:
  - Diagnostic injection:
    - 1 mL of 1% preservative-free lidocaine
  - Therapeutic injection:
    - 20 mg of Depo-Medrol®

(h) Skin preparation: Final: Alcohol prep

(i) Local anesthesia administration: Not applicable, as the joints are generally quite superficial and use of anesthetic is probably not necessary

(j) Needle placement:
  - Pierce the previously anesthetized skin and subcutaneous tissue site with the appropriate needle and direct to target. Ideally, the needle is inserted perpendicular to the joint line

(k) Aspiration: Rule out intravascular entry and confirm entry into target structure

(l) Injection: Unclamp the aspiration syringe and clamp on the injection syringe

(m) Postprocedural testing:
  - If applicable, reassess response to the aforementioned preprocedural provocative maneuver
  - If (+) response, repeat injection with therapeutic injectate:
    - Repeat steps d–f
    - Medication preparation: 20 mg of Depo-Medrol®
    - Repeat steps h–m

(n) Adhesive bandage application over needle entry site

(o) Postprocedural care discussion:
  - Symptoms may increase in the first 24–48 h related to possible steroid flare. NSAIDS may be used. Limit use of the affected finger over the next 2–3 weeks

References

1. Tallia AF, Cardone DA. Diagnostic and therapeutic injection of the wrist and hand region. Am Fam Physician 2003;67(4):745–50.
2. Raza K, Lee CY, Pilling D, Heaton S, Situnayake RD, Carruthers DM et al. Ultrasound guidance allows accurate needle placement and aspiration from small joints in patients with early inflammatory arthritis. Rheumatology (Oxford) 2003;42(8):976–9.
3. Koski JM, Hermunen H. Intra-articular glucocorticoid treatment of the rheumatoid wrist. An ultrasonographic study. Scand J Rheumatol 2001;30(5):268–70.
4. Grassi W, Lamanna G, Farina A, Cervini C. Synovitis of small joints: sonographic guided diagnostic and therapeutic approach. Ann Rheum Dis 1999;58(10):595–7.

Injection Procedure: Subungual Hematoma Drainage via Needle Trephination

1. Indications:
   (a) Diagnosis: N/A
   (b) Subungual hematoma: a collection of blood between the nail bed and nail due to bleeding from rich vascular supply within the nail bed

2. Contraindications especially pertinent to this procedure:
   (a) The following are contraindications for simple subungual hematoma evacuation (trephination) without nail removal, as nail removal allows the nail bed to be explored for any lacerations and bed repair in order to potentially optimize the cosmetic outcome
      • Crush or fracture of the nail (aka disrupted nail or nail border) [1, 2]
      • Displaced distal phalanx fracture
      • Hematoma greater than 50% of the nail bed has traditionally been believed by some as an indication for nail removal [1]. More recent studies, however, suggest that this is unnecessary in the setting of a nondisrupted nail or nail border, even if a nondisplaced distal phalanx is present [2, 3]
      • Open hemorrhage [2]

3. Possible side effects especially pertinent to this procedure:
   (a) Infection is such a possibility if there is an underling distal phalanx fracture (since this situation technically involves an open fracture) that broad spectrum antibiotics are recommended in this setting [2]
   (b) Nail deformity due to nail bed damage from needle trauma if the needle penetrates into the nail bed [1]

4. Technical details of note for this procedure (Fig. 9.4):
   (a) Preferred needle gauge; length; type: 18-gauge; 1½ in.; straight
   (b) *Need for image guidance*: No

5. Step-by-step procedure:
   (a) Informed consent
   (b) Preprocedure cleansing: Have the patient wash the affected digit and nail with soap and water
   (c) Patient positioning: Place the patient in a seated position with the hand resting on a table and the affected nail facing up
   (d) Identification and marking of injection site:
      • Identify the midportion of the subungual hematoma. This will be the needle insertion site
   (e) Skin preparation: Initial: Betadine® preparation using the no-touch technique
   (f) Skin preparation: Final: Alcohol prep pad wipe

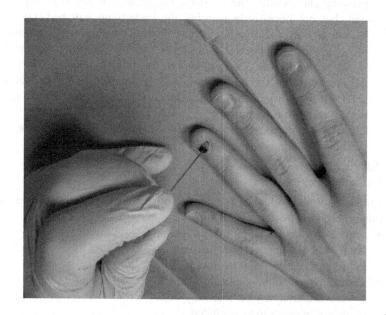

Fig. 9.4 Subungal Hematoma aspiration (trephination)

(g) Local anesthesia administration: Consider use of a digital nerve block for anesthesia of the affected digit. This will generally be needed if nail removal is necessary

(h) Clean the affected nail surface with an alcohol swab

(i) Use a flame (butane lighter or match can be used) to heat the tip of a sterile 18-gauge needle

(j) Needle placement:
- Pierce nail matrix in a location that corresponds to the base of the hematoma – this usually corresponds to the base of the nail – by gently pressing and twisting the 18-gauge needle until it is just through the nail, but not necessarily piercing the underlying nail bed. On nail puncture, you should feel a decrease in resistance to needle advancement, at which point you should stop advancing the needle and remove it. Blood should then drain through the needle entry site hole. You can then use sterile gauze to dab the blood. If satisfactory drainage is not achieved by nail puncture alone, consider gently squeezing the digit tip to express further blood
- If there is incomplete evacuation of blood and pain relief is only partial, consider repeating the procedure by puncturing a second hole

(k) *Adhesive bandage* application over needle entry site

(l) Postprocedural care discussion:

(m) Emphasis on the following considerations that are especially pertinent to this procedure:
- Elevate the involved digit to help minimize swelling
- Apply a cool compress over the bandage
- Leave bandage on for at least 12 h
- Contact physician immediately if wound becomes painful since:
  - Reevacuation may be necessary
  - Infection needs to be excluded

(n) Alternative techniques:

(o) Other drainage procedures have been described in the literature [1–3]
- Other instruments besides a needle that have been used for nail trephination include a paper clip or a commercial electric cauterizing lance [1]. The later device is contraindicated on patients wearing acrylic nails as these are flammable
- Another procedure described by Skinner involves positioning a heparinized hematocrit tube adjacent to the tip of an 18- to 21-gauge needle once a small amount of blood is noted at the tip of the needle. Capillary action then draws blood out [4]. Additional heparinized hematocrit tubes are used along with manual pressure and changing the angle of the needle to extract additional blood

References

1. Scott PM. Subungual hematoma evacuation. JAAPA 2002;15(3):63–5.
2. Pirzada A, Waseem M. Subungual hematoma. Pediatr Rev 2004;25(10):369.
3. Batrick N, Hashemi K, Freij R. Treatment of uncomplicated subungual haematoma. Emerg Med J 2003;20(1):65.
4. Skinner PB. Management of traumatic subungual hematoma. Am Fam Physician 2005; 71(5):856.

Injection Procedure

Injection Procedure:Trigger Finger Injection (aka Finger Flexor Tendon Sheath Injection)

1. Indications:
   (a) Symptomatic finger "triggering" [1]

2. Contraindications especially pertinent to this procedure:
   (a) None documented

3. Possible side effects especially pertinent to this procedure:
   (a) None documented

4. Technical details of note for this procedure (Fig. 9.5):
   (a) Preferred needle gauge; length; type: 25-gauge
   (b) Need for image guidance: No
      - In a study by Taras and Cardone [2], 95 patients with a total of 107 trigger finger injections were divided into two groups: one group with attempted intrasheath placement of the corticosteroid injection and the other group with subcutaneous placement. Of 52 attempted intrasheath injections, 24 (46%) were completely within the sheath, 19 (37%) were in the sheath and subcutaneously, and 9 (17%) were not delivered within the sheath. The response to the injection in this subgroup was good in 47% of complete intrasheath injections, 50% of both intrasheath and subcutaneous injections, and 70% of the subcutaneous injections (failed intrasheath). These data suggest that intrasheath injections for trigger digits may be less favorable than subcutaneous injection. It was noted that the intrasheath injections were dispersed more than the subcutaneous injections, which might account for the difference. Although the results of this study did not reach statistical significance, it suggests that use of imaging to ensure intrasheath injections is not warranted at this time

5. Step-by-step procedure:
   (a) Informed consent
   (b) Preprocedural testing: Not applicable
   (c) Image guidance: Optional: Ultrasound guidance
   (d) Patient positioning:
      - With the patient in a seated position, place the forearm and hand resting on the procedure table with the palm facing upward
   (e) Identification and marking of injection site:
      - If nonimage-guided:

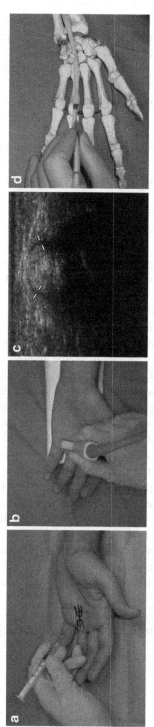

Fig. 9.5 Trigger finger injection (ultrasound guided). (**a**) Trigger finger injection–human model. (**b**) Ultrasound transducer positioning for visualizing flexor tendon and its sheath–human model. (**c**) Ultrasonogram corresponding to previous image. (**d**) Skeletal representation of trigger finger injection

- If possible, identify a tender, palpable nodule along the flexor tendon sheath, most commonly just distal to the A1 pulley of the hand if the finger is extended (near the distal end of the metacarpal). The nodule may be proximal to the A1 pulley if the finger is locked in flexion. The injectate does not need to be deposited into the nodule per se, though injection into the peritendinous sheath close to the nodule is appropriate
  - If image-guided:
    - Use ultrasound to directly visualize the tendon just proximal to the MCP joint
(f) Skin preparation: Initial: Betadine® preparation using the no-touch technique
(g) Medication preparation:
  - Diagnostic injection:
    - Not applicable

  - Therapeutic injection:
    - 40 mg of Depo-Medrol® and 0.5 mL of 1% preservative-free lidocaine
(h) Skin preparation: Final: Alcohol prep pad wipe
(i) Local anesthesia administration: Not applicable
(j) Needle placement: Pierce the previously anesthetized skin and subcutaneous tissue site with the appropriate needle and direct to the target
  - If nonimage-guided: The injection is generally performed with the needle pointing toward the fingertip (proximal to distal approach). Pierce the overlying skin and soft tissue and angle the needle into the nodule and subsequently into the tendinous sheath. When satisfactory needle position is achieved, there should be mild resistance to injection; a high level of resistance to injection may indicate that the needle is lodged in the tendon or that the bevel is abutting the tendon. If significant resistance is appreciated, draw the needle back slightly and attempt injection again. Gentle passive finger flexion may also precipitate needle movement, which can suggest that the needle is in contact with or lodged in the actual flexor tendon
  - If image-guided: Use ultrasound guidance to directly visualize needle entry into the tendon sheath
(k) Aspiration: Rule out intravascular entry and confirm entry into target structure
(l) Contrast injection: Not applicable
(m) Injection: Unclamp the aspiration syringe and clamp on the injection syringe

- If nonimage guided: The injection is generally performed with the needle pointing toward the fingertip (proximal to distal approach). Pierce the overlying skin and soft tissue and angle the needle into the nodule and subsequently into the tendinous sheath. When satisfactory needle position is achieved, there should be mild resistance to injection; a high level of resistance to injection may indicate that the needle is lodged in the tendon or that the bevel is abutting the tendon. If significant resistance is appreciated, draw the needle back slightly and attempt injection again. Gentle passive finger flexion may also precipitate needle movement, which can suggest that the needle is in contact with or lodged in the actual flexor tendon
- If image-guided: Use ultrasound guidance to directly visualize needle entry into the tendon sheath

(n) Postprocedural testing: If diagnostic injection
- If applicable, reassess response to the aforementioned preprocedural provocative maneuver

(o) If (+) response:
- Repeat steps d–f
- Medication preparation: 40 mg of Depo-Medrol®
- Repeat steps h–m

(p) Adhesive bandage application over the needle entry site
(q) Postprocedural care discussion

References

1. Tallia AF, Cardone DA. Diagnostic and therapeutic injection of the wrist and hand region. Am Fam Physician 2003;67(4):745–50.
2. Taras JS, Raphael JS, Pan WT, Movagharnia F, Sotereanos DG. Corticosteroid injections for trigger digits: is intrasheath injection necessary? J Hand Surg [Am] 1998;23(4):717–22.

Injection Procedure: Digital Nerve Block

1. Indications [1]:
   (a) Postoperative pain relief
   (b) Surgical/procedural anesthesia

2. Contraindications especially pertinent to this procedure:
   (a) Vascular insufficiency from compression of blood supply secondary to large volume injections [1]

3. Possible side effects especially pertinent to this procedure:
   (a) Damage to the digital nerve causing pain and temporary or even permanent paraesthesias [2]

5. Technical details of note for this procedure (Fig. 9.6):
   (a) Preferred needle gauge; length; type:
      • 30-gauge
      • Use of a 25–27 gauge needle has been described [1]
   (b) *Need for image guidance*: No
   (c) The use of epinephrine in the injection has been controversial in the past. It was thought that the vasoconstriction effects of the epinephrine could cause ischemia and lead to digital gangrene. Recent studies have not shown that the use of 1.5 mL of 2% lidocaine with epinephrine 1:100,000 leads to gangrene or other systemic complications. The advantage of using the epinephrine is quicker, better, and longer anesthesia. It also reduces the need for digital tourniquets used for bleeding control during longer procedures [3–5]. The theoretical risk of ischemia is not a contraindication since the vasoconstriction by epinephrine is temporary and reversible, and there have been no reported cases of ischemic injury in recent studies. Previous ischemic injury reports following digital nerve block have been attributed to thermal injuries in each case from warm soaks that occurred following the procedure [4, 5]. Nonetheless, these authors generally do not use epinephrine, as procedures performed in the scope of our practice rarely require prolonged anesthesia
   (d) The use of buffered lidocaine has been shown to provide less painful delivery and onset of anesthesia specifically in digital nerve blocks [6]
   (e) The flexor tendon sheath injection technique the authors describe in this chapter was originally described by Chiu [7]. A subsequent study showed that 1 mL of local anesthetic could be used instead of 2 mL [8]. Further modifications were described by Whetzel and colleagues, including injection at the level of the volar surface proximal to the digital crease in order to gain more reliable anesthesia [9]
   (f) The basic dorsal injection technique described here has been used or described in other studies [2, 3, 10]
   (g) The risk of nerve damage resulting from needle trauma is more significant with the dorsal approach as compared to injection in the webspace or flexor tendon sheath [2]. Injection of the flexor tendon sheath allows for injection

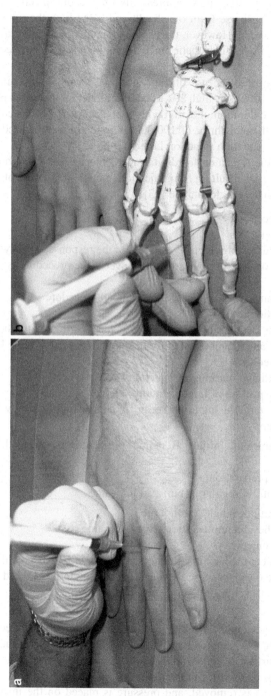

Fig. 9.6 Digital nerve block. (**a**) Digital nerve block – human model. (**b**) Skeletal representation of digital nerve block

away from the nerves and requires only one needle injection because the solution will disperse from the sheath and bathe both the ulnar and radial digital nerves [11]. However, the dorsal technique provides a faster onset of anesthesia, with less anesthetic since the solution is concentrated around the nerve [11]

(h) A study compared the use of bupivacane (0.5%), 2% lidocaine with epinephrine (1:100,000), and 2% lidocaine alone for duration of action. It found that the duration of action with bupivacaine (0.5%) lasted 24.9 h, 2% lidocaine with epinephrine (1:100,000) duration of action lasted 10.4 h, and 2% lidocaine duration of action lasted 4.9 h [12]

(i) Heating of the lidocaine for digital nerve blocks has been shown to help decrease the pain resulting from injection, though the authors of this chapter have not utilized this technique [13]

5. Step-by-step procedure:
   (a) Informed consent
   (b) Preprocedural testing: Identify and record the response to a physical examination preprocedural provocative maneuver if the procedure is a diagnostic injection
   (c) Image guidance: Not applicable; Nonguided procedure
   (d) Patient positioning:
      • Place the patient in a supine or seated position with the arm fully abducted and the elbow slightly flexed with the palm of the hand resting on a folded towel
   (e) Identification and marking of injection site
      • Visual inspection of target pending selected approach
      • Mark the target using a market or by depressing the skin with a plastic needle cap
   (f) Skin preparation: Initial: Betadine® preparation using the no-touch technique
   (g) Medication preparation:
      • 1.5 mL of 2% regular or buffered lidocaine
   (h) Skin preparation: Final: Alcohol prep
   (i) Local anesthesia administration: Not applicable
   (j) Needle placement:
      • At a point at the base of the finger, a 30-gauge 1-in. needle is inserted on each side of the proximal phalanx of the digit to be blocked
   (k) Aspiration: Rule out intravascular entry and confirm entry into target structure
   (l) Injection: Unclamp the aspiration syringe and clamp on the injecting syringe
      • While the anesthetic is slowly injected, the needle is advanced from the dorsal surface of the hand toward the palmar surface. The same technique can be used for the thumb
      • The needle is removed, and pressure is placed on the injection site to avoid hematoma formation [1]

   – Another technique has been described with a subcutaneous injection of
   2 mL of 2% lidocaine anesthetic at the A1 pulley [10]. A comparison
   of the dorsal (transmetacarpal) block, flexor tendon sheath (transthecal)
   block, and a subcutaneous block showed that the level of anesthesia for
   all three was the same. However, the flexor tendon sheath injection
   caused more pain over 48 h, and the dorsal injection requires two injections and has a slower onset of action as compared to one in the subcutaneous injection. Patients preferred the subcutaneous injection [10].
   The use of a single subcutaneous injection was also recommended in
   comparison to the modified transthecal digital block described by
   Whetzel and colleagues [9]. The two methods provided similar anesthesia, but the ease of administration and the fact that no major structures are entered make subcutaneous injection a better choice [14]
(m) Postprocedural testing: Not applicable
(n) *Adhesive bandage* application over the needle entry site
(o) Postprocedural care discussion

References

1. Waldman SD. Neural blockade and neurolytic blocks. In Lampert R, Ross A, Ruzycka A, eds. Atlas of Interventional Pain Management. Philadelphia, PA: WB Saunders, 2004:202–4.
2. Phillips JS, Gillespie PH, Logan AM. Digital nerve blocks: a cadaveric study of an unrecognized trauma? J Trauma 2005;59(3):770–2.
3. Andrades PR, Olguin FA, Calderon W. Digital blocks with or without epinephrine. Plast Reconstr Surg 2003;111(5):1769–70.
4. Wilhelmi BJ, Blackwell SJ, Miller JH, Mancoll JS, Dardano T, Tran A et al. Do not use epinephrine in digital blocks: Myth or truth? Plast Reconstr Surg 2001;107:3937.
5. Krunic AL, Wang LC, Soltani K, Weitzul S, Taylor RS. Digital anesthesia with epinephrine: an old myth revisited. J Am Acad Dermatol 2004;51(5):755–9.
6. Bartfield JM, Ford DT, Homer PJ. Buffered versus plain lidocaine for digital nerve blocks. Ann Emerg Med 1993;22(2):216–9.
7. Chiu DT. Transthecal digital block: flexor tendon sheath used for anesthetic infusion. J Hand Surg [Am] 1990;15-A:471–3.
8. Castellanos J, Ramirez C, De Sena L, Bertran C. Transthecal digital block: digital anaesthesia through the sheath of the flexor tendon. J Bone Joint Surg [Br] 2000;82(6):889.
9. Whetzel TP, Mabourakh S, Barkhordar R. Modified transthecal digital block. J Hand Surg 1997;22A(2):361.
10. Hung VS, Bodavula VK, Dubin NH. Digital anaesthesia: comparison of the efficacy and pain associated with three digital nerve block techniques. J Hand Surg [Br] 2005;30(6):581–4.
11. Sarhadi NS, Shaw-Dunn J. Transthecal digital nerve block. An anatomical appraisal. J Hand Surg [Br] 1998;23(4):490–3.
12. Thomson CJ, Lalonde DH. Randomized double-blind comparison of duration of anesthesia among three commonly used agents in digital nerve block. Plast Reconstr Surg 2006;118(2):429–32.
13. Waldbillig DK, Quinn JV, Stiell IG, Wells GA. Randomized double-blind controlled trial comparing room-temperature and heated lidocaine for digital nerve block. Ann Emerg Med 1995;26(6):677–81.
14. Brutus JP, Baeten Y, Chahidi N, Kinnen L, Ledoux P, Moermans JP. Single injection digital block: comparison between three techniques. Chir Main 2002;21(3):182–7.

Injection Procedure Templates

Injection Procedure Template: First Carpometacarpal Joint Injection

---

PROCEDURE: First Carpometacarpal (CMC) Joint Injection
Side: ☐-Right   ☐-Left   ☐-Bilateral
Procedure Type: Aspiration: ☐-Diagnostic aspiration
             Injection: ☐-Diagnostic   ☐-Therapeutic ☐-Diagnostic <u>then</u> Therapeutic
Image guidance: None unless indicated as follows- ☐-Fluoroscopy   ☐-Ultrasound
- The potential benefits and side effects of the procedure and alternative treatment options were explained to the patient, an opportunity for questions was provided, and <u>the patient signed informed consent</u>.
- ☐- If checked, the following physical examination <u>pre-procedural provocative maneuver(s)</u> was (were) performed: ☐-
_____
- The patient was positioned for the procedure and the target structure was identified.
- The overlying skin was prepped with <u>Betadine® followed by alcohol prep pad</u> after the Betadine® dried.
- ☐- If checked, the overlying skin and soft tissue was anesthetized using a <u>small amount of 1% lidocaine</u> delivered via the following needle ☐-30G1"; ☐-25G1½"; ☐-Other: _____
- The following needle was then used for the procedure:
     <u>Type</u>: Straight needle unless indicated as follows: ☐-Spinal needle; ☐-Other:_____
     <u>Gauge</u>: ☐-30; ☐-27; ☐-25; ☐-22; ☐-21; -18; -Other:_____
     <u>Length</u>: ☐-5/8"; ☐- 1"; ☐- 1 ½"; ☐- 2"; ☐- 2 ½"; ☐- 3";☐- 3½"; ☐-Other:_____
- o Image guidance if indicated above was used to confirm needle entry into target structure.
- o ☐-If checked, contrast dye was then injected and the needle position was adjusted accordingly to confirm proper placement without inadvertent intravascular entry.
- Needle was adjusted accordingly to confirm proper placement without inadvertent vascular entry.
- An attempt was made to aspirate from the structure and then the following injectate was delivered into the target structure:
   ☐-Diagnostic injection: <u>0.5 mL 2% preservative-free lidocaine</u>; ☐-Other injectate: _____
   ☐-Therapeutic injection: <u>20 mg Depo-Medrol</u> & ☐- <u>0.5 mL 1% preservative-free bupivacaine</u>
                    ☐-Other injectate:_____
- The needle was removed and an <u>adhesive bandage</u> was placed over the needle entry site.

-If the above was a <u>diagnostic injection</u>, then proceed to section immediately below.
-If above was a <u>therapeutic injection procedure, aspiration only procedure</u>, or <u>aspiration and therapeutic injection</u>, then proceed to Procedure Summary Section.

For Diagnostic Injection Procedure:
- ☐-If checked, the above listed pre-procedural physical examination provocative maneuver was repeated and pain relief was: ☐ -N/A; ☐-significant; ☐-some; ☐-equivocal; ☐-none; ☐-Other:_____
- Based on the amount of pain relief noted above:
   ☐-a therapeutic injection will be scheduled.
   ☐-a therapeutic injection will <u>not</u> be scheduled. See plan in corresponding office note.
   ☐-a therapeutic injection following the same procedure described above was done using
         ☐- <u>20 mg Depo-Medrol</u>® & ☐- <u>0.5 mL 1% preservative-free lidocaine</u>
         ☐- Other injectate:_____
- The needle was removed and an <u>adhesive bandage</u> was placed over the needle entry site.

Procedure Summary:
<u>If fluid aspirated from the target structure during the procedure:</u>
- Total volume of fluid aspirated: ___ mL; Fluid appearance: ☐- N/A; ☐-Clear yellow; ☐-Slightly cloudy; ☐-Cloudy; ☐-Purulent; ☐-Blood-tinged; ☐-Bloody; ☐-Other:_____
<u>Patient tolerance for the procedure</u>: ☐-Excellent; ☐-Good; ☐-Fair; ☐-Other:_____

<u>Additional comments regarding the procedure:</u> ☐-None; ☐Other:_____
_____

Post-Procedural Treatment Advice:
<u>Activity modification</u>: Avoid non-essential use of the structure until seen for follow up. ☐-Other:_____
_____
<u>Orthotic instructions</u>: N/A unless indicated as follows _____
<u>Modalities</u>: Apply ice over the injection site prn for 20-30 min. up to q2 hrs until seen for follow-up, unless instructed as follows: ☐- Heat; ☐-Other:_____

Injection Procedure Template: Hand MCP or IP Joint Injection

PROCEDURE: Hand MCP or IP Joint Injection
Side: ☐-Right   ☐-Left   ☐-Bilateral
Procedure Type: Aspiration: ☐-Diagnostic aspiration
         Injection: ☐-Diagnostic   ☐-Therapeutic ☐-Diagnostic <u>then</u> Therapeutic
Image guidance: None unless indicated as follows- ☐-Fluoroscopy ☐-Ultrasound

- The potential benefits and side effects of the procedure and alternative treatment options were explained to the patient, an opportunity for questions was provided, and <u>the patient signed informed consent</u>.
- ☐- If checked, the following physical examination <u>pre-procedural provocative maneuver(s)</u> was (were) performed: ☐-_____
- The patient was positioned for the procedure and the target structure was identified.
- The overlying skin was prepped with <u>Betadine® followed by alcohol prep pad</u> after the Betadine® dried.
- ☐- If checked, the overlying skin and soft tissue was anesthetized using a <u>small amount of 1% lidocaine</u> delivered via the following needle ☐-30G1"; ☐-25G1½ "; ☐-Other: _____
- The following needle was then used for the procedure:
  - <u>Type:</u> <u>Straight</u> needle unless indicated as follows: ☐-Spinal needle; ☐-Other:_____
  - <u>Gauge:</u> ☐-30; ☐-27; ☐-25; ☐-22; ☐-21; -18; -Other:_____
  - <u>Length:</u> ☐-5/8"; ☐- 1"; ☐- 1 ½ "; ☐- 2"; ☐- 2 ½"; ☐- 3";☐- 3½"; ☐-Other:_____
- ○ Image guidance if indicated above was used to confirm needle entry into target structure.
- ○ ☐-If checked, contrast dye contained in a syringe that was connected to the injection needle, was also used.
- The needle was adjusted accordingly to confirm proper placement without inadvertent vascular entry.
- An attempt was made to aspirate from the structure, and a <u>syringe containing the following injectate</u> was attached and the injection was performed into the target structure:
  - ☐-Diagnostic injection: 1 mL 1% preservative-free lidocaine; ☐-Other injectate: _____
  - ☐-Therapeutic injection: 20 mg Depo-Medrol & ☐- 1 mL 0.5% preservative-free bupivacaine
    - ☐-Other injectate: _____
- The needle was removed and an <u>adhesive bandage</u> was placed over the needle entry site.

-If the above was a <u>diagnostic injection</u>, then proceed to section immediately below.
-If above was a <u>therapeutic injection procedure</u>, <u>aspiration only procedure</u>, or <u>aspiration and therapeutic injection</u>, then proceed to Procedure Summary Section.

For Diagnostic Injection Procedure:
- ☐-If checked, the above listed pre-procedural physical examination provocative maneuver was repeated and pain relief was: ☐
  -N/A; ☐-significant; ☐-some; ☐-equivocal; ☐-none; ☐-Other:_____
- Based on the amount of pain relief noted above:
  - ☐-a therapeutic injection will be scheduled.
  - ☐-a therapeutic injection will <u>not</u> be scheduled. See plan in corresponding office note.
  - ☐-a therapeutic injection following the same procedure described above was done using
    - ☐- 40 mg Depo-Medrol® & ☐- 1 mL 1% preservative-free lidocaine
    - ☐- Other injectate: _____
- The needle was removed and an <u>adhesive bandage</u> was placed over the needle entry site.

Procedure Summary:
<u>If fluid aspirated from the target structure during the procedure:</u>
- Total volume of fluid aspirated: ___ mL; Fluid appearance: ☐- N/A; ☐-Clear yellow; ☐-Slightly cloudy; ☐-Cloudy; ☐-Purulent; ☐-Blood-tinged; ☐-Bloody; ☐-Other:_____
<u>Patient tolerance for the procedure:</u> ☐-Excellent; ☐-Good; ☐-Fair; ☐-Other:_____

<u>Additional comments regarding the procedure:</u> ☐-None; ☐Other:_____

Post-Procedural Treatment Advice:
<u>Activity modification:</u> Avoid non-essential use of the structure until seen for follow up. ☐-Other:_____

<u>Orthotic instructions:</u> N/A unless indicated as follows _____
<u>Modalities:</u> Apply ice over the injection site prn for 20-30 min. up to q2 hrs until seen for follow-up, unless instructed as follows: ☐-Heat; ☐-Other:_____

Injection Procedure Template: Subungual Hematoma Drainage

PROCEDURE: Subungual Hematoma Drainage
Side: ☐-Right   ☐-Left   ☐-Bilateral
Procedure Type: Aspiration: ☐-Diagnostic aspiration
            Injection: ☐-Diagnostic   ☐-Therapeutic   ☐-Diagnostic then Therapeutic
Image guidance: None unless indicated as follows- ☐-Fluoroscopy ☐-Ultrasound
  • The potential benefits and side effects of the procedure and alternative treatment options were explained to the patient, an
    opportunity for questions was provided, and the patient signed informed consent.
  • ☐- If checked, the following physical examination pre-procedural provocative maneuver(s) was (were) performed: ☐-
    _____
  • The patient was positioned for the procedure and the target structure was identified.
  • The overlying skin was prepped with Betadine® followed by alcohol prep pad after the Betadine® dried.
  • ☐- If checked, the overlying skin and soft tissue was anesthetized using a small amount of 1% lidocaine delivered via the
    following needle ☐-30G1"; ☐-25G1½ "; ☐-Other: _____
  • The following needle was then used for the procedure:
        Type: Straight needle unless indicated as follows: ☐-Spinal needle; ☐-Other:_____
        Gauge: ☐-30; ☐-27; ☐-25; ☐-22; ☐-21; -18; -Other:_____
        Length: ☐-5/8"; ☐- 1"; ☐- 1 ½ "; ☐- 2"; ☐- 2 ½"; ☐- 3";☐- 3½"; ☐-Other:_____
  ○ Image guidance if indicated above was used to confirm needle entry into target structure.
  ○ ☐-If checked, contrast dye contained in a syringe that was connected to the injection needle, was also used.
  • The needle was adjusted accordingly to confirm proper placement without inadvertent vascular entry.
  • An attempt was made to aspirate from the structure, and a syringe containing the following injectate was attached and the
    injection was performed into the target structure:
        ☐-Diagnostic injection: 1 mL 1% preservative-free lidocaine; ☐-Other injectate: _____
        ☐-Therapeutic injection: 40 mg Depo-Medrol® & ☐- 1 mL 0.5% preservative-free bupivacaine
                ☐-Other injectate: _____
  • The needle was removed and an adhesive bandage was placed over the needle entry site.

-If the above was a diagnostic injection, then proceed to section immediately below.
-If above was a therapeutic injection procedure, aspiration only procedure, or aspiration and therapeutic injection, then
proceed to Procedure Summary Section.

For Diagnostic Injection Procedure:
  • ☐-If checked, the above listed pre-procedural physical examination provocative maneuver was repeated and pain relief was: ☐
    -N/A; ☐-significant; ☐-some; ☐-equivocal; ☐-none; ☐-Other:_____
  • Based on the amount of pain relief noted above:
        ☐-a therapeutic injection will be scheduled.
        ☐-a therapeutic injection will not be scheduled. See plan in corresponding office note.
        ☐-a therapeutic injection following the same procedure described above was done using
                ☐- 40 mg Depo-Medrol® & ☐- 0.5 mL 1% preservative-free lidocaine
                ☐- Other injectate: _____
  • The needle was removed and an adhesive bandage was placed over the needle entry site.

Procedure Summary:
If fluid aspirated from the target structure during the procedure:
  • Total volume of fluid aspirated: ___ mL; Fluid appearance: ☐- N/A; ☐-Clear yellow; ☐-Slightly cloudy;
    ☐-Cloudy; ☐-Purulent; ☐-Blood-tinged; ☐-Bloody; ☐-Other:_____
Patient tolerance for the procedure: ☐-Excellent; ☐-Good; ☐-Fair; ☐-Other:_____

Additional comments regarding the procedure: ☐-None; ☐Other:_____
_____
_____

Post-Procedural Treatment Advice:
Activity modification: Avoid non-essential use of the structure until seen for follow up. ☐-Other:_____
_____
Orthotic instructions: N/A unless indicated as follows _____
Modalities: Apply ice over the injection site prn for 20-30 min. up to q2 hrs until seen for follow-up, unless instructed as follows: ☐-
Heat; ☐-Other:_____

Injection Procedure Template: Trigger Finger Injection

PROCEDURE: Trigger Finger Injection
Side: ☐-Right   ☐-Left   ☑-Bilateral
Procedure Type: Aspiration: ☐-Diagnostic aspiration
      Injection: ☐-Diagnostic   ☑-Therapeutic   ☐-Diagnostic <u>then</u> Therapeutic
Image guidance: None unless indicated as follows- ☐-Fluoroscopy ☐-Ultrasound
- The potential benefits and side effects of the procedure and alternative treatment options were explained to the patient, an opportunity for questions was provided, and <u>the patient signed informed consent</u>.
- ☐- If checked, the following physical examination <u>pre-procedural provocative maneuver(s)</u> was (were) performed: ☐-
  _____
- The patient was positioned for the procedure and the target structure was identified.
- The overlying skin was prepped with <u>Betadine® followed by alcohol prep pad</u> after the Betadine® dried.
- ☐- If checked, the overlying skin and soft tissue was anesthetized using a <u>small amount of 1% lidocaine</u> delivered via the following needle ☐-30G1"; ☐-25G1½ "; ☐-Other: _____
- The following needle was then used for the procedure:
      Type: <u>Straight</u> needle unless indicated as follows: ☐-Spinal needle; ☐-Other:_____
      Gauge: ☐-30; ☐-27; ☐-25; ☐-22; ☐-21; -18; -Other:_____
      Length: ☐-5/8"; ☐- 1"; ☐- 1 ½ "; ☐- 2"; ☐- 2 ½"; ☐- 3"; ☐- 3½"; ☐-Other:_____
- ○ Image guidance if indicated above was used to confirm needle entry into target structure.
- ○ ☐-If checked, contrast dye contained in a syringe that was connected to the injection needle, was also used.
- The needle was adjusted accordingly to confirm proper placement without inadvertent vascular entry.
- An attempt was made to aspirate from the structure, and a <u>syringe containing the following injectate</u> was attached and the injection was performed into the target structure:
  ☐-Diagnostic injection: <u>1 mL 1% preservative-free lidocaine</u>; ☐-Other injectate: _____
  ☐-Therapeutic injection: <u>40 mg Depo-Medrol®</u> & ☐- <u>.5 mL 1% preservative-free lidocaine</u>
      ☐-Other injectate: _____
- The needle was removed and an <u>adhesive bandage</u> was placed over the needle entry site.

-If the above was a <u>diagnostic injection</u>, then proceed to section immediately below.
-If above was a <u>therapeutic injection procedure, aspiration only procedure, or aspiration and therapeutic injection</u>, then proceed to Procedure Summary Section.

For Diagnostic Injection Procedure:
- ☐-If checked, the above listed pre-procedural physical examination provocative maneuver was repeated and pain relief was: ☐ -N/A; ☐-significant; ☐-some; ☐-equivocal; ☐-none; ☐-Other:_____
- Based on the amount of pain relief noted above:
  ☐-a therapeutic injection will be scheduled.
  ☐-a therapeutic injection will <u>not</u> be scheduled. See plan in corresponding office note.
  ☐-a therapeutic injection following the same procedure described above was done using
      ☐- <u>40 mg Depo-Medrol®</u> & ☐- <u>0.5 mL 1% preservative-free lidocaine</u>
      ☐- Other injectate: _____
- The needle was removed and an <u>adhesive bandage</u> was placed over the needle entry site.

Procedure Summary:
If fluid aspirated from the target structure during the procedure:
- Total volume of fluid aspirated: ___ mL; Fluid appearance: ☐- N/A; ☐-Clear yellow; ☐-Slightly cloudy; ☐-Cloudy; ☐-Purulent; ☐-Blood-tinged; ☐-Bloody; ☐-Other:_____
Patient tolerance for the procedure: ☐-Excellent; ☐-Good; ☐-Fair; ☐-Other:_____

Additional comments regarding the procedure: ☐-None; ☐Other:_____
_____

Post-Procedural Treatment Advice:
Activity modification: Avoid non-essential use of the structure until seen for follow up. ☐-Other:_____
_____
Orthotic instructions: N/A unless indicated as follows _____
Modalities: Apply ice over the injection site prn for 20-30 min. up to q2 hrs until seen for follow-up, unless instructed as follows: ☐-Heat; ☐-Other:_____

Injection Procedure Template: Digital Nerve Block

PROCEDURE: Digital Nerve Block
        ☐-Dorsal Approach   ☐-Flexor Sheath Approach (Transthecal Approach)
Image guidance- None unless indicated as follows: ☐- Fluoroscopy   ☐- Ultrasound
Side: ☐-Right   ☐-Left   ☐-Bilateral
- The potential benefits and side effects of the procedure were explained to the patient, an opportunity for questions was provided, then <u>the patient signed informed consent</u>.
- The following physical examination pre-procedural provocative maneuver was performed: ☐- N/A;
  ☐- _____
- The target was identified by appropriately positioning the patient.
- The overlying skin was prepped with <u>Betadine® and alcohol</u>.

For Non-Image-Guided Procedure:
- The following needle was selected for the procedure:
  ☐-30G 1" <u>straight</u>; ☐-22G 1½" <u>straight</u>; ☐-18G 1½" <u>straight</u>; ☐-Other: _____
- The above needle was attached to a 3 mL syringe containing the following injectate:
  - ☐- 1.5 mL <u>2%</u> buffered lidocaine
  - ☐- Other injectate: _____

☐-Dorsal Approach
- The above mentioned needle was inserted into the dorsal surface of the hand just ulnar to the side of the periosteum at the base of the proximal digit.
- After aspiration did not reveal blood return, the target was injected with the above mentioned solution.
- The above mentioned needle was then inserted into the dorsal surface of the hand just radial to the side of the periosteum at the base of the proximal digit.
- After aspiration did not reveal blood return, the target was injected with the above mentioned solution.

☐-Flexor Sheath Approach (Tranthecal Approach)
- The above mentioned needle was inserted into the palmar surface of the hand into the flexor tendon sheath at the palmar digital crease.
- After aspiration did not reveal blood return, the target was injected with the above mentioned solution.

- At 10 minutes after the injection, digital sensation was:
  - ☐- Absent
  - ☐- Present
    - ☐- Repeat injections of 0.5 mL buffered lidocaine were injected at 5 minute intervals with a total of _____ repeat injections.
- Total amount of buffered lidocaine given until anesthesia achieved: _____ ml
- An <u>adhesive bandage</u> was placed over the needle entry site.

Procedure Summary:
<u>Patient tolerance for the procedure</u>: ☐-Excellent ☐-Good ☐-Fair ☐-Other:_____

<u>Additional comments regarding the procedure:</u> ☐- None; Other: _____

Post-Procedural Treatment Advice:
Avoid non-essential use of the structure until seen for follow up. Apply ice for 20-30 min. up to q2 hrs prn until seen for follow-up, unless instructed as follows: _____

Part III
Lower Limb Injection Procedures

Chapter 10
The Hip

Patrick M. Foye, Christopher Castro, Todd P. Stitik, Jong H. Kim,
Mohammad Hossein Dorri, Jose Santiago Campos, Lisa Schoenherr,
Naimish Baxi, and Ladislov Habina

Introduction

Injections at the hip region are relatively common in musculoskeletal practice, due to the relatively high incidence of tendonitis, bursitis, and arthritis in this area. Injections in this region can be either diagnostic (e.g., local anesthetic blocks to more definitively determine a specific source of the patient's pain) or therapeutic (e.g., local corticosteroid injections). Probably the most common injections performed at the hip region are corticosteroid injections at the proximal lateral thigh for trochanteric bursitis +/- iliotibial band (ITB) tendonitis. Other injections in the hip region include intra-articular hip joint injections, iliopsoas bursa (psoas bursa) injections, ischial bursa injections, hamstring tendon origin site injections, and nerve blocks/injections for lateral femoral cutaneous entrapment (meralgia paresthetica).

Although this particular section focuses on injections for hip region pathology, clinicians must remember the importance of performing a comprehensive history and a comprehensive physical examination since the patient may report "hip pain," when in actuality the source of the pain may be coming from the lower back, knee, or intrapelvic pathology. It is also notable that patients will often refer to their "hip" as the upper lateral thigh (greater trochanteric region), whereas pain from the psoas bursa or the actual hip joint will often present in the groin and/or anterior-medial thigh. One author (TS) has also noted that terminology used by physicians for this body region can also be somewhat arbitrary. For example, the term hip joint injection (i.e., intra-articular injection) and trochanteric bursa injections should not be used interchangeably. In cases in which the history, physical exam, and diagnostic test results are inconclusive, a diagnostic intra-articular hip joint injection may help to differentiate hip joint pain versus pain from the sacroiliac or other regions.

The literature provides a variety of descriptions regarding how to perform each of these various injections and variable degrees of evidence regarding their effectiveness (Table 10.1). Of note, at the time of this writing, the literature does not

P.M. Foye (✉)
Department of Medicine and Rehabilitation, New Jersey Medical School, Newark, NJ, USA
e-mail: doctor.foye@gmail.com

T.P. Stitik (ed.), *Injection Procedures: Osteoarthritis and Related Conditions*,
DOI 10.1007/978-0-387-76595-2_10, © Springer Science+Business Media, LLC 2011

Table 10.1 Summary of hip region injection procedures

Injection Type	Specific structure	Meta-analysis(es)	Prospective study (Studies)	Case series/report(s)	Described in review article(s) and/or injection textbook(s)
Articulation/joint	Hip joint		X [1–3]	X	X [4–6]
Bursa	Trochanteric bursa		X [7, 8]	X	X [6, 9, 10]
	Iliopsoas bursa (psoas bursa)			X [11, 12]	X [6, 13–16]
	Ischial Bursa				X [17–19]
Nerve Blocks	Lateral femoral cutaneous nerve				X [20–22]
Tendons	Hamstring origin				X [6, 17]

The content of this table is listed within each injection type in order of descending amount of current evidence supporting its use. Except in the case of hip joint and trochanteric bursa injections, where many case series and/or reports have been reported, references are provided for all meta-analyses, prospective studies, and case series/case reports along with at least one reference to descriptions in review articles or injection textbooks. For those procedures that are only described in review articles and/or textbooks, representative references are provided.

describe an injection procedure for tendonopathy (e.g. of the gluteus medius tendon, the short hip external rotators [especially the piriformis and obturator externus], and the iliotibial band) in the region of the greater trochanter. Instead, injections into the trochanteric bursa are described, thus implying that a trochanteric bursa injection can potentially address both conditions.

Viscosupplementation injections are currently used for knee joint osteoarthritis (OA), but (at the time of this writing) similar use for hip OA has not yet been approved by the US Food and Drug Administration (FDA). However, evidence is mounting regarding the effectiveness of viscosupplementation for hip OA pain [23–26].

There is a modest but growing body of literature supporting the use of fluoroscopic guidance or ultrasound guidance in the performance of injections into various musculoskeletal regions [27]. Such image guidance may better ensure that the injectate actually reaches the target site and may minimize complications. Image guidance can be helpful for trochanteric bursal injections, which traditionally were performed using surface landmarks alone. For example, use of contrast during fluoroscopy can help ensure that the injectate is not intravascular, which would otherwise result in the injectate flowing away from the intended target site and potentially causing systemic complications such as steroid-induced hyperglycemia or anesthetic-induced toxicities. Image guidance is particularly important for deeper injections (e.g., intra-articular hip joint). Unlike the knee joint where synovial fluid aspiration can often, but not always, help confirm intra-articular placement of the needle tip, it is uncommon to blindly aspirate synovial fluid from the hip joint. In that situation, injecting a small amount of contrast under fluoroscopic guidance or use of ultrasound guidance can help confirm intra-articular placement. Accurate, intra-articular placement would seem particularly important for viscosupplementation injections (if eventually approved for use at the hip joint) since viscosupplements are generally believed to be incapable of diffusing across the joint capsule and if deposited extra-articularly would not reach the target structure. It is possible that image guidance may eventually become the gold standard, or at least the preferred method, for injections at the hip region, particularly for viscosupplementation.

There is a stark lack of published guidelines on predicting who will likely respond best to a given injection. However, one author (PMF) has found that the small percentage of lateral hip pain patients with tendon and/or a bursal calcification may experience less dramatic and less sustained improvement from local corticosteroid injections, compared with patients without such calcifications. It is likely that these patients are experiencing discomfort due to chronic tendonopathy and are therefore less likely to respond to a corticosteroid injection, an intervention best suited for acute pathology.

As is true for injections into other body regions, hip region injections have the potential for a postprocedural increase in local discomfort at the injection site as well as bleeding, bruising, and adverse reaction to the substances injected. Some complications vary by injection site. Local injections for trochanteric bursitis and/or tendonopathy appear to have very low risks of complications. Special attention to sterile technique should be used for intra-articular hip joint injections to avoid introducing bacteria that could cause a septic joint. Intra-articular hip joint injections and iliopsoas bursal injections should also strive to avoid injury to blood vessels in the groin (femoral artery and vein and profundus branch of the femoral artery) by palpation and staying lateral to these structures [13]. Intra-articular hip joint injections with corticosteroid have been reported to increase the risk of postoperative infection in patients who subsequently undergo a total hip arthroplasty (total hip replacement) [28], while a more recent study refutes this [29]. Indeed, some authors specifically advocate such hip injections for patients who are on a waiting list for surgery [4]. Nerve injuries and/or transient neural blockade are possible complications of injections into the hip joint (femoral nerve), iliopsoas bursa (femoral nerve), and trochanteric region (sciatic nerve), but usually these are avoided with proper placement [14]. One author (TPS) witnessed a temporary femoral nerve block that he believes was derived from the local anesthetic that was injected into the overlying soft tissue prior to the otherwise uneventful fluoroscopic-guided intra-articular diagnostic injection which unequivocally confirmed proper intra-articular placement.

Some of the less common injection procedures into the hip region include injections into the ischial (aka ischiogluteal or subgluteus maximus) bursa and into the common origin of the hamstring tendons. Because the hamstring tendons insert onto the ischial tuberosity, which is also the site of the ischial tuberosity bursa, chronic hamstring tendonitis (enthesitis) and ischial tuberosity bursitis can coexist. It can therefore be difficult to differentiate between these two conditions by history, physical examination, and even injection procedures as injections could potentially affect both the bursa and the hamstring origin. Some historical clues that favor bursitis as the predominant lesion include chronic sitting – the condition has been described in weavers and is therefore also known as weaver's bursitis – or acute trauma such as due to a fall onto the bursa. Historical clues that are more consistent with hamstring tendonitis include overuse activities that could potentially strain the common origin of the hamstring tendons. On physical examination, significant pain with direct palpation over the ischial tuberosity is more suggestive of bursitis, whereas pain with resisted knee flexion and/or extension is more suggestive of hamstring tendonitis. It has been the authors' collective experience that image-guidance should be used in order to maximize the probability of accurate injection. Another hip region injection procedure is used for the diagnosis and/or treatment of meralgia paresthetica. Injections in the vicinity of the lateral femoral cutaneous nerve as it passes under the inguinal ligament have been described as outlined in Table 10.1. While this injection can reportedly be done via landmark population, the authors believe that the injection can be performed more accurately using electrodiagnostic testing (EMG) guidance with or without image-guidance.

References

1. Qvistgaard E, Christensen R, Torp-Pedersen S, Bliddal H. Intra-articular treatment of hip steoarthritis: a randomized trial of hyaluronic acid, corticosteroid, and isotonic saline. Osteoarthritis Cartilage 2006;14(2):163–170.
2. Kullenberg B, Runesson R, Tuvhag R, Olsson C, Resch S. Intraarticular corticosteroid injection: pain relief in osteoarthritis of the hip? J Rheumatol 2004;31(11):2265–2268.
3. Flanagan J, Casale FF, Thomas TL, Desai KB. Intra-articular injection for pain relief in patients awaiting hip replacement. Ann R Coll Surg Eng 1988;70(3):156–157.
4. Saunders S. Hip treatments. In Law M, ed. Injection Techniques in Orthopaedic and Sports Medicine. Second edition. London: WB Saunders; 2002:70–71.

5. Waldman SD. Intra-articular injection of the hip joint. In Bralow L, Ross A, Carino M, eds. Atlas of Pain Management Injection Techniques. Philadelphia, PA: WB Saunders; 2000:201–203.

6. Kesson M, Atkins E, Davies I. The hip. In Kesson M, Atkins E, Davies I, eds. Musculoskeletal Injection Skills. New York: Butterworth Heinemann; 2002:112–127.

7. Shbeeb MI, O'Duffy JD, Michet CJ, Jr., O'Fallon WM, Matteson EL. Evaluation of glucocorticosteroid injection for the treatment of trochanteric bursitis. J Rheumatol 1996;23(12):2104–2106.

8. Cohen SP, Narvaez JC, Lebovits AH, Stojanovic MP. Corticosteroid injections for trochanteric bursitis: is fluoroscopy necessary? A pilot study. Br J Anaesth 2005;94(1):100–6.

9. Saunders S. Hip treatments. In Law M, ed. Injection Techniques in Orthopaedic and Sports Medicine. Second edition. London: W.B. Saunders; 2002:76–77.

10. Waldman SD. Trochanteric bursitis pain. In Bralow L, Ross A, Carino M, eds. Atlas of Pain Management Injection Techniques. Philadelphia, PA: WB Saunders; 2000:219–221.

11. Silver SF, Connell DG, Duncan CP. Case report 550: Snapping right iliopsoas tendon. Skeletal Radiol 1989;18(4):327–328.

12. Schaberg JE, Harper MC, Allen WC. The snapping hip syndrome. Am J Sports Med 1984;12(5):361–365.

13. Saunders S. Hip treatments. In Law M, ed. Injection Techniques in Orthopaedic and Sports Medicine. Second edition. London: WB Saunders; 2002:74–75.

14. Waldman SD. Psoas bursitis. In Ross A, Chappelle A, eds. Atlas of Uncommon Pain Syndromes: Philadelphia: WB Saunders; 2003:191–193.

15. Waldman SD. Psoas bursitis pain. In Bralow L, Ross A, Carino M, eds. Atlas of Pain Management Injection Techniques. Philadelphia, PA: WB Saunders; 2000:213–215.

16. Johnston CA, Wiley JP, Lindsay DM, Wiseman DA. Iliopsoas bursitis and tendinitis. A review. Sports Med 1998;25(4):271–283.

17. Saunders S. Hip treatments. In Law M, ed. Injection Techniques in Orthopaedic and Sports Medicine. Second edition. London: WB Saunders; 2002:80–81.

18. Waldman SD. Ischial bursitis pain. In Bralow L, Ross A, Carino M, eds. Atlas of Pain Management Injection Techniques. Philadelphia, PA: WB Saunders; 2000:207–209.

19. Waldman SD. Continuous regional analgesia. In Andjelkovic N, Chappelle A, eds. Interventional Pain Management. Second edition. Philadelphia, PA: WB Saunders; 2001:430.

20. Ferra Verdera M, Ribera Leclerc H, Garrido Pastor JP. [2 cases of paresthetic meralgia of the femoral cutaneous nerve] Rev Esp Anestesiol Reanim 2003;50(3):154–156.

21. Grossman MG, Ducey SA, Nadler SS, Levy AS. Meralgia paresthetica: diagnosis and treatment. A review. J Am Acad Orthop Surg 2001;9(5):336–44.

22. Waldman SD. Ischial bursitis pain. In Bralow L, Ross A, Carino M, eds. Atlas of Pain Management Injection Techniques. Philadelphia: WB Saunders; 2000:240–242.

23. Van Den Bekerom MP, Rys B, Mulier M. Viscosupplementation in the hip: evaluation of hyaluronic acid formulations. Arch Orthop Trauma Surg 2008;128(3):275–80.

24. Gaston MS, Tiemessen CH, Philips JE. Intra-articular hip viscosupplementation with synthetic hyaluronic acid for osteoarthritis: efficacy, safety, and relation to pre-injection radiographs. Arch Orthop Trauma Surg 2007;127(10):899–903.

25. Migliore A, Tormenta S, Massafra U, Martin Martin LS, Carloni E, Padalino C et al. 18-month observational study on efficacy of intraarticular hyaluronic acid (Hylan G-F 20) injections under ultrasound guidance in hip osteoarthritis. Reumatismo 2006;58(1):39–49.

26. Migliore A, Tormenta S, Martin Martin LS, Iannessi F, Massafra U, Carloni E et al. The symptomatic effects of intra-articular administration of hylan G-F 20 on osteoarthritis of the hip: clinical data of 6 months follow-up. Clin Rheumatol 2006;25(3):389–393.

27. Foye PM, Stitik TP. Fluoroscopic guidance during injections for osteoarthritis. Arch Phys Med Rehabil 2006;87(3):446–447.

28. Kaspar S, de V de Beer J. Infection in hip arthroplasty after previous injection of steroid. J Bone Joint Surg Br 2005;87(4):454–457.

29. Chitre AR, Fehily MJ, Bamford DJ. Total hip replacement after intra-articular injection of local anaesthetic and steroid. J Bone Joint Surg Br 2007;89(2):166–168.

Procedure Instructions

Injection Procedure: Iliopsoas Bursa Injection

1. Indications:
   (a) Iliopsoas bursitis diagnosis as pain generator or treatment
   (b) Snapping hip syndrome (patients with history of trauma or total hip arthroplasty) [1]

2. Contraindications especially pertinent to this procedure:
   (a) None documented

3. Possible side effects especially pertinent to this procedure:
   (a) Femoral nerve palsy [2]
   (b) Neurovascular injury

4. Technical details of note for this procedure (Fig. 10.1):
   (a) Preferred needle gauge; length; type:
      • Aspiration ±/- injection: 22–25-gauge, 3½-in. spinal needle [3]
   (b) Need for image guidance: Recommended
      • The use of ultrasound guidance has been recommended for iliopsoas injections, as it allows real-time verification of needle placement, while also being able to confirm the distribution of the medication. Sonography provides the added benefit of visualizing the neurovascular bundle and soft-tissue interfaces that cannot be envisioned using fluoroscopic guidance. This helps avoid these structures and prevent neurovascular injury [2]. The use of this method also allows the physician to compare the patient's symptomatic tendon with the unaffected side, taking note of any structural differences that may be present [4]. According to Adler and colleagues, a lateral approach is recommended, as the neurovascular bundle is located medial to the iliopsoas tendon, thus decreasing the possibility of injury [2].

5. Step-by-step procedure:
   (a) Informed consent
   (b) Preprocedural testing: Identify and record the response to a physical examination preprocedural provocative maneuver if the procedure is a diagnostic injection.
   (c) Image-guidance: Recommended: Ultrasound-guided procedure
   (d) Patient positioning:
      • Place the patient in a supine position.
   (e) Identification and marking of injection site:
      • Palpate the skin entry site, identifying a spot 3 fingerbreadths distal and 3 fingerbreadths lateral to the femoral pulse, and determine the most optimal needle entry site.
      • Mark the target using a marker or by depressing the skin with a plastic needle cap.

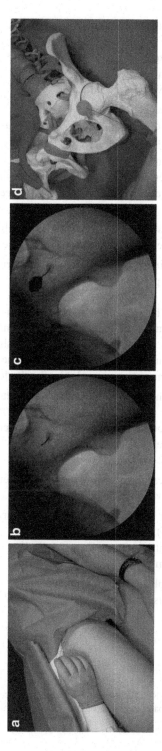

Fig. 10.1 Iliopsoas bursa injection (fluoroscopic-guided). (**a**) Iliopsoas bursa injection-human model. (**b**) Fluoroscopic image of needle entry into iliopsoas bursa. (**c**) Fluoroscopic image of iliopsoas bursogram. (**d**) Skeletal representation of iliopsoas bursa injection

(f) Skin preparation: Initial: Betadine® preparation using the no-touch technique

(g) Medication preparation:
  • Diagnostic injection:
    – 5 mL 1% preservative-free lidocaine
  • Therapeutic injection:
    – 40 mg Depo-Medrol® and 2 mL 1% preservative-free lidocaine

(h) Skin preparation: Final: Alcohol prep

(i) Local anesthesia administration:
  • Anesthetize the overlying skin and soft tissue using a *small amount of 1% lidocaine*, delivered via a *25 gauge 1½-in. needle.*

(j) Needle placement:
  • Pierce the previously anesthetized skin and subcutaneous tissue site with the appropriate needle and direct to the target.

(k) Aspiration: Rule out intravascular entry and confirm entry into bursa (if enough bursal fluid is present to allow aspiration).

(l) Contrast injection:
  • Inject the iliopsoas bursa with enough contrast to confirm entry into the target structure. Connecting the contrast dye syringe to the needle using extension tubing is recommended to prevent a shift in needle position during attachment and detachment to and from the spinal needle. Adjust needle position, if necessary, in order to clearly define an arthrogram.

(m) Injection: Unclamp the aspiration syringe and clamp on the injection syringe.
  • If resistance is encountered early during the injection, rotate the needle to dislodge the bevel from the bursal membrane.

(n) Postprocedural testing:
  • If applicable, reassess the response to the aforementioned preprocedural provocative maneuver.

(o) If (+) response, repeat injection with therapeutic injectate:
  • Repeat steps (d)–(f).
  • Medication preparation: 40 mg Depo-Medrol®.
  • Repeat steps (h)–(m).

(p) *Adhesive bandage* application over the needle entry site

(q) Postprocedural care discussion

References

1. VamLaro JP, Sauser DD, Beals RK. Iliopsoas bursa imaging. Efficacy in depicting abnormal iliopsoas tendon motion in patients with internal snapping hip syndrome. Radiology 1995;197:853–856.

2. Adler RS, Buly R, Ambrose R, Sculco T. Diagnostic and therapeutic use of sonography-guided iliopsoas peritendinous injections. AJR Am J Roentgenol 2005;185:940–943.
3. Blankenbaker D, De Smet A, Keene J. Sonography of the iliopsoas tendon and injection of the iliopsoas bursa for diagnosis and management of the painful snapping hip. Skeletal Radiol 2006;35:565–571.
4. Wank R, Miller THE, Shapiro JF. Sonographically guided injection of anesthetic for iliopsoas tendonapthy after total hip arthroplasty. J Clin Ultrasound 2004;32:354–357.

Injection Procedure: Intra-articular Hip Injection

1. Indications:
   (a) Hip joint osteoarthritis diagnosis as a pain generator (96% sensitivity) [1]
   (b) Hip joint rheumatoid arthritis diagnosis as a pain generator (87% sensitivity) [2]
   (c) Intra-articular corticosteroid injection
   (d) Intra-articular viscosupplementation injection (not currently FDA-approved)

2. Contraindications especially pertinent to this procedure:
   (a) None documented

3. Possible side effects especially pertinent to this procedure:
   (a) Femoral artery injury
   (b) Femoral nerve injury
   (c) Lateral femoral cutaneous nerve injury
   (d) Septic arthritis/purulent coxitis [3]

4. Technical details of note for this procedure (Fig. 10.2):
   (a) Preferred needle gauge; length; type:
     • Aspiration ±/- injection: 25-gauge; 3½ in.; spinal
   (b) Need for image guidance: Recommended
     • While fluoroscopic guidance is still not necessarily considered the gold standard for intra-articular hip injections, it is strongly recommended. Leopold and colleagues conducted a study in which 30 cadaver hips were injected using either an anterior or lateral approach without radiographic guidance. The specimens were dissected to identify the rate of success and proximity to neurovascular structures. The study showed that there was only a 60% success rate with an anterior approach and an 80% success rate with the lateral approach. Using the anterior approach, the femoral nerve was contacted or pierced 27% of the time and the needle was within 5 mm of the femoral nerve in 60% of the attempts. The needle was never placed within 25 mm of any neurovascular structures when using the lateral approach [4].
     • In contrast, Mauffrey and Pobbathy recommended a palpation technique in which anatomic landmarks were used in a lateral approach to the hip injection. With this method, they reported a 95% (19/20) accuracy of intra-articular placement without the use of fluoroscopic guidance. Therefore, they recommend the use of palpation of anatomic landmarks as their preferred approach [5].
     • Several studies have also shown that ultrasound is a viable alternative to fluoroscopy, giving the added benefit of being able to more readily detect joint space narrowing and osteophyte formation. These added features may aid in monitoring and predicting response to treatment [6]. The use of ultrasound guidance also allows the physician to recognize and avoid the neurovascular structures that can be injured with this procedure. Although fluoroscopic guidance can detect needle penetration onto vascular structures with the use of a contrast agent, this is not detected

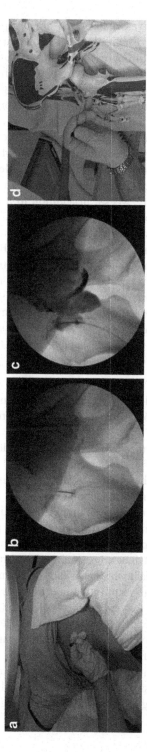

Fig. 10.2 Hip joint injection (fluoroscopic-guided). (**a**) Hip joint injection-human model. (**b**) Fluoroscopic image of needle entry through hip joint capsule. (**c**) Fluoroscopic image of contrast within the hip joint capsule. (**d**) Skeletal representation of hip joint injection

until after the blood vessel has been already penetrated. In contrast, ultrasound can allow visualization of vascular structures prior to needle placement. As is true of fluoroscopic guidance, ultrasound can also confirm accurate placement of the injection into the intra-articular space [7]. To date, no studies have been reported regarding the accuracy of ultrasound-guided intra-articular hip injections. Nonetheless, this method may become a viable alternative to fluoroscopy.

(c) Preferred corticosteroid dosage: 80 mg Depo-Medrol®
   • Robinson and colleagues conducted a study in which they compared the effectiveness of 40 mg versus 80 mg Depo-Medrol®. Based on their results, they concluded that the 80mg dose led to a statistically greater relief of stiffness at 12 weeks, in addition to a statistically significant improvement in disability at 6 and 12 weeks [8].

(d) Intra-articular hip viscosupplementation:
   • To date, viscosupplementation has only received FDA approval for use in the knee joint. While most studies refer to its effectiveness within the knee, several studies have been conducted regarding its use within the hip. Migliore and coworkers reported a statistically significant reduction of pain for up to 6 months following hip viscosupplementation (37.8% reduction in VAS). They also reported a statistically significant reduction of NSAID use 6 months after viscosupplementation (69.9% reduction) [9].

5. Step-by-step procedure:
   (a) Informed consent
   (b) Preprocedural testing: Identify and record the response to a physical examination preprocedural provocative maneuver if the procedure is a diagnostic injection.
   (c) Image guidance: Recommended: Fluoroscopic-guided procedure
   (d) Patient positioning:
      • Place the patient on the fluoroscopy table in a supine position.
   (e) Identification and marking of injection site:
      • Palpate for the femoral artery and make note of its location or mark the overlying skin. Just medial to this is the femoral nerve.
      • Palpate the anterior superior iliac spine and make note of its location or mark the overlying skin and draw a line straight down from it along the patient's upper thigh. Just medial to this line is the lateral femoral cutaneous nerve.
      • Fluoroscopy is used to identify the injection site located in between the location of the lateral femoral cutaneous nerve and the femoral nerve and above the level of the greater trochanter, but below the level of the inferior aspect of the acetabulum. This structure can sometimes be faintly seen as a shadow that traverses the femoral neck (Fig. 10.2).
      • The target injection site is through the hip joint capsule so that the needle ends up on the cortex of the femoral neck (Fig. 10.2).
      • Mark the target using a marker or by depressing the skin with a plastic needle cap.

(f) Skin preparation: Initial: Betadine® preparation using the no-touch technique
(g) Medication preparation:
- Diagnostic injection:
  - 5 mL 1% preservative-free lidocaine
- Therapeutic injection:
  - 80 mg Depo-Medrol® and 2 mL 1% preservative-free lidocaine
(h) Skin preparation: Final: Alcohol prep
(i) Local anesthesia administration:
- Anesthetize the overlying skin and soft tissue using a *small amount of 1% lidocaine* delivered via a *25 gauge 1½-in. needle.*
(j) Needle placement:
- Pierce the previously anesthetized skin and subcutaneous tissue site with the appropriate needle and direct to the target.
(k) Aspiration: Rule out intravascular entry and confirm entry into bursa (if enough bursal fluid is present to allow aspiration) or target structure.
(l) Contrast injection:
- Inject the joint with enough contrast to confirm entry into the target structure. Connecting the contrast dye syringe to the needle using extension tubing is recommended to prevent a shift in needle position during attachment and detachment to and from the spinal needle. Adjust the needle position, if necessary, in order to obtain a clearly defined arthrogram.
(m) Injection: Unclamp the aspiration syringe and clamp on the injection syringe.
- If resistance is encountered early during the injection, rotate the needle to dislodge the bevel from the side of the joint.
(n) Postprocedural testing:
- If applicable, reassess the response to the aforementioned preprocedural provocative maneuver.
(o) If (+) response, repeat injection with therapeutic injectate:
- Repeat steps (d)–(f).
- Medication preparation: 80 mg Depo-Medrol® with 2 mL 1% preservative-free lidocaine
- Repeat steps (h)–(m).
(p) *Adhesive bandage* application over the needle entry site
(q) Postprocedural care discussion

References

1. Crawford RW, Gie GA, Ling RSM, Murray DW. Diagnostic value of intra-articular anesthetic in primary osteoarthritis of the hip. J Bone Joint Surg 1998;80-B (2):279.
2. Kleiner JB, Thorne RP, Curd JG. The value of bupivicaine hip injection in the differentiation of coxarthrosis from lower extremity neuropathy. J Rheumatol 1991;18(3):422–427.

3. Broeng L, Hansen LB. Purulent coxitis after blockade treatment. Ugeskr Laeger 1991; 153(42):2962. Danish.
4. Leopold SS, Battista V, Oliverio JA. Safety and efficacy of intraarticular hip injection using anatomic landmarks. Clin Orthop Relat Res 2001;391:192–197.
5. Mauffrey C, Pobbathy Hip joint injection technique using anatomic landmarks: are we accurate? A prospective study. Internet J Orthop Surg 2006;3(1).
6. Karim Z, Brown AK, Quinn M, Wakefield RJ, Conaghan PG, Emery P et al. Ultrasound-guided steroid injections in the treatment of hip osteoarthritis: Comment on the letter by Margules. Arthritis Rheum 2004;50(1):338–9.
7. Smith J, Hurdle MF. Office-based ultrasound guided intra-articular hip injection: Technique for physiatric practice. Arch Phys Med Rehabil 2006;87:296–298.
8. Robinson P, Keenan AM, Conaghan PG. Clinical effectiveness and dose response of image-guided intra-articular corticosteroid injection for hip osteoarthritis. Rheumatology (Oxford) 2007; 46(2):285–291.
9. Migliore A, Tormenta S, Martin LS, Iannessi F, Massafra U, Carloni E et al. The symptomatic effects of intra-articular administration of hylan G-F 20 on osteoarthritis of the hip: clinical data of 6 months follow-up. Clin Rheumatol 2006;25:389–393.

Injection Procedure: Ischial Bursa Injection

1. Indications:
   (a) Differentiation of ischial bursitis ("Weaver's Bottom") from radiculopathy as the pain generator for inferior gluteal pain.
   (b) Ischial bursitis treatment

2. Contraindications especially pertinent to this procedure:
   (a) None documented.

3. Possible side effects especially pertinent to this procedure:
   (a) Trauma to the sciatic nerve is possible if the needle is directed too laterally [1].

4. Technical details of note for this procedure (Fig. 10.3):
   (a) Preferred needle gauge; length; type:
      • *Aspiration ±/- injection: 25-gauge or 22-gauge*; spinal of appropriate length depending upon body habitus
   (b) Need for image guidance: Highly recommended

5. Step-by-step procedure:
   (a) Informed consent
   (b) Preprocedural testing: Identify and record the response to a physical examination preprocedural provocative maneuver if the procedure is a diagnostic injection.
      • Sitting should be uncomfortable in patients with ischial bursitis.
   (c) Image guidance: Recommended: Fluoroscopic-guided
   (d) Patient positioning:
      • Place the patient in a prone position on the fluoroscopic table with the inferior gluteal region exposed.
      • If necessary, the patient's hip and knee can be flexed in order to bring the ischial tuberosity closer to the surface.
   (e) Identification and marking of injection site:
      • If fluoroscopic-guided:
         – Visualize the target structure by positioning the c-arm fluoroscope with the intensifier angled either caudad or cephalad so as to allow optional visualization of the structure. Then palpate deeply so as to touch the ischial tuberosity.
      • Mark the target using a marker or by depressing the skin with a plastic needle cap.
   (f) Skin preparation: Initial: Betadine® preparation using the no-touch technique
   (g) Medication preparation:
      • Diagnostic injection:
         – 4 mL of 1% preservative-free lidocaine
      • Therapeutic injection:
         – 40 mg Depo-Medrol® and 4 mL of 1% preservative-free lidocaine
   (h) Skin preparation: Final: Alcohol prep

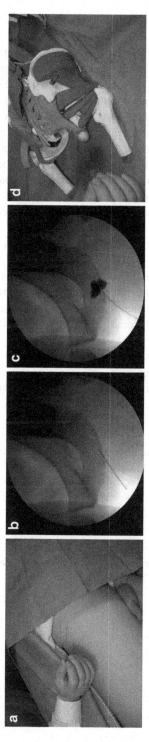

Fig. 10.3 Ischial bursa injection (fluoroscopic-guided). (**a**) Ischial bursa injection-human model. (**b**) Fluoroscopic image of needle entry into ischial bursa. (**c**) Fluoroscopic image of ischial bursogram. (**d**) Skeletal representation of ischial bursa injection

(i) Local anesthesia administration: Optional
(j) Needle placement:
- Pierce the previously anesthetized skin and subcutaneous tissue site with the appropriate needle and direct to the target.
- If nonimage-guided: Advance the needle until contact is made with the ischial tuberosity. Then withdraw the needle slightly.
- If fluoroscopic-guided: Use intermittent fluoroscopic guidance to directly visualize needle advancement onto the ischial tuberosity. Intermittent fluoroscopy can also help to prevent excessive lateral advancement of the spinal needle, which could injure the sciatic nerve.
(k) Aspiration: Rule out intravascular entry and confirm entry into bursa (if enough bursal fluid is present to allow aspiration).
(l) Injection: Unclamp the aspiration syringe and clamp on the injection syringe.
- If nonimage-guided: Maintain needle position while injecting medication.
- If fluoroscopic-guided: Use intermittent fluoroscopic guidance to visualize the injection by observing the change in the dye pattern.
- If resistance is encountered early during the injection, rotate the needle to dislodge the bevel from the surface of the ischial tuberosity.
(m) Postprocedural testing:
- If applicable, reassess the response to the aforementioned preprocedural provocative maneuver.
(n) If (+) response, repeat injection with therapeutic injectate:
- Repeat steps (d)–(f).
- Medication preparation: 40 mg Depo-Medrol®
- Repeat steps (h)–(l).
(o) Apply adhesive bandage over the needle entry site.
(p) Postprocedural care discussion

Reference

1. Waldman S. Atlas of Pain Management Injection Techniques. Philadelphia, PA: WB Saunders; 2000:242.

Injection Procedure: Lateral Femoral Cutaneous Nerve Block

1. Indications:
   (a) Differentiation of anterolateral thigh pain due to lateral femoral cutaneous neuropathy (meralgia paresthetica) from other potential sources, especially high lumbar radiculopathy
   (b) Lateral femoral diagnosis as pain generator or treatment

2. Contraindications especially pertinent to this procedure:
   (a) None documented

3. Possible side effects especially pertinent to this procedure:
   (a) Injection into the femoral artery or vein if needle placed too medially.
   (b) Penetration into peritoneal cavity and perforation of the colon if needle placed too cephalad and deep [1]

4. Technical details of note for this procedure (Fig. 10.4):
   (a) Preferred needle gauge; length; type:
      • If nonimage-guided: 25-gauge; 1½ in.; straight
      • If image-guided: 25-gauge; short; spinal
   (b) Need for image and/or EMG guidance: Optional.
      • While ultrasound guidance can help identify femoral vasculature, palpation should be sufficient to do this. An extensive review of the literature did not reveal specific studies or information regarding the use of fluoroscopic or ultrasound guidance for lateral femoral cutaneous nerve injections. The authors have some limited clinical experience with the use of EMG guidance for this procedure specifically. Specifically, a surface or needle stimulating electrode can be used in an attempt to help localize the nerve. The nerve can be stimulated on the patient, who can be asleep, to identify when he/she detects a change in or the production of paresthesias in the expected distribution of the lateral femoral cutaneous nerve in the thigh. Theoretically, by adjusting the stimulator position, one can localize the nerve location. However, if there is complete nerve impulse blockage (conduction block) at the site of pathology (generally at the inguinal ligament), this can prevent the patient from sensing paresthesia production. Alternatively, one could attempt to record a sensory nerve action potential (SNAP) from the anterolateral thigh surface; however, this is technically extremely difficult even on the uninvolved side. Furthermore, failure to record a SNAP from the clinically unaffected nerve is what leads to the performance of a diagnostic injection in the first place.

5. Step-by-step procedure:
   (a) Informed consent
   (b) Preprocedural testing: Identify and record the response to a physical examination preprocedural provocative maneuver if the procedure is a diagnostic injection.

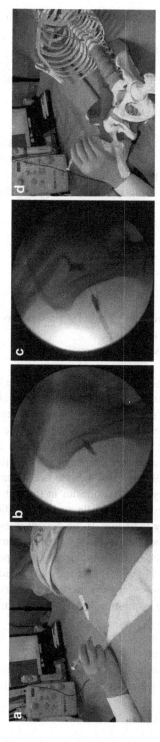

Fig. 10.4 Lateral femoral cutaneous nerve block (fluoroscopic-guided). (**a**) Lateral femoral cutaneous nerve block-human model. (**b**) Fluoroscopic image of needle entry slightly inferior and medial to anterior superior iliac spine. (**c**) Fluoroscopic image of lateral femoral cutaneous nerve block. (**d**) Skeletal representation of lateral femoral cutaneous nerve block

- In cases of meralgia paresthetica, pain can often be reproduced with standing or walking.

(c) Image guidance: Optional

(d) Patient positioning:
  - Place the patient in a supine position with the patient's anterior pelvis exposed.

(e) Identification and marking of injection site:
  - If nonimage-guided:
    - Identify the target structure by identifying the ASIS and inguinal ligament by palpation. The target site is approximately 1-in. medial to the ASIS and inferior to the inguinal ligament [2].
  - Mark the target using a marker or by depressing the skin with a plastic needle cap.

(f) Skin preparation: Initial: Betadine® preparation using the no-touch technique

(g) Medication preparation:
  - Diagnostic injection:
    - 5 mL 1% preservative-free lidocaine
  - Therapeutic injection:
    - 20 mg Depo-Medrol® and 5 mL 1% preservative-free lidocaine

(h) Skin preparation: Final: Alcohol prep

(i) Local anesthesia administration: Not applicable

(j) Needle placement:
  - If nonimage and non-EMG-guided: Insert needle perpendicular to the target site on the skin. Advance into soft tissue about 1 in.; however, depending on patient's size, additional advancement might be needed.
  - If EMG-guided: Insert needle (either EMG needle or EMG needle that has been adapted for injections) perpendicular to the target site on the skin. An electrical stimulus is delivered through the EMG needle. The stimulation can be delivered through the needle, and the patient can be asked to report if they feel paresthesias in the distribution of the lateral femoral cutaneous nerve. The needle position is adjusted as needed until the patient maximally feels this. If the patient does not report paresthesias irrespective of needle positioning and/or stimulus intensity, complete conduction block of the impulse might be present. This situation would not be compatible with the use of EMG guidance.

(k) Aspiration: Rule out intravascular entry and confirm entry into target structure.

(l) Injection: Unclamp the aspiration syringe and clamp on the injection syringe.
  - Monitor for symptoms of increased pain, which could suggest needle contact with the nerve.
  - If resistance is encountered early during the injection, rotate the needle to dislodge the bevel from direct contact with the nerve.

(m) Postprocedural testing:
  • If applicable, reassess the response to the same aforementioned preprocedural provocative maneuver.

(n) If (+) response, repeat injection with therapeutic injectate:
  • Repeat steps (d)–(f).
  • Medication preparation: 20 mg Depo-Medrol®
  • Repeat steps (h)–(l).

(o) *Adhesive bandage* application over the needle entry site

(p) Postprocedural care discussion:
  • Emphasize to the patient the need to avoid factors that may be contributing to the neuropathy. These factors can include wearing tight clothing and/or belts that can compress the lateral femoral cutaneous nerve at the inguinal ligament region.

References

1. Waldman SD. Ischial bursitis pain. In Bralow L, Ross A, Carino M, eds. Atlas of Pain Management Injection Techniques. Philadelphia, PA: WB Saunders; 2000:242.
2. Lennard T, Shin D. Pain Procedures in Clinical Practice. Second edition. Philadelphia, PA: Hanley and Belfus; 2000:115.

Injection Procedure: Trochanteric Bursa Injection

1. Indications:
    (a) Differentiation of trochanteric bursitis from other potential causes of lateral hip region/thigh pain, especially referred or radicular lumbar pain and iliotibial band tendonitis without coexistent trochanteric bursitis.
    (b) Trochanteric bursitis diagnosis as pain generator or treatment

2. Contraindications especially pertinent to this procedure:
    (a) None

3. Possible side effects especially pertinent to this procedure:
    (a) Necrotizing fasciitis [1]

4. Technical details of note for this procedure (Fig. 10.5):
    (a) Preferred needle gauge; length; type:
        • Aspiration ±/- injection: 25-gauge; 2–3½ in. spinal
    (b) Need for image guidance: Recommended
        • Fluoroscopic guidance is recommended for injections into the trochanteric bursa. In a study aimed at determining the accuracy of physicians attempting blind trochanteric bursa injections for patients experiencing hip pain, attending physicians obtained a bursagram only 53% of the time on the first attempt [2]. In comparison, fellows were accurate in their placement 46% on the first attempt, and resident physicians only obtained a bursagram 32% of the time with the first attempt. The need for fluoroscopic guidance is likely to be especially important in obese patients. In cases where there is chronic pain, injecting the point of maximal tenderness can often lead to minimal relief, as the patient may have developed peripheral sensitization, where the tenderness is felt at a site other than at the pain generator [3].
        • Ultrasound guidance can instead be used.

5. Step-by-step procedure:
    (a) Informed consent
    (b) Preprocedural testing: Identify and record the response to a physical examination preprocedural provocative maneuver if the procedure is a diagnostic injection.
    (c) Image guidance: Recommended: Fluoroscopic-guided or ultrasound-guided procedure.
    (d) Patient positioning:
        • Place the patient in a lateral recumbent position, with the affected side up on the table. While some recommend that the hip be flexed at a 30–50° angle and the knee flexed at a 60–90° angle [4], the authors have not found hip and knee flexion to offer any advantage over the hip and knee being kept in a neutral position.
    (e) Identification and marking of injection site:

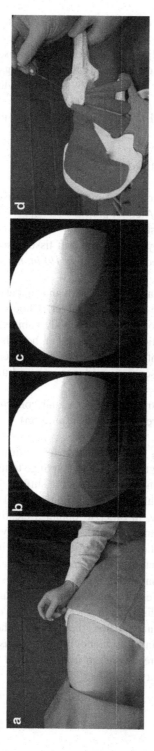

Fig. 10.5 Greater trochanteric bursa injection (fluoroscopic-guided). (**a**) Greater trochanteric bursa injection-human model. (**b**) Fluoroscopic image of needle entry into greater trochanteric bursa. (**c**) Fluoroscopic image of greater trochanteric bursogram. (**d**) Skeletal representation of greater trochanteric bursa injection

- Rotate the c-arm fluoroscope so that it is placed in an AP or PA position relative to the patient.
- Use fluoroscopy to adjust the position of a fluoroscopic metallic marker on the skin so that it corresponds to the underlying trochanteric process.
- Mark the target using a marker or by depressing the skin with a plastic needle cap.

(f) Skin preparation: Initial: Betadine® preparation using the no-touch technique
(g) Medication preparation:
- Diagnostic injection:
  - 5 mL 1% preservative-free lidocaine
- Therapeutic injection:
  - 80 mg Depo-Medrol® and 1 mL 1% preservative-free lidocaine

(h) Skin preparation: Final: Alcohol prep
(i) Local anesthesia administration:
- Anesthetize the overlying skin and soft tissue using a *small amount of 1% lidocaine* delivered via a *25 gauge 1½-in. needle.*

(j) Needle placement:
- Pierce the previously anesthetized skin and subcutaneous tissue site with the appropriate needle and direct to target. (Choose the needle length that is most appropriate for the patient's body habitus. The required needle length can vary significantly depending on body habitus.)
- Attempt to make contact with the tip of the trochanteric process. Use intermittent fluoroscopic guidance to adjust needle position accordingly.

(k) Aspiration: Rule out intravascular entry and confirm entry into bursa (if enough bursal fluid is present to allow aspiration).
(l) Contrast injection:
- Inject the bursa with enough contrast to confirm entry into the target structure. Connecting the contrast dye syringe to the needle using extension tubing is recommended to prevent a shift in needle position during attachment and detachment to and from the spinal needle. Adjust needle position, if necessary, in order to obtain a clearly defined bursagram. Obtaining a bursagram can be difficult and may require a significant amount of adjustment of needle position. It is not uncommon for the dye pattern to reveal injection into the tensor fascia lata below or above the gluteus medius tendon. If this occurs, the needle should be repositioned so that subsequent dye injection does not reveal further uptake into those tendons. At times, a discrete bursagram cannot be obtained and one must settle for a dye pattern that bathes the greater trochanteric region without showing evidence of intravascular or intratendinous uptake. Alternatively, the contrast might spread either in front or behind the trochanter without showing a definite bursagram.

(m) Injection: Unclamp the aspiration syringe and clamp on the injection syringe.
- If resistance is encountered early during the injection, rotate the needle to dislodge the bevel from the side of the joint.

(n) Postprocedural testing:
- If applicable, reassess response to the aforementioned preprocedural provocative maneuver.

(o) If (+) response, repeat injection with therapeutic injectate:
- Repeat steps (d)–(f).
- Medication preparation: 80 mg Depo-Medrol®
- Repeat steps (h)–(m).

(p) *Adhesive bandage* application over the needle entry site

(q) Postprocedural care discussion

References

1. Hofmeister E, Engelhardt S. Necrotizing fasciitis as complication of injection into greater trochanteric bursa. Am J Orthop 2001;30(5):426–427.
2. Cohen SP, Narvaez JC, Lebovits AH, Stojanovic MP. Corticosteroid injections for trochanteric bursitis: is fluoroscopy necessary? A pilot study. Br J Anaesth 2005;94(1):100–106.
3. Foye P, Stitik T, Nadler S. Trochanteric Bursitis. E-medicine. 2006 June.
4. Cardone DA, Tallia AF. Diagnostic and therapeutic injection of the hip and knee. Am Fam Physician 2003;67(10):2147–2152.

Injection Procedure Templates

Injection Procedure Template: Iliopsoas Bursa Injection

PROCEDURE: Iliopsoas Bursa Injection
Side: ☐-Right   ☐-Left   ☐-Bilateral
Procedure Type: Aspiration: ☐-Diagnostic aspiration
                    Injection: ☐-Diagnostic   ☐-Therapeutic   ☐-Diagnostic then Therapeutic
Image guidance: None unless indicated as follows- ☐-Fluoroscopy ☐-Ultrasound

- The potential benefits and side effects of the procedure and alternative treatment options were explained to the patient, an opportunity for questions was provided, and the patient signed informed consent.
- ☐- If checked, the following physical examination pre-procedural provocative maneuver(s) was (were) performed: ☐-
  _____
- The patient was positioned for the procedure and the target structure was identified.
- The overlying skin was prepped with Betadine® followed by alcohol prep pad after the Betadine® dried.
- ☐- If checked, the overlying skin and soft tissue was anesthetized using a small amount of 1% lidocaine delivered via the following needle ☐-30G1"; ☐-25G1½"; ☐-Other: _____
- The following needle was then used for the procedure:
    Type: Straight needle unless indicated as follows: ☐-Spinal needle; ☐-Other:_____
    Gauge: ☐-30; ☐-27; ☐-25; ☐-22; ☐-21; -18; Other: _____
    Length: ☐-5/8"; ☐- 1"; ☐- 1 ½"; ☐- 2"; ☐- 2 ½"; ☐- 3";☐- 3½"; ☐-Other:_____
- o   Image guidance if indicated above was used to confirm needle entry into target structure.
- o   ☐-If checked, contrast dye was then injected and the needle position was adjusted accordingly to confirm proper placement without inadvertent intravascular entry.
- Needle was adjusted accordingly to confirm proper placement without inadvertent vascular entry.
- An attempt was made to aspirate from the structure and then the following injectate was delivered into the target structure:
    ☐-Diagnostic injection: 5 mL 1% preservative-free lidocaine; ☐-Other injectate: _____
    ☐-Therapeutic injection: 40 mg Depo-Medrol® & ☐- 2 mL 1% preservative-free bupivacaine
          ☐-Other injectate: _____
- The needle was removed and an adhesive bandage was placed over the needle entry site.

-**If the above was a diagnostic injection, then proceed to section immediately below.**
-**If above was a therapeutic injection procedure, aspiration only procedure, or aspiration and therapeutic injection, then proceed to Procedure Summary Section.**

For Diagnostic Injection Procedure:
- ☐-If checked, the above listed pre-procedural physical examination provocative maneuver was repeated and pain relief was: ☐-
  N/A; ☐-significant; ☐-some; ☐-equivocal; ☐-none; ☐-Other:_____
- Based on the amount of pain relief noted above:
    ☐-a therapeutic injection will be scheduled.
    ☐-a therapeutic injection will not be scheduled. See plan in corresponding office note.
    ☐-a therapeutic injection following the same procedure described above was done using
          ☐- 40 mg Depo-Medrol® & ☐- 2 mL 1% preservative-free lidocaine
          ☐- Other injectate:_____
- The needle was removed and an adhesive bandage was placed over the needle entry site.

Procedure Summary:
If fluid aspirated from the target structure during the procedure:
- Total volume of fluid aspirated: ____ mL; Fluid appearance: ☐- N/A; ☐-Clear yellow; ☐-Slightly cloudy;
    ☐-Cloudy; ☐-Purulent; ☐-Blood-tinged; ☐-Bloody; ☐-Other:_____
Patient tolerance for the procedure: ☐-Excellent; ☐-Good; ☐-Fair; ☐-Other:_____

Additional comments regarding the procedure: ☐-None; ☐Other:_____
_____

Post-Procedural Treatment Advice:
Activity modification: Avoid non-essential use of the structure until seen for follow up. ☐-Other:_____

Orthotic instructions: N/A unless indicated as follows _____
Modalities: Apply ice over the injection site prn for 20-30 min. up to q2 hrs until seen for follow-up, unless instructed as follows: ☐-
Heat; ☐-Other:_____

Injection Procedure Template: Intra-Articular Hip Injections

PROCEDURE: Intra-articular Hip Injections
Side: ☐-Right   ☐-Left   ☐-Bilateral
Procedure Type: Aspiration: ☐-Diagnostic aspiration
           Injection: ☐-Diagnostic   ☐-Therapeutic   ☐-Diagnostic then Therapeutic
Image guidance: None unless indicated as follows- ☐-Fluoroscopy   ☐-Ultrasound
* The potential benefits and side effects of the procedure and alternative treatment options were explained to the patient, an opportunity for questions was provided, and the patient signed informed consent.
* ☐- If checked, the following physical examination pre-procedural provocative maneuver(s) was (were) performed: ☐
  _____
* The patient was positioned for the procedure and the target structure was identified.
* The overlying skin was prepped with Betadine® followed by alcohol prep pad after the Betadine® dried.
* ☐- If checked, the overlying skin and soft tissue was anesthetized using a small amount of 1% lidocaine delivered via the following needle ☐-30G1"; ☐-25G1½"; ☐-Other:_____
* The following needle was then used for the procedure:
       Type: Straight needle unless indicated as follows: ☐-Spinal needle; ☐-Other:_____
       Gauge: ☐-30; ☐-27; ☐-25; ☐-22; ☐-21; -18; Other:_____
       Length: ☐-5/8"; ☐- 1"; ☐- 1 ½"; ☐- 2"; ☐- 2 ½"; ☐- 3"; ☐- 3½"; ☐-Other:_____
o Image guidance if indicated above was used to confirm needle entry into target structure.
o ☐-If checked, contrast dye was then injected and the needle position was adjusted accordingly to confirm proper placement without inadvertent intravascular entry.
* Needle was adjusted accordingly to confirm proper placement without inadvertent vascular entry.
* An attempt was made to aspirate from the structure and then the following injectate was delivered into the target structure:
  ☐-Diagnostic injection: 5 mL 1% preservative-free lidocaine; ☐-Other injectate: _____
  ☐-Therapeutic injection: 80 mg Depo-Medrol® & ☐- 2 mL 1% preservative-free lidocaine
              ☐-Other injectate: _____
* The needle was removed and an adhesive bandage was placed over the needle entry site.

-If the above was a **diagnostic injection**, then proceed to section immediately below.
-If above was a **therapeutic injection procedure, aspiration only procedure,** or **aspiration and therapeutic injection,** then proceed to Procedure Summary Section.

For Diagnostic Injection Procedure:
* ☐-If checked, the above listed pre-procedural physical examination provocative maneuver was repeated and pain relief was: ☐-N/A; ☐-significant; ☐-some; ☐-equivocal; ☐-none; ☐-Other:_____
* Based on the amount of pain relief noted above:
  ☐-a therapeutic injection will be scheduled.
  ☐-a therapeutic injection will not be scheduled. See plan in corresponding office note.
  ☐-a therapeutic injection following the same procedure described above was done using
          ☐- 80 mg Depo-Medrol® & ☐- 2 mL 1% preservative-free lidocaine
          ☐- Other injectate: _____
* The needle was removed and an adhesive bandage was placed over the needle entry site.

Procedure Summary:
If fluid aspirated from the target structure during the procedure:
* Total volume of fluid aspirated: ___ mL; Fluid appearance: ☐- N/A; ☐-Clear yellow; ☐-Slightly cloudy;
  ☐-Cloudy; ☐-Purulent; ☐-Blood-tinged; ☐-Bloody; ☐-Other:_____
Patient tolerance for the procedure: ☐-Excellent; ☐-Good; ☐-Fair; ☐-Other:_____

Additional comments regarding the procedure: ☐-None; ☐Other:_____
_____
_____

Post-Procedural Treatment Advice:
Activity modification: Avoid non-essential use of the structure until seen for follow up. ☐-Other:_____
_____
Orthotic instructions: N/A unless indicated as follows _____
Modalities: Apply ice over the injection site prn for 20-30 min. up to q2 hrs until seen for follow-up, unless instructed as follows: ☐-Heat; ☐-Other:_____

Injection Procedure Template: Ischial Bursa

PROCEDURE: Ischial bursa (Ischiogluteal Bursa; Subgluteus Maximus Bursa) Injection
Side: ☐-Right   ☐-Left   ☐-Bilateral
Procedure Type: Aspiration: ☐-Diagnostic aspiration
Injection: ☐-Diagnostic   ☐-Therapeutic   ☐-Diagnostic then Therapeutic
Image guidance: None unless indicated as follows- ☐-Fluoroscopy   ☐-Ultrasound
- The potential benefits and side effects of the procedure and alternative treatment options were explained to the patient, an opportunity for questions was provided, and the patient signed informed consent.
- ☐- If checked, the following physical examination pre-procedural provocative maneuver(s) was (were) performed: ☐-
  _____
- The patient was positioned for the procedure and the target structure was identified.
- The overlying skin was prepped with Betadine® followed by alcohol prep pad after the Betadine® dried.
- ☐- If checked, the overlying skin and soft tissue was anesthetized using a small amount of 1% lidocaine delivered via the following needle ☐-30G1"; ☐-25G1½ "; ☐-Other: _____
- The following needle was then used for the procedure:
  Type: Straight needle unless indicated as follows: ☐-Spinal needle; ☐-Other:_____
  Gauge: ☐-30; ☐-27; ☐-25; ☐-22; ☐-21; -18; Other:_____
  Length: ☐-5/8"; ☐- 1"; ☐- 1 ½"; ☐- 2"; ☐- 2 ½"; ☐- 3"; ☐- 3½"; ☐-Other:_____
o Image guidance if indicated above was used to confirm needle entry into target structure.
o ☐-If checked, contrast dye was then injected and the needle position was adjusted accordingly to confirm proper placement without inadvertent intravascular entry.
- Needle was adjusted accordingly to confirm proper placement without inadvertent vascular entry.
- An attempt was made to aspirate from the structure and then the following injectate was delivered into the target structure:
  ☐-Diagnostic injection: 4 mL 1% preservative-free lidocaine; ☐-Other injectate: _____
  ☐-Therapeutic injection: 40 mg Depo-Medrol® & ☐- 4 mL 1% preservative-free lidocaine
  ☐-Other injectate:_____
- The needle was removed and an adhesive bandage was placed over the needle entry site.

-If the above was a **diagnostic injection**, then proceed to section immediately below.
-If above was a **therapeutic injection procedure, aspiration only procedure,** or **aspiration and therapeutic injection,** then proceed to Procedure Summary Section.

For Diagnostic Injection Procedure:
- ☐-If checked, the above listed pre-procedural physical examination provocative maneuver was repeated and pain relief was: ☐- N/A; ☐-significant; ☐-some; ☐-equivocal; ☐-none; ☐-Other:_____
- Based on the amount of pain relief noted above:
  ☐-a therapeutic injection will be scheduled.
  ☐-a therapeutic injection will not be scheduled. See plan in corresponding office note.
  ☐-a therapeutic injection following the same procedure described above was done using
  ☐- 40 mg Depo-Medrol® & ☐- 4 mL 1% preservative-free lidocaine
  ☐- Other injectate:_____
- The needle was removed and an adhesive bandage was placed over the needle entry site.

Procedure Summary:
If fluid aspirated from the target structure during the procedure:
- Total volume of fluid aspirated: ___ mL; Fluid appearance: ☐- N/A; ☐-Clear yellow; ☐-Slightly cloudy; ☐-Cloudy; ☐-Purulent; ☐-Blood-tinged; ☐-Bloody; ☐-Other:_____
Patient tolerance for the procedure: ☐-Excellent; ☐-Good; ☐-Fair; ☐-Other:_____

Additional comments regarding the procedure: ☐-None; ☐Other:_____

Post-Procedural Treatment Advice:
Activity modification: Avoid non-essential use of the structure until seen for follow up. ☐-Other:_____

Orthotic instructions: N/A unless indicated as follows _____
Modalities: Apply ice over the injection site prn for 20-30 min. up to q2 hrs until seen for follow-up, unless instructed as follows: ☐-Heat; ☐-Other:_____

Injection Procedure Template: Lateral Femoral Cutaneous Nerve Block

---

PROCEDURE: Lateral Femoral Cutaneous Nerve Block
Side: ☐-Right   ☐-Left   ☐-Bilateral
Procedure Type: Aspiration: ☐-Diagnostic aspiration
              Injection: ☐-Diagnostic   ☐-Therapeutic ☐-Diagnostic then Therapeutic
Image guidance: None unless indicated as follows- ☐-Fluoroscopy ☐-Ultrasound

- The potential benefits and side effects of the procedure and alternative treatment options were explained to the patient, an opportunity for questions was provided, and the patient signed informed consent.
- ☐- If checked, the following physical examination pre-procedural provocative maneuver(s) was (were) performed: ☐-
  _____
- The patient was positioned for the procedure and the target structure was identified.
- The overlying skin was prepped with Betadine® followed by alcohol prep pad after the Betadine® dried.
- ☐- If checked, the overlying skin and soft tissue was anesthetized using a small amount of 1% lidocaine delivered via the following needle ☐-30G1"; ☐-25G1½ "; ☐-Other: _____
- The following needle was then used for the procedure:
    Type: Straight needle unless indicated as follows: ☐-Spinal needle; ☐-Other:_____
    Gauge: ☐-30; ☐-27; ☐-25; ☐-22; ☐-21; -18; Other: _____
    Length: ☐-5/8"; ☐- 1"; ☐- 1 ½"; ☐- 2"; ☐- 2 ½"; ☐- 3";☐- 3½"; ☐-Other:_____
- o Image guidance if indicated above was used to confirm needle entry into target structure.
- o ☐-If checked, contrast dye was then injected and the needle position was adjusted accordingly to confirm proper placement without inadvertent intravascular entry.
- Needle was adjusted accordingly to confirm proper placement without inadvertent vascular entry.
- An attempt was made to aspirate from the structure and then the following injectate was delivered into the target structure:
    ☐-Diagnostic injection: 5 mL 1% preservative-free lidocaine; ☐-Other injectate: _____
    ☐-Therapeutic injection: 20 mg Depo-Medrol® & ☐- 5 mL 1% preservative-free lidocaine
              ☐-Other injectate: _____
- The needle was removed and an adhesive bandage was placed over the needle entry site.

-If the above was a diagnostic injection, then proceed to section immediately below.
-If above was a therapeutic injection procedure, aspiration only procedure, or aspiration and therapeutic injection, then proceed to Procedure Summary Section.

For Diagnostic Injection Procedure:
- ☐-If checked, the above listed pre-procedural physical examination provocative maneuver was repeated and pain relief was: ☐-N/A; ☐-significant; ☐-some; ☐-equivocal; ☐-none; ☐-Other:_____
- Based on the amount of pain relief noted above:
    ☐-a therapeutic injection will be scheduled.
    ☐-a therapeutic injection will not be scheduled. See plan in corresponding office note.
    ☐-a therapeutic injection following the same procedure described above was done using
              ☐- 20 mg Depo-Medrol® & ☐- 5 mL 1% preservative-free lidocaine
              ☐- Other injectate: _____
- The needle was removed and an adhesive bandage was placed over the needle entry site.

Procedure Summary:
If fluid aspirated from the target structure during the procedure:
- Total volume of fluid aspirated: ___ mL; Fluid appearance: ☐- N/A; ☐-Clear yellow; ☐-Slightly cloudy; ☐-Cloudy; ☐-Purulent; ☐-Blood-tinged; ☐-Bloody; ☐-Other:_____
Patient tolerance for the procedure: ☐-Excellent; ☐-Good; ☐-Fair; ☐-Other:_____

Additional comments regarding the procedure: ☐-None; ☐Other:_____
_____
_____

Post-Procedural Treatment Advice:
Activity modification: Avoid non-essential use of the structure until seen for follow up. ☐-Other:_____

Orthotic instructions: N/A unless indicated as follows _____
Modalities: Apply ice over the injection site prn for 20-30 min. up to q2 hrs until seen for follow-up, unless instructed as follows: ☐-Heat; ☐-Other:_____

Injection Procedure Template: Trochanteric Bursa Injection

PROCEDURE: Trochanteric Bursa Injection
Side: ☐-Right   ☐-Left   ☐-Bilateral
Procedure Type: Aspiration: ☐-Diagnostic aspiration
                 Injection: ☐-Diagnostic   ☐-Therapeutic ☐-Diagnostic <u>then</u> Therapeutic
Image guidance: None unless indicated as follows- ☐-Fluoroscopy ☐-Ultrasound

- The potential benefits and side effects of the procedure and alternative treatment options were explained to the patient, an opportunity for questions was provided, and <u>the patient signed informed consent</u>.
- ☐- If checked, the following physical examination <u>pre-procedural provocative maneuver(s)</u> was (were) performed: ☐-
  _____
- The patient was positioned for the procedure and the target structure was identified.
- The overlying skin was prepped with <u>Betadine® followed by alcohol prep pad</u> after the Betadine® dried.
- ☐- If checked, the overlying skin and soft tissue was anesthetized using a <u>small amount of 1% lidocaine</u> delivered via the following needle ☐-30G1"; ☐-25G1½ "; ☐-Other: _____
- The following needle was then used for the procedure:
  - Type: Straight needle unless indicated as follows: ☐-Spinal needle; ☐-Other:_____
  - Gauge: ☐-30; ☐-27; ☐-25; ☐-22; ☐-21; -18; -Other:_____
  - Length: ☐-5/8"; ☐- 1"; ☐- 1 ½"; ☐- 2"; ☐- 2 ½"; ☐- 3";☐- 3½"; ☐-Other:_____
- ○ Image guidance if indicated above was used to confirm needle entry into target structure.
- ○ ☐-If checked, contrast dye was then injected and the needle position was adjusted accordingly to confirm proper placement without inadvertent intravascular entry.
- Needle was adjusted accordingly to confirm proper placement without inadvertent vascular entry.
- An attempt was made to aspirate from the structure and then the following injectate was delivered into the target structure:
  ☐-Diagnostic injection: <u>5 mL 1% preservative-free lidocaine</u>; ☐-Other injectate: _____
  ☐-Therapeutic injection: <u>80 mg Depo-Medrol®</u> & ☐- <u>1 mL 1% preservative-free lidocaine</u>
  ☐-Other injectate: _____
- The needle was removed and an <u>adhesive bandage</u> was placed over the needle entry site.

-If the above was a <u>diagnostic injection</u>, then proceed to section immediately below.
-If above was a <u>therapeutic injection procedure</u>, <u>aspiration only procedure</u>, or <u>aspiration and therapeutic injection</u>, then proceed to Procedure Summary Section.

For Diagnostic Injection Procedure:
- ☐-If checked, the above listed pre-procedural physical examination provocative maneuver was repeated and pain relief was: ☐- N/A; ☐-significant; ☐-some; ☐-equivocal; ☐-none; ☐-Other:_____
- Based on the amount of pain relief noted above:
  ☐-a therapeutic injection will be scheduled.
  ☐-a therapeutic injection will <u>not</u> be scheduled. See plan in corresponding office note.
  ☐-a therapeutic injection following the same procedure described above was done using
    ☐- <u>80 mg Depo-Medrol®</u> & ☐- <u>1 mL 1% preservative-free lidocaine</u>
    ☐- Other injectate:_____
- The needle was removed and an <u>adhesive bandage</u> was placed over the needle entry site.

Procedure Summary:
If fluid aspirated from the target structure during the procedure:
- Total volume of fluid aspirated: ___ mL; Fluid appearance: ☐- N/A; ☐-Clear yellow; ☐-Slightly cloudy; ☐-Cloudy; ☐-Purulent; ☐-Blood-tinged; ☐-Bloody; ☐-Other:_____
Patient tolerance for the procedure: ☐-Excellent; ☐-Good; ☐-Fair; ☐-Other:_____

Additional comments regarding the procedure: ☐-None; ☐Other:_____

Post-Procedural Treatment Advice:
Activity modification: Avoid non-essential use of the structure until seen for follow up. ☐-Other:_____

Orthotic instructions: N/A unless indicated as follows _____
Modalities: Apply ice over the injection site prn for 20-30 min. up to q2 hrs until seen for follow-up, unless instructed as follows: ☐-Heat; ☐-Other:_____

Chapter 11
The Knee and Its Region

Todd P. Stitik, Jong H. Kim, Christopher Castro,
Mohammad Hossein Dorri, Jose Santiago Campos,
Lisa Schoenherr, Naimish Baxi, and Ladislov Habina

Introduction

Knee region injections as a group are generally accepted as being one of the most frequently performed musculoskeletal office-based injection procedures. This is supported by a survey of primary care physicians, which found them to be the third most common office-based injection procedure after shoulder region injections and lateral epicondyle injections [1]. A study from an outpatient physiatric musculoskeletal medicine practice found that knee region injections ($n = 244$; knee joint = 181; suprapatellar bursa = 51; pes anserine bursa = 12) were the most frequent office-based injection procedure, as they represented 54.8% of the total joint and soft tissue (other than trigger point injections) injection and/or aspiration procedures performed during a 2-year time period [2].

Knee Region Procedures

In addition to injections into the knee joint (both directly through the joint capsule and indirectly via the suprapatellar bursa, which communicates with the joint), various other knee region injection and aspiration procedures have been described (Table 11.1).

These procedures include those into other structures such as the pes anserine bursa, prepatellar bursa, superficial and deep infrapatellar bursae, iliotibial band, hamstring bursa, aspiration +/- injections into popliteal cysts, injections into the medial and lateral coronary ligaments that attach the menisci to the tibia, injections at tendon insertion sites of the quadriceps and patellar tendons, injections at the musculotendinous junction of the popliteus tendon, and injection of the tibiofibular articulation.

T.P. Stitik (✉)
Department of Physical Medicine and Rehabilitation, New Jersey Medical School,
Newark, NJ, USA
e-mail: todd.stitik@gmail.com

T.P. Stitik (ed.), *Injection Procedures: Osteoarthritis and Related Conditions*,
DOI 10.1007/978-0-387-76595-2_11, © Springer Science+Business Media, LLC 2011

Table 11.1 Summary of knee region injection procedures (The content of this table is listed within each injection type in order of descending amount of current evidence supporting its use. Except in the case of intra-articular knee joint and suprapatellar bursa injections where there is an extensive amount of literature, references are provided for all meta-analyses, prospective studies, and case series/case reports along with at least one reference to descriptions in review articles or injection textbooks. For those procedures that are only described in review articles and/or textbooks, representative references are provided)

Injection type	Specific structure	Meta-analysis(es)	Prospective study (Studies)	Case series/report(s)	Described in review article(s) and/or injection textbook(s)
Articulation/joint	Knee joint	X	X	X	X
	Tibiofibular joint (aka superior tibiofibular joint)				X [3, 4]
Bursa	Suprapatellar[a]	X	X	X	X
	Pes anserine		X [5]	X [6]	X [3]
	Tibial collateral (aka MCL) ligament bursae[b] (Voshell's bursa)			X [7]	X [8]
	Prepatellar				X [3]
	Superficial (subcutaneous) infrapatellar				X [3]
	Deep (subtendinous) infrapatellar				X [3]
	Iliotibial band				X [3]
Cyst	Popliteal (aka. Baker's cyst or bursa interposed between the medial head of gastrocnemius and posterior aspect medial femoral condyle)				X [3]

Structure	Subtype			
Fat pad	Anterior (aka Infrapatellar or Hoffa's fat pad)		X [9]	
Ligament	Coronary			X [3]
	MCL			X [3]
Plica	Medial plica	X [10]		X [8, 11]
Tendon: insertion site	Patellar (aka infrapatellar)	X [12]		X [3]
	Quadriceps (aka suprapatellar or quadriceps expansion)			X [3]
	Semimembranous insertion +/- oblique popliteal ligament insertion			X [3]
	Hamstring tendonitis: semitendinosus and/or semimembranosus			X [3]
Tendon musculotendinous junction	Popliteus		X [13]	

a Literature on knee joint injections includes procedures performed via the suprapatellar approach to injecting a knee

b It was originally described that "numerous bursa (usually five) are interposed between the deep middle capsular ligament and the superficial collateral ligament," [8, 14, 15] divisions of the MCL. Standard anatomy texts, however, do not describe the existence of bursa (e) deep to the MCL [16, 17]

The amount of literature on these injections varies widely. For example, while there is a large body of literature, including major meta-analyses on knee joint corticosteroid and viscosupplementation injection procedures, procedures such as coronary ligament, tibiofibular joint, and hamstring bursa injections are only described in the context of articles and/or injection textbooks that describe how to do the procedure, but actual results from these injections are not reported in the literature, even as case reports.

While other knee region bursal structures [e.g., the fibular collateral ligament bursa (i.e., LCL bursa or fibular collateral ligament-biceps femoris bursa) and the semimembranosus bursa] [3, 18, 19] have been implicated as causing symptomatology, no reports or descriptions of injection procedures into them were found. When reviewing anatomical descriptions of these structures, it should be noted that, although some sources refer to the fibular collateral ligament bursa and the biceps femoris bursa as one bursa (thus the fibular collateral ligament-biceps femoris bursa [20, 21]), others depict these as two distinct bursae [16]. In contrast, injections into the medial collateral ligament (i.e., MCL, tibial collateral ligament, or Voshell's bursa) have been described and have personally been performed by the senior author (TS) [7, 8]. For the purposes of this current book, only those procedures that the authors of this text have actually performed are described in the individual procedure chapters.

Injection Accuracy

Despite the relatively superficial location of the knee joint, studies on injection accuracy have been quite surprising and humbling [22, 23]. For example, Jackson and colleagues reported a 71–93% accuracy rate for 240 intra-articular knee injections by one experienced orthopedist [22]. Using contrast arthrograms, Jones and coworkers found inadvertent extra-articular knee injection placement in nearly 29% of injections and uncertainty in placement in an additional 19% [23].

Given the documented problems with injection accuracy, various techniques have been taught and described over the years in an attempt to improve accuracy. For example, Green's sign (detection of an audible swish with passive knee flexion and extension after the injection of a combination of 1 ml of air and corticosteroid) was described in a letter to the editor as a method of confirming that accurate intra-articular placement had been achieved [24]. Glattes and colleagues then formally studied this method in 20 knees and found 100% specificity [25]. While the authors acknowledge that this method can not help guide an injection, as it can only be applied after the injection needle has been removed, it can be used as a teaching tool that provides immediate feedback.

Another, somewhat more cumbersome, method to confirm accurate intra-articular placement is mini air-arthrography [26]. This technique involves the injection of 5 ml of air into the knee joint through the needle that was used to place medication. On subsequent lateral and anterior–posterior radiographs, correct intra-articular placement can be verified by a sharply defined shadow of air in the suprapatellar pouch, while extra-articular air will be diffusely spread in the surrounding tissue.

In contrast to these methods of determining if an injection was properly placed after it had been already performed, ultrasound confirmation of intra-articular air injection during knee injections was described by Qvistgaard and colleagues as a real-time method of confirming accurate placement during an injection [27]. As described in greater detail later in this chapter, the senior author (TS) has taught viscosupplementation knee injections using fluoroscopic guidance in order to provide immediate feedback to the physician performing the injection. More recently the senior author is transitioning to ultrasound guidance.

Intra-articular Knee Injection Instruction

In part because of the documented difficulties with accurate knee injections noted previously, the senior author (TS) has a particular interest in teaching intra-articular knee injections. In addition to the teaching experiences mentioned in Chap. 1, he teaches these injections as part of his clinical practice to fellows, residents, and medical students who rotate through the outpatient division of the Department of Physical Medicine and Rehabilitation. Their exposure to these injections includes hands-on care of outpatients who present for a knee aspirations and/or corticosteroid injections. This most typically includes patients with knee osteoarthritis (OA) and patients or college athletes who have suffered a knee injury.

The fellows, residents, and medical students also directly participate in a weekly knee viscosupplementation clinic. During this clinic, ultrasound guidance is used so that the physician trainee can directly visualize exact needle placement during the injection. The senior author (TS) is also aware of a colleague who routinely uses ultrasound guidance for knee viscosupplementation injections [28]. While it is presently unclear whether image guidance, either in the form of fluoroscopy or ultrasound, will become the gold standard by which viscosupplementation will be performed or will only regularly be used into patients with very poor anatomic landmarks, it is becoming clear that relatively painless and extremely accurate injections are crucial for viscosupplementation. This is particularly true given the need for multiple injections (e.g., 3 or 5 weekly knee injections with Hyalgan® (Sanofi-Aventis, Bridgewater, NJ, USA) [sodium hyaluronate] performed into the knees of a patient with bilateral knee OA for a total of 6 or 10 injections) and the need for extreme accuracy with viscosupplementation, as visco-supplements cannot diffuse into the knee joint if they are inadvertently placed extra-articularly. Furthermore, one viscosupplementation preparation is available as a one injection regimen (Synvisc-One™ Gynzyme Corporation, Cambridge, MA, USA). Injection accuracy with this preparation will be particularly important. Although extreme accuracy for knee injections is less crucial for corticosteroids as these are believed to be capable of diffusion into the joint if inadvertently injected extra-articularly, it is likely preferable for accurate injection. In cases of arthrocentesis, the need for accurate needle placement into the joint is self-evident.

Cadaveric Instruction

The senior author also directed a cadaver-based knee injection CME workshop [29]. During this hands-on workshop, cadaver knee joints were filled with various volumes of Betadine® (Purdue-Pharma LP, Stamford, CT, USA), and participants practiced aspirating the knees using the suprapatellar, retropatellar, and parapatellar approaches that are described later in this section within the intra-articular knee injection and viscosupplementation procedure instructions. A live knee injection demonstration was also performed during the workshop.

Teaching knee injections using cadavers has also been utilized at New Jersey Medical School by the senior author and one of his colleagues (Patrick M. Foye, MD), who is the director of medical student education for the Department of PM&R at the same institution. A published survey documented that this teaching approach was very well received by the students, as it helped to bridge the gap between traditional cadaver dissections and clinical medicine [30].

The senior author coproduced an instructional knee injection CD along with one of his orthopedic colleagues [31]. This CD is used in conjunction with a synthetic knee injection workshop that the author has presented nationally in order to train physicians, physicians in training, physician assistants, and nurse practitioners.

Summary and Conclusion

Knee region aspiration and/or injection procedures are commonly performed as a part of musculoskeletal medicine practices. They are the most intensely studied type of procedure both in terms of efficacy and accuracy. This scrutiny has occurred in part due to the practice of viscosupplementation, a procedure being performed with increased frequency on a patient population whose numbers are rapidly increasing.

References

1. Gormley GJ, Corrigan M, Steele WK, Stevenson M, Taggart AJ. Joint and soft tissue injections in the community: questionnaire survey of general practitioners' experiences and attitudes. Ann Rheum Dis 2003;62(1):61–64.
2. Stitik TP, Foye PM, Nadler SF, Chen B, Schoenherr L, Von Hagen S. Injections in patients with osteoarthritis and other musculoskeletal disorders: use of synthetic injection models for teaching physiatry residents. Am J Phys Med Rehabil 2005;84:550–559.
3. Waldman SD. Knee Pain Syndromes. In Ross A, Chappelle A, eds. Atlas of Uncommon Pain Syndromes. Philadelphia, PA: WB Saunders, 2003:209–230.
4. Stephanie Saunders. Knee Treatments. In Law M, ed. Injection Techniques in Orthopaedic and Sports Medicine. Second edition. London: WB Saunders, 2002:84–99.
5. Calvo-Alén J, Rua-Figueroa I, Erausquin C. Tratamiento de la bursitis anserina: infiltración local con corticoides frente a AINE: estudio prospectivo [Anserine bursitis treatment: local corticosteroid injection against NSAID: a prospective study] [Spanish]. Rev Esp Reumatol 1993;20:13–15.
6. Kang I, Han SW. Anserine bursitis in patients with osteoarthritis of the knee. South Med J 2000;93(2):207–209.
7. Kerlan RK, Glousman RE. Tibial collateral ligament bursitis. Am J Sports Med 1988;16(4):344–346.
8. Kerlan RK, Glousman RE. Injections and techniques in athletic medicine. Clin Sports Med 1989;8(3):541–560.
9. Duri ZA, Aichroth PM, Dowd G. The fat pad. Clinical observations. Am J Knee Surg 1996;9(2):55–66.
10. Rovere GD, Adair DM. Medial synovial shelf plica syndrome. Treatment by intraplical steroid injection. Am J Sports Med 1985;13(6):382–386.
11. Millard RS, Dillingham MF. Peripheral Joint Injections. In Weinstein SM, Kraft GH, eds. Physical Medicine and Rehabilitation Clinics of North America. Philadelphia, PA: WB Saunders, 1995:841–849.
12. Fredberg U, Bolvig L, Pfeiffer-Jensen M, Clemmensen D, Jakobsen BW, Stengaard-Pedersen K. Ultrasonography as a tool for diagnosis, guidance of local steroid injection and, together with pressure algometry, monitoring of the treatment of athletes with chronic jumper's knee and Achilles tendinitis: a randomized, double-blind, placebo-controlled study. Scand J Rheumatol 2004;33(2):94–101.
13. Petsche TS, Selesnick FH. Popliteus tendinitis: tips for diagnosis and management. Phys Sportsmed 2002;30(8):27–31.
14. Brantigan OC, Voschell AF. The tibial collateral ligament: its function, its bursae and its relation to medial meniscus. J Bone Joint Surg 1943;25:121–131.
15. Cailliet R. Structural Anatomy. In Cailliet R ed. Knee Pain and Disability. Philadelphia, PA: FA Davis Company, 1973:11.
16. Netter FH. In Netter FH, Dalley II AF, eds. Atlas of Human Anatomy. Second edition. East Hanover, NJ: Novartis, 1997: plates 472–473.
17. Craft RC. Lower Limb Joint. In Craft RC ed. A Textbook of Human Anatomy. Second edition. New York: Wiley; 1979:421–437.
18. Lanier BE. Acute calcific bursitis in the region of the fibular head. A case report. Clin Orthop Relat Res 1970;69:159–161.
19. Hendryson IE. Bursitis in the region of the fibular collateral ligament. J Bone Joint Surg 1946;28:446–450.
20. LaPrade RF, Hamilton CD. The fibular collateral ligament-biceps femoris bursa. An anatomic study. Am J Sports Med 1997;25(4): 439–443.

21. McCarthy CL, McNally EG. The MRI appearance of cystic lesions around the knee. Skelet Radiol 2004;33(4):187–209.
22. Jackson DW, Evans NA, Thomas BM. Accuracy of needle placement into the intra-articular space of the knee. J Bone Joint Surg Am 2002;84-A(9):1522–1527.
23. Jones A, Regan M, Ledingham J, Pattrick M, Manhire A, Doherty M. Importance of placement of intra-articular steroid injections. BMJ 1993;307:1329–1330.
24. Gardner A, Datta A, Green M. Steroid injection of the knee – is it in yet? Green's sign. Ann R Coll Surg Engl 2003;85(6):428.
25. Glattes RC, Spindler KP, Blanchard GM, Rohmiller MT, McCarty EC, Block JA. Simple, accurate method to confirm placement of intra-articular knee injection. Am J Sports Med 2004;32(4):1029–1031.
26. Bliddal H. Placement of intra-articular injections verified by mini air-arthrography. Ann Rheum Dis 1999;58:641–3.
27. Qvistgaard E, Kristoffersen H, Terslev L, Danneskiold-Samsøe B, Torp-Pedersen S, Bliddal H.Guidance by ultrasound of intra-articular injections in the knee and hip joints. Osteoarthritis Cartilage 2001;9(6):512–517.
28. John Cianca MD. Personal conversation, November 11, 2006.
29. CME. "A Hands-On Cadaveric Knee Injection Workshop for the Primary Care Physician Who Manages Patients with Osteoarthritis of the Knee" UMDNJ-NJMS CME-sponsored lecture/ workshop, Teaneck, NJ 11/29/00.
30. Foye PM, Stitik TP, Campagnolo DI, Nadler SF, Chen B. "Bedside Teaching at the Gurney: Results of Cadaver-based Anatomy Teaching for PM&R Residents." Presented 3/1/00–3/4/00. Association of Academic Physiatrists (AAP) 36 annual Educational Conference, San Diego, California.
31. Stitik TP, Axe MJ. Injection Techniques Educator: Techniques for Administering Intra-articular Injections of Hyalgan® (sodium hyaluronate) for the Treatment of Osteoarthritis Knee Pain. Sanofi-Aventis, Inc. [11/3/06 date of production]

Procedure Instructions

Injection Procedure: Iliotibial Band Injection

1. Indications:
   (a) Iliotibial band friction syndrome (ITBFS) [1]

2. Contraindications especially pertinent to this procedure:
   (a) None documented

3. Possible side effects especially pertinent to this procedure:
   (a) Iliotibial band rupture: No documented cases of this exist, but this theoretically could occur
   (b) Previous injections. Repeat injections should be avoided due to the risk of tendon rupture. The exact number of injections that increases the risk is not known with certainty

4. Technical details of note for this procedure (Fig. 11.1):
   (a) Preferred needle gauge: 25 gauge [2]
   (b) Need for image guidance: No
   - No studies have been published to date regarding the accuracy and need for image guidance when performing iliotibial band injections. Instead, palpation of anatomical landmarks is used to identify the needle entry site. Cardone and Schwellnus recommend palpation along the lateral thigh, following the iliotibial band to the insertion point at Gerdy's tubercle, and then injecting the point of maximal tenderness [2]. In contrast, Gunter and Tallia recommend a posterior approach, in which the needle is "directed at 90° to the long axis of the body and medial to the posterior border of the iliotibial band," and the solution is then injected at the "point of maximal tenderness just lateral to the lateral femoral condyle tubercle." [1]

5. Step-by-step procedure:
   (a) Obtain informed consent after explaining potential benefits and side effects of the procedure to the patient
   (b) Preprocedural testing:
   - Identify and record the response to a physical examination preprocedural provocative maneuver if the procedure is a diagnostic injection
   (c) Image guidance: Not applicable
   - Nonguided procedure described later in this section
   (d) Patient positioning:
   - Place the patient in a lateral recumbent position, with the affected side up on the table, and the knee flexed to approximately 30°
   (e) Identification and marking of injection site:
   - Palpate the skin entry site along the lateral thigh, identifying the iliotibial band and following it to its insertion point at Gerdy's tubercle

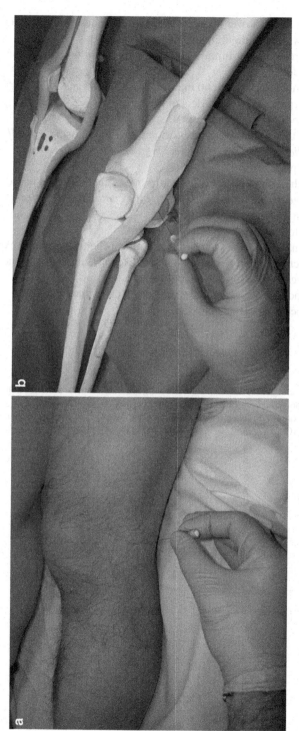

Fig. 11.1 Iliotibial band injection. (**a**) Iliotibial band injection. (**b**) Skeletal representation of iliotibial band injection

- Mark the spot over the point of maximal tenderness with a plastic needle cap with or without image guidance
(f) Skin preparation: Initial: Betadine® preparation using the no-touch technique
(g) Medication preparation: 40 mg of Depo-Medrol® and 1 ml of 1% lidocaine
(h) Skin preparation: Final: Alcohol prep
(i) Local anesthesia administration:
  - Anesthetize the overlying skin and soft tissue using a *small amount of 1% lidocaine,* delivered via a *25-gauge needle*
(j) Needle placement:
(k) Pierce the previously anesthetized skin/and subcutaneous tissue site with a *25-gauge needle attached to the syringe containing the injectate*
(l) Contrast injection: Not applicable
(m) Aspiration to rule out intravascular entry
(n) Injection: Some degree of resistance during the injection is to be expected, but the injection should not be continued if excessive resistance is encountered
(o) Postprocedural testing: Not applicable
(p) Apply adhesive *bandage* over the needle entry site
(q) Postprocedural care discussion

References

1. Gunter P, Schwellnus MP. Local corticosteroid injection in iliotibial band friction syndrome in runners: a randomized controlled trial. Br J Sports Med 2004;38:269–272.
2. Cardone DA, Tallia AF. Diagnostic and therapeutic injection of the hip and knee. Am Fam Phys 2003;67(10):2147–2152.

Injection Procedure: Intra-Articular Knee Aspiration and/or Corticosteroid Injection

1. Indications:
   (a) Osteoarthritis
   (b) Rheumatoid arthritis, including juvenile rheumatoid arthritis [1]
   (c) Symptomatic meniscal tear without definite surgical indication
   (d) Synovitis: e.g., due to other arthropathy or injury

2. Contraindications especially pertinent to this procedure:
   (a) None documented

3. Possible side effects especially pertinent to this procedure:
   (a) Local pain
   (b) Local joint irritation if use of air to help confirm accurate placement [2]
   (c) Septic arthritis [3]
   (d) Skin and soft tissue necrosis along needle track (specific concern with triamcinolone hexacetonide, which has been withdrawn from some European countries) [4]

4. Technical details of note for this procedure (Figs. 11.2, 11.3, 11.4):
   (a) Preferred corticosteroid:
   - A variety of corticosteroid preparations are available and used for intra-articular knee injections. While most physicians choose their corticosteroids based on personal preference, Pyne and colleagues performed a comparative study of triamcinolone hexacetonide and methylprednisolone acetate to compare their effectiveness. Triamcinolone hexacetonide provided significantly greater relief at week 3 (32.9 mm vs. 13.7 mm improvement from baseline). Conversely, methylprednisolone was more effective at relieving pain into the eighth week (18.3 mm vs. 7.6 mm improvement from baseline), though these results did not reach statistical significance ($p = 0.17$) [4]
   (b) Preferred needle gauge: Range of 18-gauge–*25-gauge*
   - 18-gauge preferred if attempting to aspirate effusion
   - 25-gauge can be used if only performing injection without aspiration
   - Needle length generally ranges from 1.5 to 2 in. depending upon body habitus
   (c) Injection approach: Three major knee injection approaches have been described throughout the literature. These approaches include the suprapatellar bursa entry, retropatellar (aka capsular) entry, and the parapatellar entry. The needle entry site varies depending upon the injection approach. To help understand this, the patella can be thought of as the face of a clock (Fig. 11.5). The needle entry sites correspond to the following clock positions:
   - Suprapatellar bursa approach: 11:00 or 1:00 (Fig. 11.6)

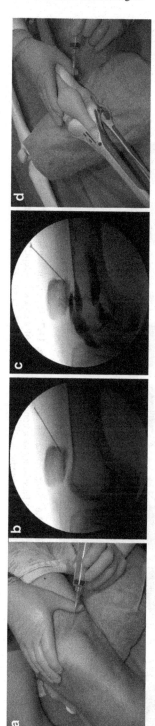

Fig. 11.2 Intra-articular suprapatellar bursa approach: Knee joint aspiration and/or injection (fluoroscopic-guided). (**a**) intra-articular suprapatellar bursa approach knee joint aspiration – human model. (**b**) Fluoroscopic image of needle entry into suprapatellar bursa. (**c**) Fluoroscopic image of knee joint arthrogram. (**d**) Skeletal representation of intra-articular suprapatellar bursa approach knee joint aspiration and/or injection

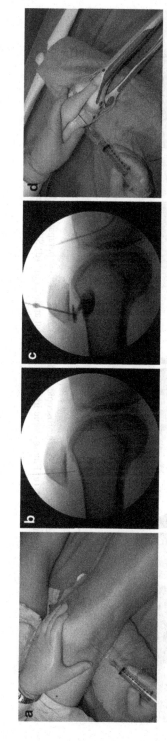

Fig. 11.3 Intra-articular retropatellar knee joint aspiration and/or injection (fluoroscopic-guided). (**a**) intra-articular retropatellar knee joint injection – human model. (**b**) Fluoroscopic image of needle entry into knee joint. (**c**) Fluoroscopic image of knee joint arthrogram. (**d**) Skeletal representation of intra-articular retropatellar knee joint aspiration and/or injection

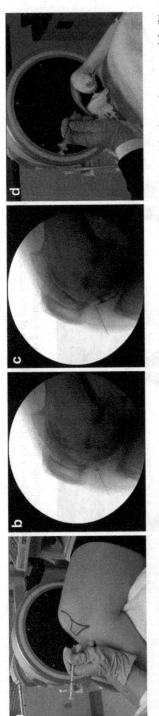

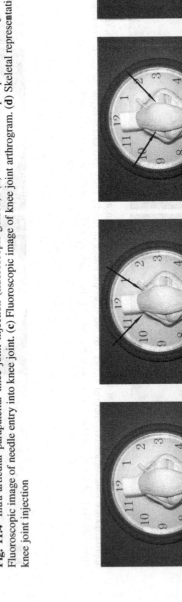

Fig. 11.4 Intra-articular parapatellar knee joint injection (fluoroscopic-guided). (**a**) Intra-articular parapatellar knee joint injection – human model. (**b**) Fluoroscopic image of needle entry into knee joint. (**c**) Fluoroscopic image of knee joint arthrogram. (**d**) Skeletal representation of intra-articular parapatellar knee joint injection

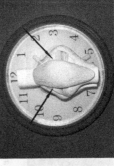

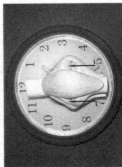

Fig. 11.5 Knee: Face of clock concept

Fig. 11.6 Suprapatellar bursa approach: Face of a clock concept: 11:00 or 1:00 needle position

Fig. 11.7 Retropatellar approach: Face of a clock concept: 10:00 or 2:00 needle position

Fig. 11.8 Parapatellar approach: Face of a clock concept: 7:00 or 5:00 needle position

- Retropatellar (aka capsular) approach: 10:00 or 2:00: Rather than placing the needle at the midportion of the patella (i.e., 3:00 or 9:00), sensory innervation is less dense in these more proximal locations [5] (Fig. 11.7)
- Parapatellar approach: 7:00 or 5:00 (Fig. 11.8)

(d) Because all three approaches can be performed on either the medial or lateral sides of the knee, a total of six different approaches are possible. The decision as to which approach to chose is dependent upon several factors including whether or not an effusion is present, the relative size of the effusion, the patient's body habitus, the range of motion of the knee, the physician's experience level. General guidelines regarding knee effusions and injection site selection are as follows:

- Suprapatellar bursa approach: If a very large effusion is present, the suprapatellar burse can be distended enough so that it is relatively easy for the needle to puncture the skin and subcutaneous tissue that overlie the bursa (Fig. 11.9). In contrast, if no or minimal effusion is present, the bursal walls are essentially collapsed and needle entry into the bursa is very difficult even with ultrasound guidance
- Retropatellar (aka capsular) approach: In the presence of a moderately large or small effusion, this approach is preferable as the needle can be navigated between the overlying patella and underlying femoral condoyle so as to puncture the joint capsule and synovial membrane (Fig. 11.10)
- Parapatellar approach: This approach is best when the intent is to perform an injection without a knee aspiration. The approach allows for the needle rest up against the medial or lateral femoral condyle within the joint space (Fig. 11.11). It is relatively poor for aspirating a knee as the needle generally enters the joint above the level of a small effusion which would pool by gravity at the bottom of the joint. With this approach, the patient can be either supine with the knee bent as much as possible or seated with the knee bent at 90° and the leg dangling over the side of the exam table

(e) Need for image guidance: Optional

- Studies have shown only fair accuracy of needle placement into the knee joint using a nonimage-guided approach. Injection accuracy becomes more difficult in the cases of "dry" osteoarthritis, in which the patient has no clinically detectable effusion [2]. Jackson and colleagues documented different accuracies, depending upon the injection approach that was used without radiographic guidance [6]:
  - Anterolateral approach: 71%
  - Anteromedial approach: 75%
  - Lateral midpatellar injection: 93%
- In a separate study, Jones and coworkers determined via postinjection radiographs used to assess for intra-articular contrast placement that only 66% of their injections were definitely intra-articular [7]
- Waddell and colleagues found that real-time fluoroscopy increased the injection accuracy to 100% [8]

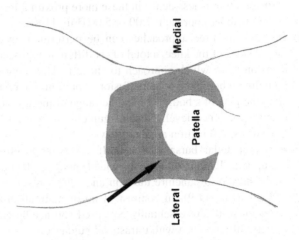

Fig. 11.9 Suprapatellar bursa approach. Needle pathway into distended bursa

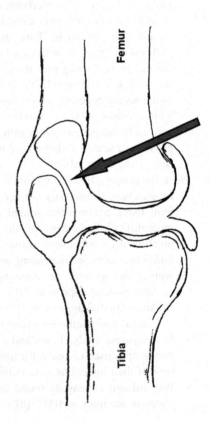

Fig. 11.10 Retropatellar Approach. Navigation of needle

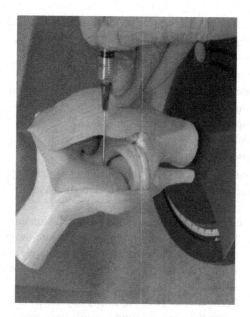

Fig. 11.11 Parapatellar approach: Oblique view

- Bliddal described a technique known as mini-air arthrography, in which postprocedure radiographs were taken after a 5 ml bolus of air was given at the time of an injection in order to determine if placement was actually intra-articular [2]. Because this technique retrospectively looks at placement of the injection, it does not prevent inadvertent extra-articular injection. However, it could potentially be used as a teaching tool and a quality assurance method for studies involving intra-articular injections

5. Step-by-step procedure:
   (a) Informed consent
   (b) Preprocedural testing: Identify and record the response to a physical examination preprocedural provocative maneuver if the procedure is a diagnostic injection
   (c) Image guidance: Optional: fluoroscopic or ultrasound guidance
   (d) Patient positioning:
     - Place the patient in a supine position with the affected knee positioned depending upon the injection approach to be used as follows:
       – Suprapatellar bursa approach: slightly flexed with a rolled pillow or towel underneath the popliteal space [9]
       – Retropatellar (aka capsular) approach: slightly flexed with a rolled pillow or towel underneath the popliteal space [9]
       – Parapatellar approach:
         ▪ Patient supine with knee flexed as much as possible with a buttress under it

- Alternatively, a seated position with the leg dangling (foot not supported) over the side of the exam table can be used for the parapatellar approach

(e) Identification and marking of injection site:
- As discussed previously, the needle entry site varies depending upon the chosen injection approach:
  - Suprapatellar bursa approach
  - Retropatellar (aka capsular) approach
  - Parapatellar approach
- More exact identification of the injection site then depends upon whether the procedure is being done with image guidance:
  - If nonimage-guided:
    - Use palpation to identify the proposed skin entry site as follows:
      ○ *Suprapatellar bursa approach*: Palpate the proximal medial or proximal lateral patellar corner and move away approximately 1 finger breadth (so that the needle does not contact the patella upon entry)
      ○ *Retropatellar (aka capsular) approach*: Use a hand to attempt to "milk" synovial fluid towards the opposite side in an attempt to detect the fluid by palpation. Once the fluid is detected, try to palpate the side of the patella at approximately the 10:00 or 2:00 positions as discussed previously and move away from the side of the patella approximately 1 finger breadth (so that the needle does not contact the patella upon entry). It is believed by some that the lateral approach offers several advantages [5]
  - If the subcutaneous fat layer is thicker than usual, the lateral aspect of the joint is generally much closer to the body surface compared to the medial aspect
  - The medial side contains a pyramid-shaped fat pad beneath the medial patellar facet independent of the overall body fat. The fat pad is very sensitive to needle contact and causes significant discomfort [10]. Finally, because the amount of synovial fluid is much smaller than the overall potential space volume, most of the fluid might drop into the lateral gutter
  - *Parapatellar approach*: Palpate for the "soft spot of the knee" – the center of a triangle formed by the meniscus overlying the tibial edge of the joint line (floor), the patellar tendon (side), and the femoral condyle (other side) (Fig. 11.12). If the needle is directed too low, grittiness consistent with inadvertent meniscal tissue penetration will be felt. If the needle is directed too much towards the midline, it can encounter the patellar tendon and/or the underlying fat pad which is particularly prominent along the medial aspect of the joint. Fat pad penetration will be readily perceived by the patient as being very painful [10]. Ultimately, the goal is to position the needle so that it gently abuts the underlying femoral condyle without forcibly impaling it

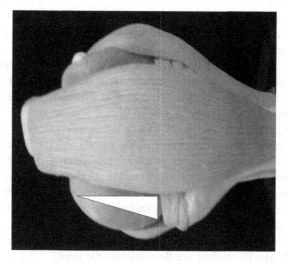

Fig. 11.12 Parapatellar approach: Soft spot of the knee

- If image-guided:
  - Use image guidance along with palpation to directly visualize the underlying target
    - Mark the target using a marker or by depressing the skin with a plastic needle cap
(f) Skin preparation- initial: Betadine® preparation using the no-touch technique
(g) Medication preparation: 1 ml 1% preservative-free lidocaine
(h) Skin preparation: Final: Alcohol prep
(i) Local anesthesia administration:
- Anesthetize the overlying skin and soft tissue using a *small amount of 1% lidocaine* delivered via a *25-gauge* needle. As the needle is advanced, deliver small amounts of lidocaine in order to anesthetize the tissue leading up to the target. As you advance the needle, pay particular attention to the angle that is needed to pass the needle to the target structure without inadvertently impaling other structures. For those procedures during which fluid aspiration is to be subsequently performed, the larger aspirating needle will ideally need to be advanced along the same tissue plane as was the anesthesia needle
- Because the parapatellar approach should be used when the intent is only for injection without fluid aspiration (e.g., a corticosteroid or viscosupplementation injection in a patient with knee OA but without a palpable effusion), at times, the syringe attached to the 25 gauge needle used to deliver the anesthetic can simply be unclamped and the injectate syringe can be attached, and the injectate delivered without having to switch to another needle

(j) Needle placement:
- Pierce the previously anesthetized skin/and subcutaneous tissue site with the appropriate needle and direct to the target
    - Suprap`atellar bursa approach: Direct the needle through the skin and subcutaneous tissue. Use care not to strike the corner of the patella. Subsequent aspiration of bursal fluid will signify needle entry into the bursa
    - Retropatellar approach: Direct the needle carefully into the space between the undersurface of the patella and the underlying condyle without striking either structure. It is often very helpful to have an assistant or to use the other hand to tilt the patella towards the needle and upwards in order to create additional space between the undersurface of the patella and the underlying condyle (Fig. 11.13). On occasion, needle entry through the joint capsule can be detected by a sudden sense of decreased resistance. The subsequent aspiration of fluid will confirm needle entry into the joint
    - Parapatellar approach: If the needle used to deliver the local anesthetic did not reach the underlying condyle or if the physician wishes to attempt fluid aspiration using the parapatellar approach, the needle used for aspiration or injection is directed through the soft spot of the knee along the same tissue plane as for the local anesthetic needle until it gently abuts against the underlying condyle
    - Aspiration: Rule out intravascular entry (all approaches) and confirm entry into bursa or joint space (if suprapatellar bursa or retropatellar approach and enough bursal or joint fluid respectively present to allow aspiration). Fluid aspiration using the parapatellar approach is usually unsuccessful as the needle generally enters above the level of synovial fluid

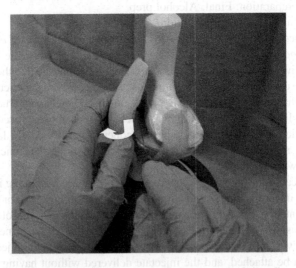

Fig. 11.13 Retropatellar approach. Tilting of patella to create space for needle entry

(k) Contrast injection: Not applicable unless fluoroscopic-guided
(l) Injection: Unclamp the aspiration syringe and clamp on the injection syringe
   • If resistance is encountered early during the injection, rotate the needle to dislodge the bevel from the side of the bursa (suprapatellar bursa approach), the joint capsule (retropatellar approach), or the condyle (parapatellar approach)
(m) Postprocedural testing:
   • If applicable, reassess the response to the aforementioned preprocedural provocative maneuver
(n) If (+) response, repeat injection with therapeutic injectate:
   • Repeat steps (d)–(f)
   • Medication preparation: 80 mg Depo-Medrol® and 2 ml 1% preservative-free lidocaine
   • Repeat steps (h)–(m)
(o) *Adhesive bandage* application over the needle entry site
(p) Postprocedural care discussion

References

1. Heuck C, Wolthers OD, Herlin T. Growth-suppressive effect of intra-articular glucocorticoids detected by knemometry. Hormone Res 1999;52:95–96.
2. Bliddal H. Placement of intra-articular injections verified by mini-air arthrography. Ann Rheum Dis 1999;58:641–643.
3. Charalambous CP, Tryfonidis M, Sadiq S, Hirst P, Paul A. Septic arthritis following intra-articular steroid injection of the knee–a survey of current practice regarding antiseptic technique used during intra-articular steroid injection of the knee. Clin Rheumatol 2003;22(6):386–90.
4. Pyne D, Ioannou Y, Mootoo R, Bhanji A. Intra-articular steroids in knee osteoarthritis: a comparative study of triamcinolone hexacetonide and methylprednisolone acetate. Clin Rheumatol 2004;23:116–120.
5. Roberts WN. Primer: pitfalls of aspiration and injection. Nat Clin Pract Rheumatol 2007;3(8):464–472.
6. Jackson DW, Evans NA, Thomas BM. Accuracy of needle placement of intra-articular steroid injections. J Bone Joint Surgery Am 2002;84:1522–1527.
7. Jones A, Regan M, Ledingham J, Pattrick M, Manhire A, Doherty M. Importance of placement of intra-articular steroid injections. BMJ 1993;307:1329–1330.
8. Waddell D, Estey D, Bricker DC, Marsala A. Viscosupplementation under fluoroscopic control. Am J Med Sports 2001;3:237–241,249.
9. Cardone DA, Tallia AF. Diagnostic and therapeutic injection of the hip and knee. American Family Physician 2003;67(10):2147–2152.
10. Dye SF, Vaupel GL, Dye CC. Conscious neurosensory mapping of the internal structures of the human knee without intraarticular anesthesia. Am J Sports Med 1998; 26: 773–777.

Injection Procedure: Intra-Articular Knee Viscosupplementation

1. Indications:
   (a) Knee osteoarthritis

2. Contraindications especially pertinent to this procedure:
   (a) Hypersensitivity to eggs, feathers, avian proteins, or chickens [1]

3. Possible side effects especially pertinent to this procedure:
   (a) Local injection site pain
   (b) Postinjection synovitis [2]
   (c) Septic arthritis [3]

4. Technical details of note for this procedure (See Figures from previous section on Intra-articular Knee Aspiration and/or Corticosteroid Injection):
   (a) Preferred needle gauge: 18-gauge–*25-gauge* [1]
      • Larger bore needle if palpable knee effusion present
   (b) *Need for fluoroscopic guidance*: Optional
      • Many of the same studies aimed at determining the accuracy of needle placement into the intra-articular space for knee corticosteroid injections hold true for knee viscosupplementation. These studies have suggested that these injections are surprisingly inaccurate without the use of radiographic guidance. Jackson and colleagues showed an accuracy of 71% via an anterolateral approach, 75% using an anteromedial approach, and 93% accuracy with a lateral midpatellar injection without the use of radiographic guidance [4]. In a separate study by Jones and coworkers, it was determined that 66% of injections were intra-articular, while 33% were extra-articular [5]
      • While it has been shown repeatedly that blind intra-articular injections are relatively inaccurate, Waddell and colleagues proved that using real-time fluoroscopy increased the accuracy of the injections to 100% [3]. The intra-articular placement of hyaluronic acid has been hypothesized to be important, as it is believed that inflammatory reactions to viscosupplements are more common when injected into the extra-articular space [6]

5. Step-by-step procedure:
   (a) Informed consent
   (b) Preprocedural testing: Identify and record the response to a physical examination preprocedural provocative maneuver if the procedure is a diagnostic injection
   (c) Image guidance: Optional: Fluoroscopic
   (d) Patient positioning: As in Intra-articular Knee Aspiration and/or Corticosteroid Injection, previous section
   (e) Identification and marking of injection site:
      • Mark the target using a marker or by depressing the skin with a plastic needle cap
   (f) Skin preparation: Initial: Betadine® preparation using the no-touch technique

(g) Medication preparation:
  - Hyalgan® (sodium hyaluronate 20 mg/2 ml) or other injectate
(h) Skin preparation: Final: Alcohol prep
(i) Local anesthesia administration:
  - Anesthetize the overlying skin and soft tissue using a *small amount of 1% lidocaine* delivered via a 25-guage needle
(j) Needle Placement:
  - Pierce the previously anesthetized skin and subcutaneous tissue site with appropriate needle and direct to target
(k) Aspiration: Rule out intravascular entry and to confirm entry into synovium (if enough synovial fluid is present to allow aspiration) or target structure
(l) Contrast injection:
  - Inject the joint with enough contrast in order to confirm entry into the target structure
  - Connecting the contrast dye syringe to the needle using extension tubing is recommended to prevent a shift in needle position during attachment and detachment to and from the spinal needle
  - Adjust the needle position, if necessary, in order to obtain a clearly defined arthrogram
(m) Injection: Unclamp the aspiration syringe and clamp on the injection syringe
(n) Postprocedural testing:
  - If applicable, reassess response to the aforementioned preprocedural provocative maneuver
(o) Repeat injection with therapeutic injectate if bilateral:
  - Repeat steps (h)–(m)
(p) *Adhesive bandage* application over the needle entry site
(q) Postprocedural care discussion

References

1. Leopold SS, Redd BB, Warme WJ, Wehrle PA, Pettis PD, Shott S. Corticosteroid compared with hyaluronic acid injections for the treatment of osteoarthritis of the knee. J Bone Joint Surg 2003;85-A:1197–1203.
2. Albert C, Brocq O, Gerard D, Roux C, Euller-Ziegler L. Septic knee arthrtits after intr-articular hyaluronate injection. Two case reports. Joint, Bone, Spine:revue du rhumatisme 2006;3(2): 205–207.
3. Waddell D, Estey D, Bricker DC, Marsala A. Viscosupplementation under fluoroscopic control. Am J Med Sports 2001;3(4):327–241, 249.
4. Jackson DW, Evans NA, Thomas BM. Accuracy of needle placement of intra-articular steroid injections. J Bone Joint Surgery Am 2002;84:1522–1527.
5. Jones A, Regan M, Ledingham J, Patrick M, Manhire A, Doherty M. Importance of placement of intrarticular steroid injections. BMJ 1995;307:1329–1330.
6. Bliddal H. Placement of intra-articular injections verified by mini-air arthrography. Ann Rheum Dis 1999;58:641–643.

Injection Procedure: Closed-Needle Knee Joint Lavage

Background: While the term knee joint lavage generally refers to arthroscopic lavage, it is also possible to perform needle lavage. Lavage removes debris such as microscopic or macroscopic fragments of cartilage, calcium phosphate crystals, and other inflammatory mediators in synovial fluid.

1. Indications: the removal of particulate matter and debris associated with any of the following conditions:
   (a) Chondrocalcinosis [1]
   (b) Osteoarthritis (Efficacy of lavage in knee osteoarthritis remains controversial.)
   (c) Rheumatoid arthritis [1]

2. Contraindications especially pertinent to this procedure:
   (a) None documented

3. Possible side effects especially pertinent to this procedure:
   (a) Discomfort from joint distension
   (b) Published reports have not otherwise described complications specifically attributable to the lavage

4. Technical details of note for this procedure (Fig. 11.14):
   (a) Preferred needle gauge; length; type: 14 gauge *or 16 gauge* [5]
      • The literature on preferred needle gauge size is very limited. Lavage with a small-bore cannula (e.g., 18- or 20-gauge needles) has been shown to produce no greater benefit than aspiration of the joint [2]. Dawes and colleagues also compared joint lavage, using a 14-gauge needle, with aspiration and injection of saline in a group of 20 patients; both groups improved at the third month and there was no statistical difference between them [3]
   (b) Note that techniques vary more for this procedure than for other knee joint injection procedures. A wide selection of needle size, volume of saline injected, and type of irrigants have been previously described [7–9]
   (c) Need for image guidance: Optional
      • The use of fluoroscopic and/or ultrasound guidance for knee joint lavage has not been reported in the literature. In contrast to other intra-articular injection procedures, image guidance is not necessary for knee lavage because successful entry into the knee joint should be readily apparent upon injection of saline solution, as resistance to the initial injection would indicate improper needle position

5. Step-by-step procedure:
   (a) Informed consent
   (b) Preprocedural testing: N/A
   (c) Image guidance: Optional: Fluoroscopic or ultrasound guidance
   (d) Patient positioning:

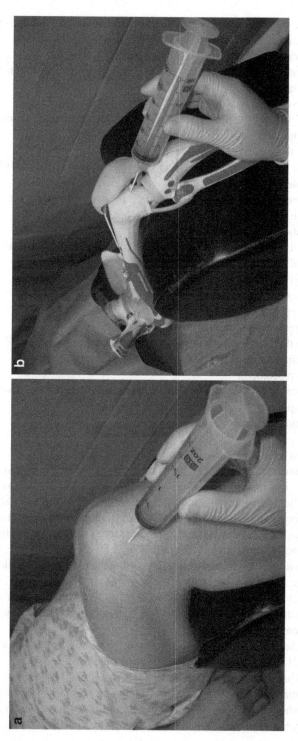

Fig. 11.14 Knee joint lavage. (**a**) Knee joint lavage – human model. (**b**) Skeletal representation of knee joint lavage

- Place the patient in a supine position and slightly flex the affected knee with a rolled pillow or towel underneath the popliteal space

(e) Identification and marking of injection site:
  - Palpate the skin entry site, and determine the most optimal needle entry site based upon:
    - Overlying skin integrity
    - If there is effusion: consider suprapatellar bursa or retropatellar approach
    - If there is no effusion: consider parapatellar approach
  - Mark the target using a marker or by depressing the skin with a plastic needle cap

(f) Skin preparation: Initial: Betadine® preparation using the no-touch technique

(g) Medication preparation:
  - Small amount of 1% lidocaine for skin/soft tissue anesthesia
  - 15 ml preservative-free lidocaine
  - 50 ml sterile preservative-free saline
  - 80 mg of Depo-Medrol®

(h) Skin preparation: Final: Alcohol prep

(i) Local anesthesia administration:
  - Anesthetize the overlying skin and soft tissue using a *small amount of 1% lidocaine* delivered via a *25-gauge*

(j) Needle placement:
  - Pierce the previously anesthetized skin and subcutaneous tissue site with the appropriate needle and direct to the target

(k) Aspiration: Rule out intravascular entry and confirm entry into target structure

(l) Contrast injection
  - If fluoroscopic guidance: Inject the joint with enough contrast to confirm entry into the target structure. Connecting the contrast dye syringe to the needle using extension tubing is recommended to prevent a shift in needle position during attachment and detachment to and from the needle. Adjust the needle position, if necessary, in order to obtain a clearly defined arthrogram

(m) Injection: Unclamp the aspiration syringe and clamp on the injection syringe:
  - Inject the joint with *15 ml of preservative-free 1% lidocaine* in order to anesthetize the joint capsule so as to more comfortably allow knee joint distension
  - Unclamp the syringe from the extension tubing and attach a syringe to inject the *50 ml of sterile preservative-free saline:*
    - The optimal total amount of fluid that should be used to lavage the knee is unclear. In one study, including rheumatoid arthritis patients who received lavage with 5 or 10 l of saline, these patients recovered better than those who received either 0.5 or 1 l of saline [6]. Since

there was no significant difference between the 5 and 10 1 dose, administrating 5 1 of saline appears most practical. In knee osteoarthritis patients, Vad and coworkers performed needle lavage using 500 ml of saline, delivered in ten exchanges of 50 ml injectate [10]

- Instill the 50 ml and then either:
  - Aspirate the knee (using the same syringe attached to the needle via extension tubing). In order to aspirate the saline, one may further flex or extend the patient's knee. The senior author (TS) had an interesting experience where he initially instilled a knee with 50 ml of saline, but was then unable to aspirate this out until the knee position was slightly altered
  - Instill as much saline as tolerable by the patient [4]. Because maximum distension is important, the senior author (TS) prefers this approach at the time of this writing. Aspirate the saline as above
- Note the quantity and appearance of fluid aspirated after the first fluid exchange cycle
- Optional: After the last saline exchange has been made, unclamp the syringe from the extension tubing, attach a *syringe* containing 80 mg of *Depo-Medrol®*, and inject this in to the joint

(n) *Adhesive bandage* application over the needle entry site
(o) Postprocedural care discussion

References

1. Livesley PJ, Doherty M, Needoff M, Moulton A. Arthroscopic lavage of osteoarthritic knees. J Bone Joint Surg 1991;73-B:922–926.
2. Fitzgerald O, Hanly J, Callan A, McDonald K, Molony J, Bresnihan B. Effects of joint lavage on knee synovitis in rheumatoid arthritis. Br J Rheumatol 1985;24:6–10.
3. Lindsay DJ, Ring EF, Coorey PF, Jayson MI. Synovial irrigation in rheumatoid arthritis. Acta Rheumatol Scand 1971;17(3):169–174.
4. Dawes PT, Kirlew C, Haslock I. Saline washout for knee osteoarthritis: results of a controlled study. Clin Rheumatol 1987;6(1):61–63.
5. Ravaud P, Moulinier L, Giraudeau B, Ayral X, Guerin C, Noel E et al. Effects of joint lavage and steroid injection in patients with osteoarthritis of the knee. Arthritis Rheum 1999;42(3):475–482.
6. Jackson DW, Evans NA, Thomas BM. Accuracy of needle placement of intra-articular steroid injections. J Bone Joint Surgery Am 2002;84:1522–1527.
7. Jones A, Regan M, Ledingham J, Pattrick M, Manhire A, Doherty M. Importance of placement of intra-articular steroid injections. BMJ 1993;307:1329–1330.
8. Tanaka N, Sakahashi H, Sato E, Hirose K, Ishii S. Effects of needle-arthroscopic lavage with different volumes of fluid on knee synovitis in rheumatoid arthritis. Clin Rheumatol 2002;21: 4–9.
9. Vad V, Bhat AL, Sculco TP, Wickiewicz TL. Management of knee osteoarthritis: knee lavage combined with hylan versus hylan alone. Arch Phys Med Rehabil 2003;84:634–637.
10. Schumacher HR. Aspiration and injection therapies for joints. Arthritis Rheum 2003;49(3): 413–420.

Injection Procedure: Pes Anserine Injection

1. Indications:
   (a) Pes anserine bursitis
      - Primary due to direct trauma or repetitive friction
      - Secondary due to altered lower limb alignment (especially varus knee deformity) associated with osteoarthritis
   (b) Pes anserine tendonitis (i.e., tendonitis of the sartorius, gracilis and/or semi-membranosus tendons at insertion sites)

2. Contraindications especially pertinent to this procedure:
   (a) None documented

3. Possible side effects especially pertinent to this procedure:
   (a) None documented

4. Technical details of note for this procedure (Fig. 11.15):
   (a) Preferred needle gauge: 25 gauge [1]
   (b) Need for image guidance: Optional
      - There are no documented studies evaluating the accuracy of injections into the pes anserine bursa or the need for image guidance. Cardone and Tallia recommend palpating anatomical landmarks prior to injection [1]. At the present time, the authors of this book agree and specifically suggest identifying the tendinous borders of the sartorius, gracilis, and semitendinosus muscles, whose conjoined insertions make up the pes anserine. Once identified, these tendons can be followed to their insertions, at which the point of maximal tenderness can be injected. However, ultrasound guidance rather than simple palpation may ultimately prove to be more accurate

5. Step-by-step procedure:
   (a) Informed consent
   (b) Preprocedural testing: Identify and record the response to a physical examination preprocedural provocative maneuver if the procedure is a diagnostic injection
      - Although resisted knee flexion should theoretically cause the semitendinosus tendon to compress the underlying bursa and exacerbate pes anserine bursitis, the authors have found this maneuver to be inconsistent. Under these circumstances, pain associated with ambulation may need to be used as the provocative maneuver
   (c) Image guidance: Optional
   (d) Patient positioning:
      - Place the patient in a supine position and slightly flex the affected knee with a rolled pillow or towel underneath the popliteal space
   (e) Identification and marking of injection site:
      - Palpate the skin entry site. Identify the tendinous borders of the sartorius, gracilis, and semitendinosus muscles, whose conjoined insertions make up the pes anserine

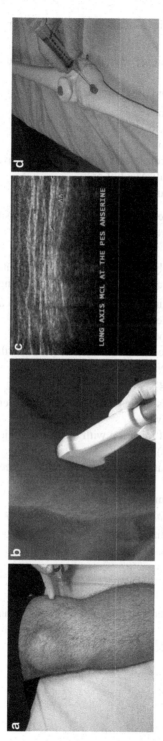

Fig. 11.15 Pes anserine bursa injection (ultrasound-guided). (**a**) Pes anserine bursa injection – human model. (**b**) Ultrasound transducer positioning for visualizing pes anserine bursa – human model. (**c**) Ultrasound corresponding to previous image. (**d**) Skeletal representation of pes anserine bursa injection

- Mark the target using a marker or by depressing the skin with a plastic needle cap
(f) Skin preparation: Initial: Betadine® preparation using the no-touch technique
(g) Medication preparation:
  - Diagnostic injection
    - 2 ml 1% preservative-free lidocaine
  - Therapeutic injection
    - 40 mg Depo-Medrol® and 1 ml 1% preservative-free lidocaine
(h) Skin preparation: Final: Alcohol prep
(i) Local anesthesia administration: Optional

  - Anesthetize the overlying skin and soft tissue using a *small amount of 1% lidocaine,* delivered via a *25-gauge needle*
(j) Needle placement:
  - Pierce the previously anesthetized skin and subcutaneous tissue site with a *25-gauge needle* attached to a syringe containing the injectate

(k) Aspiration: Rule out inadvertent intravascular entry and confirm entry into target structure (if able to aspirate bursal fluid)
(l) Contrast injection: Not applicable
(m) Injection: If resistance is encountered early during the injection, rotate the needle to dislodge the bevel from the bursal wall
(n) Postprocedural testing:
  - If applicable, reassess response to the aforementioned preprocedural provocative maneuver
(o) If (+) response, repeat injection with therapeutic injectate:
  - Repeat steps (d)–(f)
  - Medication preparation: 1 ml of preservative-free lidocaine and 40 mg Depo-Medrol®
  - Repeat steps (h)–(m)
(p) *Adhesive bandage* application over the needle entry site
(q) Postprocedural care discussion

Reference

1. Cardone D, Tallia AF. Diagnostic and therapeutic injection of the hip and knee. Am Fam Phys 2003;67(10):2147–2152.

Injection Procedure: Popliteal/Baker Cyst Injections

1. Indications:
   (a) Popliteal cyst

2. Contraindications especially pertinent to this procedure:
   (a) None documented

3. Possible side effects especially pertinent to this procedure:
   (a) Neurovascular damage to tibial nerve and/or popliteal artery/vein [1]
   (b) Popliteal cyst rupture

4. Technical details of note for this procedure (Fig. 11.16):
   (a) Preferred needle gauge: 18 gauge
   (b) Need for image guidance: Recommended
      • According to Grassi and colleagues, ultrasound can be a useful tool in detecting popliteal cysts and determining their contents. Based on the characteristics of the cyst, aspiration and corticosteroid injection may be an appropriate mode of treatment. Under sonographic guidance, it is easier to avoid neurovascular damage and assure appropriate needle placement, especially in patients with loculated cysts [1]. There have not been many studies comparing the accuracy or efficacy of popliteal cyst injections with or without sonographic guidance

5. Step-by-step procedure:
   (a) Informed consent
   (b) Preprocedural testing: Not applicable
   (c) Image guidance: Recommended: Ultrasound-guided procedure
   (d) Patient positioning: Place the patient in a prone position with a rolled pillow or towel underneath the front of the knee
   (e) Identification and marking of injection site:
      • Palpate the skin entry site, identifying the point of maximal tenderness. (The posterior-medial aspect of the knee joint has been found to be the most common location for popliteal cysts to develop.) [2]
      • Mark the target using a marker or by depressing the skin with a plastic needle cap
   (f) Skin preparation: Initial: Betadine® preparation using the no-touch technique
   (g) Medication preparation:
      • 40 mg of Depo-Medrol® and 0.5 ml of 1% lidocaine
   (h) Skin preparation: Final: Alcohol prep
   (i) Local anesthesia administration:
      • Anesthetize the overlying skin and soft tissue using a *small amount of 1% lidocaine* delivered via a *25-gauge or 30-gauge needle*

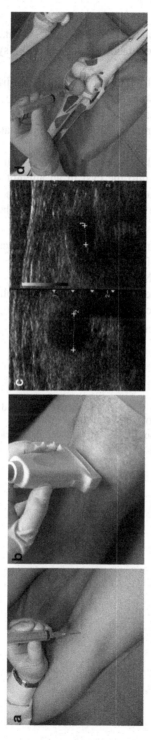

Fig. 11.16 Popliteal cyst aspiration (ultrasound-guided). (**a**) Popliteal cyst aspiration – human model. (**b**) Ultrasound transducer positioning for visualizing popliteal cyst – human model. (**c1**). Ultrasonogram corresponding to previous image. (**c2**). Ultrasonogram after partial cyst aspiration. (**d**) Skeletal representation of popliteal cyst aspiration

(j) Needle Placement:
  - Pierce the previously anesthetized skin and subcutaneous tissue site with the appropriate needle attached to an aspirating syringe and direct into the target

(k) Aspiration: Rule out intravascular entry and confirm entry into cyst (if enough cyst fluid is present to allow aspiration)

(l) Aspiration and Injection:
  - Aspirate all of the contents within the cyst and take note of the amount and color of the fluid aspirated
  - On occasion, the fluid is extremely viscous and may require injection of sterile normal saline into the cyst in an attempt to dilute its contents. Alternatively, a 16-gauge needle or angiocath can be used if available

(m) Injection: Unclamp the aspiration syringe and clamp on the injection syringe
  - If resistance is encountered early during the injection, rotate the needle to dislodge the bevel from the side of the cyst

(n) Postprocedural testing: Not applicable

(o) Repeat injection with therapeutic injectate: Not applicable

(p) *Adhesive bandage* application over the needle entry site

(q) Postprocedural care discussion

References

1. Grassi W, Farina A, FilippumLi E, Cervini C. Sonographically guided procedures in rheumatology. Semin Arthritis Rheum 2001;30(5):347–353.
2. Labropoulos N, Shifrin DA, Paxinos O. New insights into the development of popliteal cysts. Br J Surg 2004;91(10):1313–1318.

Injection Procedure: Prepatellar Bursa Aspiration/Injection

1. Indications:
   (a) Prepatellar bursitis: diagnosis as pain generator or treatment

2. Contraindications especially pertinent to this procedure:
   (a) None documented

3. Possible side effects especially pertinent to this procedure:
   (a) None

4. Technical details of note for this procedure (Fig. 11.17):
   (a) Preferred needle gauge:
      - Aspiration ±/– injection: 18 gauge
      - Injection only: 25 gauge
   (b) Need for image guidance: Optional
      - Ultrasound guidance can be used for this procedure if palpation does not definitively detect a bursal effusion

5. Step-by-step procedure:
   (a) Informed consent
   (b) Preprocedural testing: Not applicable
   (c) Image guidance: Optional: ultrasound guidance
   (d) Patient positioning:
      - Place the patient in a supine position and slightly flex the affected knee slightly with a rolled pillow or towel underneath the popliteal space
   (e) Identification and marking of injection site:
      - If nonimage-guided:
         - Palpate for a bursal effusion
      - If ultrasound-guided:
         - Directly visualize the underlying bursa
         - Mark the target using a marker or by depressing the skin with a plastic needle cap
   (f) Skin preparation: Initial: Betadine® preparation using the no-touch technique
   (g) Medication preparation:
      - Therapeutic injection:
         - 40 mg Depo-Medrol® and 0.5 ml 1% preservative-free lidocaine
   (h) Skin preparation: Final: Alcohol prep
   (i) Local anesthesia administration: Optional
      - Anesthetize the overlying skin and soft tissue using a *small amount of 1% lidocaine* delivered via a *25-gauge* or 30-gauge needle
   (j) Needle placement:
      - Direct the needle attached to an aspiration syringe in a zig-zag direction, to prevent leakage of the reaccumulated fluid through a needle tract that can develop if the needle is directed straight through the tissue, into the

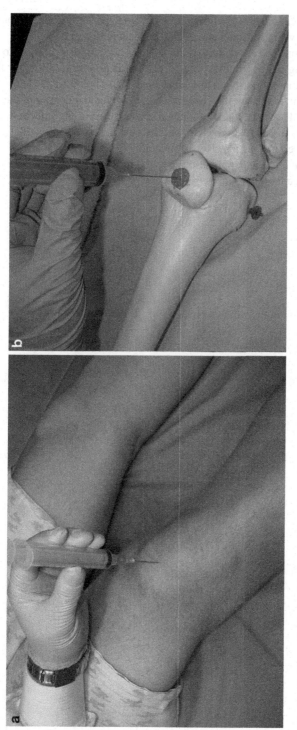

Fig. 11.17 Prepatellar bursa aspiration. (**a**) Prepatellar bursa aspiration – human model. (**b**) Skeletal representation of Prepatellar bursa aspiration

prepatellar bursa by trying to detect needle entry into the bursa or by direct visualization if ultrasound guidance was used

(k) Aspiration: Rule out intravascular entry and confirm entry into bursa by aspirating out any bursal fluid (if enough is present to allow for this)

(l) Contrast injection: Not applicable

(m) Injection: Unclamp the aspiration syringe and clamp on the injection syringe. If resistance is encountered early during the injection, rotate the needle to dislodge the bevel from the bursal wall

(n) Postprocedural testing: Not applicable

(o) *Adhesive bandage* application over the needle entry site

(p) Postprocedural care discussion

Injection Procedure: Tibiofibular Joint (Proximal) Injection

1. Indications:
   (a) Diagnosis: Evaluation of nonspecific lateral knee pain
   (b) Treatment: Osteoarthritis of the proximal tibiofibular joint [1]

2. Contraindications especially pertinent to this procedure:
   (a) None documented

3. Possible side effects especially pertinent to this procedure:
   (a) Theoretical possibility of iatrogenic peroneal nerve injury

4. Technical details of note for this procedure (Fig. 11.18):
   (a) Preferred needle gauge: 25 gauge
   (b) Need for image guidance: Recommended

5. Step-by-step procedure:
   (a) Informed consent
   (b) Preprocedural testing: Identify and record the response to a physical examination preprocedural provocative maneuver if the procedure is a diagnostic one
     • Flexion and medial rotation of the knee can often provoke pain [1]
   (c) Image guidance: Recommended: Fluoroscopic or ultrasound guidance
   (d) Patient positioning: Supine
   (e) Identification and marking of injection site:
     • If nonimage-guided: Identify the target structure visually and by palpation
     • If fluoroscopic-guided: Visualize the target structure by obliquely rotating the c-arm fluoroscope intensifier towards the affected joint until the joint space is optimally seen. Cephalad-caudad tilting might also be needed
     • If ultrasound-guided: Use the ultrasound transducer to image the underlying target structure
     • Mark the target using a marker or by depressing the skin with a plastic needle cap
   (f) Skin preparation: Initial: Betadine® preparation using the no-touch technique
   (g) Medication preparation:
     • Diagnostic injection:
       – 2 ml 2% preservative-free Lidocaine
     • Therapeutic injection:
       – 40 mg Depo-Medrol® and 1.0 ml 1% preservative-free lidocaine
   (h) Skin preparation: Final: Alcohol prep pad wipe
   (i) Local anesthesia administration:
     • Not generally required because target structure is close to the skin surface

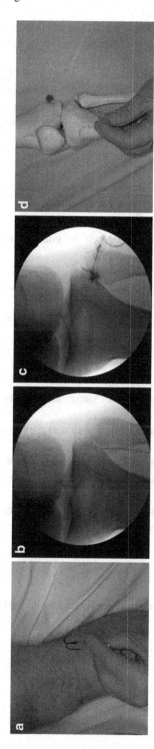

Fig. 11.18 Proximal tibiofibular joint injection (fluoroscopic-guided). (**a**) Proximal tibiofibular joint injection – human model. (**b**) Fluoroscopic image of needle entry into proximal tibiofibular joint. (**c**) Fluoroscopic image of proximal tibiofibular joint arthrogram. (**d**) Skeletal representation of proximal tibiofibular joint injection

390

T.P. Stitik et al.

(j) Needle placement: Pierce the previously anesthetized skin and subcutaneous tissue site with a *25-gauge needle* attached to a syringe containing the injectate
- If nonimage-guided: The needle is directed in an oblique direction towards the midportion of the joint [1]. The needle is then advanced through skin and subcutaneous tissue into the joint space
- If fluoroscopic-guided: Use intermittent fluoroscopic guidance to directly visualize needle entry into the joint
- If ultrasound-guided: Use ultrasound to directly visualize needle placement into the joint

(k) Aspiration: Rule out intravascular entry and to confirm entry into joint (if enough joint fluid is present to allow aspiration)

(l) Contrast injection (only for fluoroscopic guidance):
- Inject a small amount of contrast to confirm entry into the target structure

(m) Injection:
- If nonimage-guided: Inject medication. Rotate the needle if there is a high amount of resistance
- If fluoroscopic-guided: Use intermittent fluoroscopic guidance to visualize the dye pattern
- If ultrasound-guided: Use ultrasound guidance to directly visualize the injection

(n) Postprocedural testing: If diagnostic injection:
- Reassess the response to the same aforementioned preprocedural provocative maneuver

(o) If positive response, repeat injection with therapeutic injectate
- Repeat steps (d)–(f)
- Medication preparation for therapeutic injection: 40 mg Depo-Medrol® and 1.0 ml 1% preservative-free lidocaine
- Repeat steps (h)–(m)

(p) Application of adhesive bandage over the needle entry site

(q) Postprocedural care discussion

Reference

1. Waldman S. Atlas of Pain Management Injection Techniques. Philadelphia, PA: WB Saunders; 2000:252–253.

Injection Procedures Templates

Injection Procedure Template: Iliotibial Band Injection
Injection Procedure Template: Intra-articular Knee Injection

PROCEDURE: Iliotibial Band Injection
☐-Right   ☐-Left   ☐-Bilateral
Procedure Type: Aspiration: ☐-Diagnostic aspiration
               Injection: ☐-Diagnostic   ■-Therapeutic   ■-Diagnostic then Therapeutic
Image guidance: None unless indicated as follows- ■-Fluoroscopy ■-Ultrasound
- The potential benefits and side effects of the procedure and alternative treatment options were explained to the patient, an opportunity for questions was provided, and the patient signed informed consent.
- ■- If checked, the following physical examination pre-procedural provocative maneuver(s) was (were) performed: ■-_____
- The patient was positioned for the procedure and the target structure was identified.
- The overlying skin was prepped with Betadine® and alcohol.
- ■- If checked, the overlying skin and soft tissue was anesthetized using a small amount of 1% lidocaine delivered via the following needle ■-30G1"; ■-25G1½ "; ■-Other: _____
- The following needle was then used for the procedure:
      Type: Straight needle unless indicated as follows: ■-Spinal needle; ■-Other:_____
      Gauge: ■-30; ■-27; ■-25; ■-22; ■-21; -18; -Other:_____
      Length: ■-5/8"; ■- 1"; ■- 1 ½"; ■- 2"; ■- 2 ½"; ■- 3";■- 3½"; ■-Other:_____
- o   Image guidance if indicated above was used to confirm needle entry into target structure.
- o   ■-If checked, contrast dye was then injected and the needle position was adjusted accordingly to confirm proper placement without inadvertent intravascular entry.
- Needle was adjusted accordingly to confirm proper placement without inadvertent vascular entry.
- An attempt was made to aspirate from the structure and then the following injectate was delivered into the target structure:
      ■-Diagnostic injection: 3 mL 1% preservative-free lidocaine
      ■-Therapeutic injection: 40 mg Depo-Medrol® & 1 mL 1% preservative-free lidocaine
      ■- Other injectate: _____
- Visual inspection was used to confirm entry into the target structure. The needle position was adjusted as needed such that aspiration did not reveal blood return. Then the above solution was injected into the target structure.
- An adhesive bandage was placed over the needle entry site.

-If the above was a **diagnostic injection,** then proceed to section immediately below.
-If above was a **therapeutic injection procedure, aspiration only procedure,** or **aspiration and therapeutic injection,** then proceed to Procedure Summary Section.

For Diagnostic Injection Procedure:
- ■-If checked, the above listed pre-procedural physical examination provocative maneuver was repeated and pain relief was: ■-N/A; ■-significant; ■-some; ■-equivocal; ■-none; ■-Other:_____
- Based on the amount of pain relief noted above:
      ■-a therapeutic injection will be scheduled.
      ■-a therapeutic injection will not be scheduled. See plan in office note below.
      ■-a therapeutic injection following the same procedure described above was done using:
            ■- 40 mg Depo-Medrol® & 1 mL 1% preservative-free lidocaine
            ■- Other injectate: _____

Procedure Summary:
If fluid aspirated from the target structure during the procedure:
- Total volume of fluid aspirated: ___ mL; Fluid appearance: ■- N/A; ■-Clear yellow; ■-Slightly cloudy; ■-Cloudy; ■-Purulent; ■-Blood-tinged; ■-Bloody; ■-Other:_____
Patient tolerance for the procedure: ■-Excellent; ■-Good; ■-Fair; ■-Other:_____

Additional comments regarding the procedure: ■-None; ■Other:_____

Post-Procedural Treatment Advice:
Activity modification: Avoid non-essential use of the structure until seen for follow up. ■-Other:_____
Orthotic instructions: N/A unless indicated as follows _____
Modalities: Apply ice over the injection site prn for 20-30 min. up to q2 hrs until seen for follow-up, unless instructed as follows: ■-Heat; ■-Other:_____

Injection Procedure Template: Intra-articular Viscosupplementation

PROCEDURE: Intra-articular Knee Injection
Side: ☐-Right   ☐-Left   ☐-Bilateral
Procedure Type: Aspiration: ☐-Diagnostic aspiration
          Injection: ☐-Diagnostic   ☐-Therapeutic   ☐-Diagnostic <u>then</u> Therapeutic
Image guidance: None unless indicated as follows- ☐-Fluoroscopy   ☐-Ultrasound
- The potential benefits and side effects of the procedure and alternative treatment options were explained to the patient, an opportunity for questions was provided, and <u>the patient signed informed consent</u>.
- ☐- If checked, the following physical examination <u>pre-procedural provocative maneuver(s)</u> was (were) performed: ☐-_____
- The patient was positioned for the procedure and the target structure was identified.
- The overlying skin was prepped with <u>Betadine® followed by alcohol prep pad</u> after the Betadine® dried.
- ☐ If checked, the overlying skin and soft tissue was anesthetized using a <u>small amount of 1% lidocaine</u> delivered via the following needle ☐-30G1"; ☐-25G1½"; ☐-Other: _____
- The following needle was then used for the procedure:
  <u>Type</u>: Straight needle unless indicated as follows: ☐-Spinal needle; ☐-Other:_____
  <u>Gauge</u>: ☐-30; ☐-27; ☐-25; ☐-22; ☐-21; -18; -Other: _____
  <u>Length</u>: ☐-5/8"; ☐- 1"; ☐- 1 ½"; ☐- 2"; ☐- 2 ½"; ☐- 3"; ☐- 3½"; ☐-Other:_____
- ○ Image guidance if indicated above was used to confirm needle entry into target structure.
- ○ ☐-If checked, contrast dye was then injected and the needle position was adjusted accordingly to confirm proper placement without inadvertent intravascular entry.
- Needle was adjusted accordingly to confirm proper placement without inadvertent vascular entry.
- An attempt was made to aspirate from the structure and then the following injectate was delivered into the target structure:
  ☐-Diagnostic injection: <u>5 mL 1% preservative-free lidocaine</u>; ☐-Other injectate: _____
  ☐-Therapeutic injection: <u>80 mg Depo-Medrol®</u> & ☐- <u>2 mL 1% preservative-free lidocaine</u>
          ☐-Other injectate: _____
- The needle was removed and an <u>adhesive bandage</u> was placed over the needle entry site.

-If the above was a <u>diagnostic injection</u>, then proceed to section immediately below.
-If above was a <u>therapeutic injection procedure</u>, <u>aspiration only procedure</u>, or <u>aspiration and therapeutic injection</u>, then proceed to Procedure Summary Section.

For Diagnostic Injection Procedure:
- ☐-If checked, the above listed pre-procedural physical examination provocative maneuver was repeated and pain relief was: ☐-N/A; ☐-significant; ☐-some; ☐-equivocal; ☐-none; ☐-Other:_____
- Based on the amount of pain relief noted above:
  ☐-a therapeutic injection will be scheduled.
  ☐-a therapeutic injection will <u>not</u> be scheduled. See plan in corresponding office note.
  ☐-a therapeutic injection following the same procedure described above was done using
        ☐- <u>80 mg Depo-Medrol®</u> & ☐- <u>1 mL 1% preservative-free lidocaine</u>
        ☐- Other injectate:_____
- The needle was removed and an <u>adhesive bandage</u> was placed over the needle entry site.

Procedure Summary:
<u>If fluid aspirated from the target structure during the procedure:</u>
- Total volume of fluid aspirated: ___ mL; Fluid appearance: ☐- N/A; ☐-Clear yellow; ☐-Slightly cloudy; ☐-Cloudy; ☐-Purulent; ☐-Blood-tinged; ☐-Bloody; ☐-Other:_____
<u>Patient tolerance for the procedure</u>: ☐-Excellent; ☐-Good; ☐-Fair; ☐-Other:_____

<u>Additional comments regarding the procedure</u>: ☐-None; ☐Other:_____

Post-Procedural Treatment Advice:
<u>Activity modification</u>: Avoid non-essential use of the structure until seen for follow up. ☐-Other:_____

<u>Orthotic instructions</u>: N/A unless indicated as follows _____
<u>Modalities</u>: Apply ice over the injection site prn for 20-30 min. up to q2 hrs until seen for follow-up, unless instructed as follows: ☐-Heat; ☐-Other:_____

Injection Procedure Template: Popliteal/Baker Cyst Injections

PROCEDURE: Intra- Articular Knee Viscosupplementation
Side: ☐-Right   ☐-Left   ☐-Bilateral
Procedure Type: Aspiration: ☐-Diagnostic aspiration
                Injection: ☐-Therapeutic
Image guidance: None unless indicated as follows- ☐-Fluoroscopy ☐-Ultrasound
- The potential benefits and side effects of the procedure and alternative treatment options were explained to the patient, an opportunity for questions was provided, and <u>the patient signed informed consent</u>.
- ☐- If checked, the following physical examination <u>pre-procedural provocative maneuver(s)</u> was (were) performed: ☐-
- The patient was positioned for the procedure and the target structure was identified.
- The overlying skin was prepped with <u>Betadine®</u> <u>followed by alcohol prep pad</u> after the Betadine® dried.
- ☐- If checked, the overlying skin and soft tissue was anesthetized using a <u>small amount of 1% lidocaine</u> delivered via the following needle ☐-30G1"; ☐-25G1½ "; ☐-Other: _____
- The following needle was then used for the procedure:
    Type: Straight needle unless indicated as follows: ☐-Spinal needle; ☐-Other: _____
    <u>Gauge:</u> ☐-30; ☐-27; ☐-25; ☐-22; ☐-21; -18; -Other: _____
    <u>Length:</u> ☐-5/8"; ☐- 1"; ☐- 1 ½"; ☐- 2"; ☐- 2 ½"; ☐- 3"; ☐- 3½"; ☐-Other: _____
- ○ Image guidance if indicated above was used to confirm needle entry into target structure.
- ○ ☐-If checked, contrast dye was then injected and the needle position was adjusted accordingly to confirm proper placement without inadvertent intravascular entry.
- Needle was adjusted accordingly to confirm proper placement without inadvertent vascular entry.
- An attempt was made to aspirate from the structure and then the following injectate was delivered into the target structure:
    ☐-Therapeutic injection: 40 mg Hyalgan (sodium hyaluronate 20mg/2ml) or
                ☐-Other injectate: _____
- The needle was removed and an <u>adhesive bandage</u> was placed over the needle entry site.

Procedure Summary:
If fluid aspirated from the target structure during the procedure:
- Total volume of fluid aspirated: ___ mL; Fluid appearance: ☐- N/A; ☐-Clear yellow; ☐-Slightly cloudy; ☐-Cloudy; ☐-Purulent; ☐-Blood-tinged; ☐-Bloody; ☐-Other: _____
Patient tolerance for the procedure: ☐-Excellent; ☐-Good; ☐-Fair; ☐-Other: _____

Additional comments regarding the procedure: ☐-None; ☐Other: _____

Post-Procedural Treatment Advice:
Activity modification: Avoid non-essential use of the structure until seen for follow up. ☐-Other: _____

Orthotic instructions: ☐-N/A; ☐-Other: _____
Modalities: Apply the following modality for 20-30 min. up to q2 hrs prn until seen for follow-up, unless otherwise instructed- ☐-Ice; ☐-Heat; ☐-Other: _____

Injection Procedure Template: Prepatellar Bursa Aspiration/Injection

PROCEDURE: **Closed-Needle Knee Joint Lavage**
Side: ☐-Right   ☐-Left   ☐-Bilateral
Procedure Type: Aspiration: ☐-Diagnostic aspiration
                Injection: ☐-Diagnostic   ☐-Therapeutic   ☐-Diagnostic <u>then</u> Therapeutic
Image guidance: None unless indicated as follows- ☐-Fluoroscopy   ☐-Ultrasound

- The potential benefits and side effects of the procedure and alternative treatment options were explained to the patient, an opportunity for questions was provided, and <u>the patient signed informed consent</u>.
- ☐- If checked, the following physical examination <u>pre-procedural provocative maneuver(s)</u> was (were) performed: ☐-_____
- The patient was positioned for the procedure and the target structure was identified.
- The overlying skin was prepped with <u>Betadine® followed by alcohol prep pad</u> after the Betadine® dried.
- ☐- If checked, the overlying skin and soft tissue was anesthetized using a <u>small</u> amount of 1% <u>lidocaine</u> delivered via the following needle ☐-30G1"; ☐-25G1½ "; ☐-Other: _____
- The following needle was then used for the procedure:
  <u>Type</u>: Straight needle unless indicated as follows: ☐-Spinal needle; ☐-Other:_____
  <u>Gauge</u>: ☐-30; ☐-27; ☐-25; ☐-22; ☐-21; -18; -Other: _____
  <u>Length</u>: ☐-5/8"; ☐- 1"; ☐- 1 ½"; ☐- 2"; ☐- 2 ½"; ☐- 3";☐- 3½"; ☐-Other:_____
- ○ Image guidance if indicated above was used to confirm needle entry into target structure.
- ○ ☐-If checked, contrast dye was then injected and the needle position was adjusted accordingly to confirm proper placement without inadvertent intravascular entry.
- Needle was adjusted accordingly to confirm proper placement without inadvertent vascular entry.
- An attempt was made to aspirate from the structure and then the following injectate was delivered into the target structure:
  ☐-Diagnostic injection: <u>1 mL 1% preservative-free lidocaine</u>; ☐-Other injectate: _____
  ☐-Therapeutic injection: <u>80 mg Depo-Medrol®</u> & ☐- <u>15 mL 1% preservative-free lidocaine</u>
          ☐-Other injectate: _____
- The needle was removed and an <u>adhesive bandage</u> was placed over the needle entry site.

-If the above was a <u>diagnostic injection</u>, then proceed to section immediately below.
-If above was a <u>therapeutic injection procedure</u>, <u>aspiration only procedure</u>, or <u>aspiration and therapeutic injection</u>, then proceed to Procedure Summary Section.

For Diagnostic Injection Procedure:
- ☐-If checked, the above listed pre-procedural physical examination provocative maneuver was repeated and pain relief was: ☐-N/A; ☐-significant; ☐-some; ☐-equivocal; ☐-none; ☐-Other:_____
- Based on the amount of pain relief noted above:
  ☐-a therapeutic injection will be scheduled.
  ☐-a therapeutic injection will <u>not</u> be scheduled. See plan in corresponding office note.
  ☐-a therapeutic injection following the same procedure described above was done using
          ☐- <u>40 mg Depo-Medrol®</u> & ☐- <u>0.5 mL 1% preservative-free lidocaine</u>
          ☐- Other injectate:_____
- The needle was removed and an <u>adhesive bandage</u> was placed over the needle entry site.

Procedure Summary:
<u>If fluid aspirated from the target structure during the procedure:</u>
- Total volume of fluid aspirated: _____ mL; Fluid appearance: ☐- N/A; ☐-Clear yellow; ☐-Slightly cloudy;
  ☐-Cloudy; ☐-Purulent; ☐-Blood-tinged; ☐-Bloody; ☐-Other:_____
<u>Patient tolerance for the procedure</u>: ☐-Excellent; ☐-Good; ☐-Fair; ☐-Other:_____

<u>Additional comments regarding the procedure</u>: ☐-None; ☐Other:_____
_____

Post-Procedural Treatment Advice:
<u>Activity modification</u>: Avoid non-essential use of the structure until seen for follow up. ☐-Other:_____

<u>Orthotic instructions</u>: N/A unless indicated as follows _____
<u>Modalities:</u> Apply ice over the injection site prn for 20-30 min. up to q2 hrs until seen for follow-up, unless instructed as follows: ☐-Heat; ☐-Other:_____

Injection Procedure Template: Tibiofibular Joint (Proximal) Injection

---

PROCEDURE: Pes Aneserine Injection
Side: ☐-Right   ☐-Left   ☐-Bilateral
Procedure Type: Aspiration: ☐-Diagnostic aspiration
        Injection: ☐-Diagnostic   ☐-Therapeutic ☐-Diagnostic then Therapeutic
Image guidance: None unless indicated as follows- ☐-Fluoroscopy ☐-Ultrasound
- The potential benefits and side effects of the procedure and alternative treatment options were explained to the patient, an opportunity for questions was provided, and the patient signed informed consent.
- ☐- If checked, the following physical examination pre-procedural provocative maneuver(s) was (were) performed: ☐-_____
- The patient was positioned for the procedure and the target structure was identified.
- The overlying skin was prepped with Betadine® followed by alcohol prep pad after the Betadine® dried.
- ☐- If checked, the overlying skin and soft tissue was anesthetized using a small amount of 1% lidocaine delivered via the following needle ☐-30G1"; ☐-25G1½ "; ☐-Other: _____
- The following needle was then used for the procedure:
  Type: Straight needle unless indicated as follows: ☐-Spinal needle; ☐-Other:_____
  Gauge: ☐-30; ☐-27; ☐-25; ☐-22; ☐-21; -18; -Other:_____
  Length: ☐-5/8"; ☐- 1"; ☐- 1 ½"; ☐- 2"; ☐- 2 ½"; ☐- 3";☐- 3½"; ☐-Other:_____
- ○ Image guidance if indicated above was used to confirm needle entry into target structure.
- ○ ☐-If checked, contrast dye was then injected and the needle position was adjusted accordingly to confirm proper placement without inadvertent intravascular entry.
- Needle was adjusted accordingly to confirm proper placement without inadvertent vascular entry.
- An attempt was made to aspirate from the structure and then the following injectate was delivered into the target structure:
  ☐-Diagnostic injection: 2 mL 1% preservative-free lidocaine; ☐-Other injectate: _____
  ☐-Therapeutic injection: 40 mg Depo-Medrol® & ☐- 1 mL 1% preservative-free lidocaine
          ☐-Other injectate: _____
- The needle was removed and an adhesive bandage was placed over the needle entry site.

-If the above was a diagnostic injection, then proceed to section immediately below.
-If above was a therapeutic injection procedure, aspiration only procedure, or aspiration and therapeutic injection, then proceed to Procedure Summary Section.

For Diagnostic Injection Procedure:
- ☐-If checked, the above listed pre-procedural physical examination provocative maneuver was repeated and pain relief was: ☐-N/A; ☐-significant; ☐-some; ☐-equivocal; ☐-none; ☐-Other:_____
- Based on the amount of pain relief noted above:
  ☐-a therapeutic injection will be scheduled.
  ☐-a therapeutic injection will not be scheduled. See plan in corresponding office note.
  ☐-a therapeutic injection following the same procedure described above was done using
          ☐- 40 mg Depo-Medrol® & ☐- 1 mL 1% preservative-free lidocaine
          ☐- Other injectate: _____
- The needle was removed and an adhesive bandage was placed over the needle entry site.

Procedure Summary:
If fluid aspirated from the target structure during the procedure:
- Total volume of fluid aspirated: ____ mL; Fluid appearance: ☐- N/A; ☐-Clear yellow; ☐-Slightly cloudy; ☐-Cloudy; ☐-Purulent; ☐-Blood-tinged; ☐-Bloody; ☐-Other:_____
Patient tolerance for the procedure: ☐-Excellent; ☐-Good; ☐-Fair; ☐-Other:_____
Additional comments regarding the procedure: ☐-None; ☐Other:_____

Post-Procedural Treatment Advice:
Activity modification: Avoid non-essential use of the structure until seen for follow up. ☐-Other:_____

Orthotic instructions: N/A unless indicated as follows _____
Modalities: Apply ice over the injection site prn for 20-30 min. up to q2 hrs until seen for follow-up, unless instructed as follows: ☐-Heat; ☐-Other:_____

Chapter 12
The Ankle and the Foot

Patrick M. Foye, Christopher Castro, Peter P. Yonclas, Todd P. Stitik, Mohammad Hossein Dorri, Jong H. Kim, Jose Santiago Campos, Lisa Schoenherr, Naimish Baxi, and Ladislav Habina

Introduction

In many general musculoskeletal practices, injections into the foot and ankle regions are not as commonly performed as are injections into other body regions. For example, in a 2-year musculoskeletal injection teaching study, injections into the foot/ankle region were the least commonly performed (1.6% of the total) [1]. Perhaps one reason for the relative paucity of injections into the foot and ankle regions is the principle that injections into the foot should generally be avoided if possible in diabetic patients. In addition, aspiration/injection procedures have not been proven to be of benefit as part of the typical treatment algorithm for typical soft tissue ankle injuries such as the usual (inversion) ankle sprain, one of the most common musculoskeletal conditions involving the foot/ankle region [2]. Furthermore, injections into this body region can be quite uncomfortable. Finally, it has traditionally been taught that corticosteroid injection procedures should be avoided into regions of weight-bearing tendons, particularly the posterior tibial tendon and the Achilles tendon regions. In contrast to their comparatively smaller incidence in general musculoskeletal practice, these injections obviously play a potentially large role in the practice of orthopedic foot/ankle surgeons and podiatrists both for therapeutic purposes and by offering diagnostic information, particularly when arthrodesis or other surgical interventions are being considered [3–5].

The use of image guidance, with either fluoroscopy or ultrasound, has been advocated as a way of increasing the injection accuracy into the foot and ankle region [6–8]. The authors have found fluoroscopic guidance to be particularly useful for ankle joint injections in osteoarthritis patients given the altered anatomy, including variable degrees of joint space narrowing.

The ankle joint (tibiotalar joint) may be a source of pain due to osteoarthritis, rheumatoid arthritis, acute injury, or chronic instability. Ankle joint corticosteroid injections are sometimes performed as part of the management of patients with

P.M. Foye (✉)
Department of Medicine and Rehabilitation, New Jersey Medical School, Newark, NJ, USA
e-mail: doctor.foye@gmail.com

T.P. Stitik (ed.), *Injection Procedures: Osteoarthritis and Related Conditions*,
DOI 10.1007/978-0-387-76595-2_12, © Springer Science+Business Media, LLC 2011

osteoarthritis, rheumatoid arthritis, or other inflammatory arthropathies. For osteoarthritis, the use of viscosupplementation has shown some preliminary positive results as an alternative to corticosteroid injections [9, 10]. One of the authors (TS) has personally performed ankle viscosupplementation in a limited number of patients with encouraging results [11]. In doing so, fluoroscopic guidance was used, given the absolute necessity of intra-articular placement of the viscosupplement and the potential technical difficulty due to joint space narrowing in the osteoarthritic ankle joint. As noted previously, a meta-analysis concluded that there was insufficient evidence that joint aspiration or injection was of benefit in the setting of acute soft tissue trauma such as an ankle sprain [2]. The possibility that intra-articular injections impair ankle proprioception was refuted in a study of 22 healthy volunteers who received ankle joint lidocaine injections [12]. In rheumatoid arthritis, the safety of intra-articular tumor necrosis factor alpha (TNF-alpha) antagonists into the ankle joints of two patients was evaluated, and no noticeable adverse events were found [13]. Chemical synovectomy achieved through injection of a radioactive material into the joint has been described for use in patients with rheumatoid arthritis, hemophilic synovitis, and pigmented villonodular synovitis (PVNS) [14–19]. Severe complications, however, have been reported following intra-articular injection of the yttrium 90 isotope into the ankle joint for diffuse PVNS [18]. Another method of chemical synovectomy, intra-articular injection of osmic acid, has been studied for patients with corticosteroid-resistant arthritis in the knee and for arthropathy in Von Willebrand's Disease of the knee and ankle [20]. The use of intra-articular methylprednisolone, bupivacaine, and morphine as a method of pain reduction after ankle arthroscopy was found to reduce pain, joint swelling, time of immobilization, duration of sick leave, and hasten return to sports [21]. Some benefits from the intra-articular administration of the hormone somatostatin were reported on in a limited number of athletes with nonspecific arthrosynovitis or tendinitis of the ankle or knee [22].

The first MTP joint is frequently affected by gout and osteoarthritis. In an acute gouty flare, the joint capsule can be significantly swollen. The capsular distension associated with the swollen joint theoretically should allow for easier aspiration compared to a nonswollen joint. A case series, however, found that aspiration using a 29-gauge needle yielded little difference in successful aspiration rates between asymptomatic (89%) and inflamed joints (93%) [23]. It has been reasoned that aspiration of gouty crystals might provide sufficient pain relief without the necessity for concomitant injection of corticosteroids [24]. The value of selective use of corticosteroid injections into an osteoarthritic joint has been reported [25]. While gout and osteoarthritis primarily affect the first MTP joint, the remaining MTP joints can also be affected by inflammatory arthropathies, especially rheumatoid arthritis. Corticosteroid injections as a treatment for synovitis affecting these joints have been studied [26]. There was also previous interest in injection of Erbium 169 for radioactive synoviortheses [27]. One of the authors has administered a viscosupplement intra-articularly into the MTP joint of a collegiate basketball player with posttraumatic osteoarthritis.

The intertarsal joints can be a source of pain especially in the setting of acute injury and posttraumatic degenerative changes. There is scant literature on injections into intertarsal joints, including the talonavicular and the calcaneocuboid joints. Retrospective studies have reported on a limited number of injections, using fluoroscopic or CT scan guidance, into various joints including the talocalcaneonavicular, calcaneocuboid, calcaneonavicular, navicular-cuneiform, and fifth metatarsocuboid joints [5, 28].

The subtalar joint can be a source of pain, especially in rheumatoid arthritis patients. A beneficial effect from corticosteroid injections into the subtalar joints of patients with rheumatoid arthritis has been reported [29]. Subtalar joint corticosteroid injections have also been studied in children with juvenile idiopathic arthritis (juvenile chronic arthritis) and were found to be effective and accurate when performed using fluoroscopic guidance [30, 31]. In a prospective study of 55 patients, fluoroscopic-guided subtalar joint injections using an anterolateral approach were found to be more accurate than injections performed using a posterior talocalcaneal/posterior subtalar approach [32].

Depending upon the injury grade, a typical (aka usual) ankle sprain involves the anterior talofibular ligament with or without involvement of the calcaneofibular ligament +/- the posterior talofibular ligament. Hyaluronic acid injections in the vicinity of the lateral ankle ligaments (aka periarticular injections) were studied in the setting of a typical inversion ankle sprain [33]. This one randomized controlled trial found that this intervention, combined with usual care, was more effective than the combination of placebo injection and usual care, in terms of reduced pain and more rapid return to sports, and was associated with fewer adverse events.

Plantar fasciitis, the most common cause of adult heel pain, likely involves a degenerative tear of part of the origin of the fascia from the calcaneus. Corticosteroid injections for plantar fasciitis have traditionally been a mainstay of conservative treatment. Both clinical and ultrasonographic anatomic benefits have been documented [34–36]. While extracorporeal shock wave treatment has been a more recently described treatment, whether the prior injection of cortisone affects the likelihood of a positive response to this treatment is unclear [37, 38]. Complications of corticosteroid injections have included plantar fascia rupture, injury to the lateral plantar nerve, sterile abscess formation, and calcaneal osteomyelitis [39–43]. Ultrasound guidance has been proposed as a way of improving outcomes from the injections [44, 45]. There is also one report of technetium scintigraphy to help localize the steroid injection site in resistant cases of plantar fasciitis [46]. Newer potential methods of treatment that are still under investigation include the injection of autologous blood [47, 48]. One of the authors (TS) performed an autologous blood injection into one patient with plantar fasciitis, with very good benefit.

Subfascial injections of botulinum toxin were shown to be efficacious in two prospective studies and a retrospective review of patients with plantar fasciitis [49–51]. One case report showed benefit in a patient with spasticity and plantar fasciitis from the combination of a botox injection into the gastrocnemius and an autologous blood injection into the plantar fascia [52].

The two sesamoid bones in the foot are located within the flexor hallucis brevis tendon underneath the first metatarsal head. Disorders of the sesamoid bones include inflammation (sesamoiditis), arthritis, and fracture (either traumatic or stress-induced). Diagnostic local anesthetic and corticosteroid injections for sesamoiditis have been described in injection textbooks, but no peer-review articles on this topic have been published in the literature at the time of this writing [53, 54].

Retrocalcaneal bursitis (aka Achilles bursitis) is an inflammation of the bursa located between the posterior aspect of the calcaneus and the anterior aspect of the Achilles tendon where it inserts on the calcaneus. An ultrasound-guided technique for corticosteroid injections of the retrocalcaneal bursa and the tibialis posterior tendon sheath in patients with chronic inflammatory arthropathy has been described [54, 55]. Reports in the literature on aspiration/injection of the retrocalcaneal bursa are otherwise quite limited. Two cadaveric studies examined the bursa and the bursal fluid, respectively [56, 57].

Morton neuroma (aka Morton's neuralgia, Morton's metatarsalgia, interdigital neuropathy of the foot, interdigital neuritis, or plantar interdigital neuroma) involves perineural fibrosis of a branch of the common plantar digital nerves especially frequently between the third and fourth metatarsal heads and leads to intermittent pain and paresthesias. In addition, the intermetatarsal bursa, which overlies the nerve, may also compress the nerve if the bursa is inflamed [58]. The diagnosis is generally based on history and physical examination, especially the squeeze test. Initial conservative treatment is often attempted and can include a corticosteroid injection into the affected webspace. Literature on the success of this approach is limited, but the results were favorable [58–60]. However, a Cochrane database systematic review concluded that there is insufficient evidence with which to assess the effectiveness of this nonsurgical intervention [61]. A case of hyperpigmentation, thinning of the skin, and subcutaneous fat atrophy that developed at the site of the injection perhaps due to the injection being delivered too superficially has been reported [62]. More recently, an ultrasound-guided approach has been described for corticosteroid injections, alcohol injections, and sclerosing solution injections [63–65]. Chemical neurolysis via serial injections of dilute alcohol, serial injections of a sclerosing solution containing alcohol, as well as electrical stimulation-guided phenol injections were also found to be a safe and effective treatment option [64–67]. The utility of a diagnostic block as a predictor of subsequent surgical outcome has yielded mixed results [68, 69].

Sinus tarsi syndrome can be defined as pain originating from the lateral entrance (sinus tarsi) into the subtalar joint. Local anesthetic injections into the sinus tarsi have been reported to be useful as a diagnostic procedure [70, 71]. Although corticosteroid injections for this condition have been described, there are no peer-reviewed published studies supporting their use [70, 71]. A variant of sinus tarsi syndrome, in which the patient complains of pain on the medial aspect of the hindfoot in conjunction with the typical lateral pain, has been coined the "canalis tarsi syndrome." Injections into this region concomitantly with those into the sinus tarsi have been described [72]. Injections using landmark palpation or fluoroscopy are probably advantageous over ultrasound guidance which can be difficult to visualize the needle.

Posterior tibial tendon sheath injections under ultrasound guidance have been reported within a case series for patients with posterior tibial tendon dysfunction [7]. Good efficacy without complications was noted. Other peer-reviewed literature pertaining to injections in this body region is lacking at the time of this writing.

Literature on injection procedures for patients with tarsal tunnel syndrome is scant. Aspiration of tarsal tunnel cysts under ultrasound guidance has been reported within a case series [7]. Good efficacy without complications was noted. A case report described the injection of lidocaine into the tarsal tunnel of a patient with paraplegia and presumed tarsal tunnel syndrome as a method of diminishing the flexor-withdrawal reflex which was interfering with sleep and causing severe pain after hot baths [73]. Other peer-reviewed literature pertaining to injections in this body region is lacking at the time of this writing. At least one injections textbook has described posterior tibial nerve blocks at the ankle using local anesthetic and corticosteroid as a method of treating the symptoms associated with tarsal tunnel syndrome [74]. However, there are no peer-reviewed publications on this topic. Hydrodissection under ultrasound guidance offers a potential non-surgical treatment that is in need of validation.

The literature provides a variety of descriptions regarding how to perform the various injections described in this chapter and variable degrees of evidence regarding their effectiveness (Table 12.1).

Table 12.1 Summary of foot–ankle region injection procedures

Injection type	Specific structure	Meta-analysis(es)	Prospective study (studies)	Case series/ report(s)	Described in review article(s) and/or injection textbook(s)
Articulation/joint	Ankle (tibiotalar) joint	[2]	[9, 10, 14, 15, 21]	[1, 13, 17–20, 22]	[75]
	1st MTP			[23]	[24, 25, 75]
	MTP- other			[26, 27]	
	Intertarsal joints			[5, 28]	
	Talocalcaneonavicular				
	Calcaneocuboid				
	Talonavicular				
	Calcaneonavicular				
	Calcaneocuboid				
	Navicular-cuneiform				
	5th Metatarsocuboid				
	Subtalar (talocalcaneal) joint			[29–31]	
Bursa	Retrocalcaneal (aka Achilles bursa)				[55]
Ligament					
Morton's Neuroma		[61]	[58, 64, 68, 69]	[59, 60, 62–64, 67, 76]	[75]
Periarticular region			[33]		
Plantar fascia			[34–36, 44, 47–50, 51]	[37, 39–43, 45, 46, 51, 52]	[75]
Sesamoids					[53, 54]

(continued)

Table 12.1 (continued)

Injection type	Specific structure	Meta-analysis(es)	Prospective study (studies)	Case series/report(s)	Described in review article(s) and/or injection textbook(s)
Sinus tarsi				[70–72]	
Tarsal tunnel				[7]	[74, 75]
Tendon sheath	Peroneal tendon			[32]	
	Posterior tibial tendon			[7]	[55]
Tendon (intratendinous)	Achilles Tendon			[77, 78]	
Tendon sheath (paratendon)	Achilles Tendon			[79]	
	Posterior tibial tendon			[55]	[80]

References

1. Stitik TP, Foye PM, Nadler SF, Chen B, Schoenherr L, Van Hagen S. Injections in patients with osteoarthritis and other musculoskeletal disorders: use of synthetic injection models for teaching physiatry residents. Am J Phys Medicine Rehabil 2005;84:550–9.
2. Ogilvie-Harris DJ, Gilbart M. Treatment modalities for soft tissue injuries of the ankle: a critical review. Clin J Sport Med 1995;5(3):175–86.
3. Khoury NJ, el-Khoury GY, Saltzman CL, Brandser EA. Intraarticular foot and ankle injections to identify source of pain before arthrodesis. AJR Am J Roentgenol 1996;167(3):669–73.
4. Lucas PE, Hurwitz SR, Kaplan PA, Dussault RG, Maurer EJ. Fluoroscopically guided injections into the foot and ankle: localization of the source of pain as a guide to treatment – prospective study. Radiology 1997;204(2):411–5.
5. Mitchell MJ, Bielecki D, Bergman AG, Kursunoglu-Brahme S, Sartoris DJ, Resnick D. Localization of specific joint causing hindfoot pain: value of injecting local anesthetics into individual joints during arthrography. AJR Am J Roentgenol 1995;164(6):1473–6.
6. Newman JS. Diagnostic and therapeutic injections of the foot and ankle. Semin Roentgenol 2004;39(1):85–94.
7. Sofka CM, Adler RS. Ultrasound-guided interventions in the foot and ankle. Semin Musculoskelet Radiol 2002;6(2):163–8.
8. Fredberg U, van Overeem Hansen G, Bolvig L. Placement of intra-articular injections verified by ultrasonography and injected air as contrast medium. Ann Rheum Dis 2001;60:542.
9. Sun SF, Chou YJ, Hsu CW, Hwang CW, Hsu PT, Wang JL et al. Efficacy of intra-articular hyaluronic acid in patients with osteoarthritis of the ankle: a prospective study. Osteoarthritis Cartilage 2006;14(9):867–74.
10. Salk RS, Chang TJ, D'Costa WF, Soomekh DJ, Grogan KA. Sodium hyaluronate in the treatment of osteoarthritis of the ankle: a controlled, randomized, double-blind pilot study. J Bone Joint Surg Am 2006;88(2):295–302.
11. Stitik TP, Lin GMSIV, Foye PM, Schoenherr L. A novel ankle osteoarthritis treatment? Fluoroscopic-Guided Viscosupplementation. Submitted to the 65th Annual Meeting of the American Academy of PM&R, 2005.
12. Down S, Waddington G, Adams R, Thomson M. Movement discrimination after intra-articular local anaesthetic of the ankle joint. Br J Sports Med 2007;41(8):501–5.
13. Bliddal H, Terslev L, Qvistgaard E, Recke P, Holm CC, Danneskiold-Samsoe B, Savnik A, Torp-Pedersen S. Safety of intra-articular injection of etanercept in small-joint arthritis: an

uncontrolled, pilot-study with independent imaging assessment. Joint Bone Spine 2006; 73(6):714–7.

14. Göbel D, Gratz S, von Rothkirch T, Becker W. Chronic polyarthritis and radiosynoviorthesis: a prospective, controlled study of injection therapy with erbium 169 and rhenium 186. Z Rheumatol 1997;56(4):207–13.

15. Göbel D, Gratz S, von Rothkirch T, Becker W, Willert HG. Radiosynoviorthesis with rhenium-186 in rheumatoid arthritis: a prospective study of three treatment regimens. Rheumatol Int 1997;17(3):105–8.

16. Barnes CL, Shortkroff S, Wilson M, Sledge CB. Intra-articular radiation treatment of rheumatoid synovitis of the ankle with dysprosium-165 ferric hydroxide macroaggregates. Foot Ankle Int 1994;15(6):306–10.

17. Gilbert MS, Radomisli TE. Therapeutic options in the management of hemophilic synovitis. Clin Orthop Relat Res 1997;(343):88–92.

18. Bickels J, Isaakov J, Kollender Y, Meller I. Unacceptable complications following intra-articular injection of yttrium 90 in the ankle joint for diffuse pigmented villonodular synovitis. J Bone Joint Surg Am 2008;90(2):326–8.

19. Shabat S, Kollender Y, Merimsky O, Isakov J, Flusser G, Nyska M et al. The use of surgery and yttrium 90 in the management of extensive and diffuse pigmented villonodular synovitis of large joints. Rheumatology (Oxford) 2002;41(10):1113–8.

20. Salis G, Molho P, Verrier P, Stieltjes N, Vassilieff D, Ounnoughène N et al. Nonsurgical synovectomy in the treatment of arthropathy in Von Willebrand's Disease. Rev Rhum Engl Ed 1998;65(4):232–7.

21. Rasmussen S, Kehlet H. Intraarticular glucocorticoid, morphine and bupivacaine reduces pain and convalescence after arthroscopic ankle surgery: a randomized study of 36 patients. Acta Orthop Scand 2000;71(3):301–4.

22. Russo S, Mangrella M, Vitagliano S, Russo P, Berrino L. Local administration of somatostatin in joint diseases in athletes. Minerva Med 1997;88(6):265–70.

23. Sivera F, Aragon R, Pascual E. First metatarsophalangeal joint aspiration using a 29-gauge needle. Ann Rheum Dis 2008;67(2):273–5. Epub 2007 Jun 8.

24. Scott PM. Arthrocentesis to diagnose and treat acute gouty arthritis in the great toe. JAAPA 2000;13(10):93–6.

25. Boxer MC. Osteoarthritis involving the metatarsophalangeal joints and management of metatarsophalangeal joint pain via injection therapy. Clin Podiatr Med Surg 1994;11(1):125–32.

26. Trepman E, Yeo SJ. Nonoperative treatment of metatarsophalangeal joint synovitis. Foot Ankle Int 1995;16(12):771–7.

27. Bouvier M, Bouysset M, Bonvoisin B, Diaine A, Lejeune E. Erbium 169 synoviortheses and infiltrations of triamcinolone hexacetonide in metatarsophalangeal arthritis of chronic inflammatory rheumatism. Rev Rhum Mal Osteoartic 1983;50(4):267–71.

28. Saifuddin A, Abdus-Samee M, Mann C, Singh D, Angel JC. CT guided diagnostic foot injections. Clin Radiol 2005;60(2):191–5.

29. Beaudet F, Dixon AS. Posterior subtalar joint synoviography and corticosteroid injection in rheumatoid arthritis. Ann Rheum Dis 1981;40(2):132–5.

30. Cahill AM, Cho SS, Baskin KM, Beukelman T, Cron RQ, Kaye RD et al. Benefit of fluoroscopically guided intraarticular, long-acting corticosteroid injection for subtalar arthritis in juvenile idiopathic arthritis. Pediatr Radiol 2007;37(6):544–8. Epub 2007 Apr 17.

31. Remedios D, Martin K, Kaplan G, Mitchell R, Woo P, Rooney M. Juvenile chronic arthritis: diagnosis and management of tibio-talar and sub-talar disease. Br J Rheumatol 1997; 36(11):1214–7.

32. Ruhoy MK, Newberg AH, Yodlowski ML, Mizel MS, Trepman E. Subtalar joint arthrography. Semin Musculoskelet Radiol 1998;2(4):433–438.

33. Petrella RJ, Petrella MJ, Cogliano A. Periarticular hyaluronic acid in acute ankle sprain. Clin J Sport Med 2007;17(4):251–7.

34. Genc H, Saracoglu M, Nacir B, Erdem HR, Kacar M. Long-term ultrasonographic follow-up of plantar fasciitis patients treated with steroid injection. Joint Bone Spine 2005;72(1):61–5.
35. Chigwanda PC. A prospective study of Plantar fasciitis in Harare. Cent Afr J Med 1997;43(1):23–5.
36. Tsai WC, Wang CL, Tang FT, Hsu TC, Hsu KH, Wong MK. Treatment of proximal plantar fasciitis with ultrasound-guided steroid injection. Arch Phys Med Rehabil 2000;81(10):1416–21.
37. Ogden J, Alvarez RG, Cross GL, Jaakkola JL. Plantar fasciopathy and orthotripsy: the effect of prior cortisone injection. Foot Ankle Int 2005;26(3):231–3.
38. Melegati G, Tornese D, Bandi M, Caserta A. The influence of local steroid injections, body weight and the length of symptoms in the treatment of painful subcalcaneal spurs with extracorporeal shock wave therapy. Clin Rehabil 2002;16(7):789–94.
39. Acevedo JI, Beskin JL. Complications of plantar fascia rupture associated with corticosteroid injection. Foot Ankle Int 1998;19(2):91–7.
40. Sellman JR. Plantar fascia rupture associated with corticosteroid injection. Foot Ankle Int 1994;15(7):376–81.
41. Snow DM, Reading J, Dalal R. Lateral plantar nerve injury following steroid injection for plantar fasciitis. Br J Sports Med 2005;39(12):e41; discussion e41.
42. Buccilli TA Jr, Hall HR, Solmen JD. Sterile abscess formation following a corticosteroid injection for the treatment of plantar fasciitis. J Foot Ankle Surg 2005;44(6):466–8.
43. Gidumal R, Evanski P. Calcaneal osteomyelitis following steroid injection: a case report. Foot Ankle 1985;6(1):44–6.
44. Tsai WC, Hsu CC, Chen CP, Chen MJ, Yu TY, Chen YJ. Plantar fasciitis treated with local steroid injection: comparison between sonographic and palpation guidance. J Clin Ultrasound 2006;34(1):12–6.
45. Kane D, Greaney T, Bresnihan B, Gibney R, FitzGerald O. Ultrasound guided injection of recalcitrant plantar fasciitis. Ann Rheum Dis 1998;57(6):383–4.
46. Dasgupta B, Bowles J. Scintigraphic localisation of steroid injection site in plantar fasciitis. Lancet 1995;346(8987):1400–1.
47. Kiter E, Celikbas E, Akkaya S, Demirkan F, Kiliç BA. Comparison of injection modalities in the treatment of plantar heel pain: a randomized controlled trial. J Am Podiatr Med Assoc 2006;96(4):293–6.
48. Lee TG, Ahmad TS. Intralesional autologous blood injection compared to corticosteroid injection for treatment of chronic plantar fasciitis. A prospective, randomized, controlled trial. Foot Ankle Int 2007;28(9):984–90.
49. Babcock MS, Foster L, Pasquina P, Jabbari B. Treatment of pain attributed to plantar fasciitis with botulinum toxin a: a short-term, randomized, placebo-controlled, double-blind study. Am J Phys Med Rehabil 2005;84(9):649–54.
50. Placzek R, Deuretzbacher G, Meiss AL. Treatment of chronic plantar fasciitis with Botulinum toxin A: preliminary clinical results. Clin J Pain 2006;22(2):190–2.
51. Placzek R, Hölscher A, Deuretzbacher G, Meiss L, Perka C. Treatment of chronic plantar fasciitis with botulinum toxin A – an open pilot study on 25 patients with a 14-week-follow-up. Z Orthop Ihre Grenzgeb 2006;144(4):405–9.
52. Logan LR, Klamar K, Leon J, Fedoriw W. Autologous blood injection and botulinum toxin for resistant plantar fasciitis accompanied by spasticity. Am J Phys Med Rehabil 2006;85(8):699–703.
53. Kesson M, Atkins E, Davies I. The ankle and foot. In Kesson M, Atkins E, Davies I, eds. Musculoskeletal Injection Skills. New York, NY: Butterworth Heinemann; 2002:160–1.
54. Waldman SD. Sesamoiditis Pain Syndrome. Atlas of Pain Management Injection Techniques. Philadelphia, PA: WB Saunders company; 2007:579–82.
55. Brophy DP, Cunnane G, Fitzgerald O, Gibney RG. Technical report: ultrasound guidance for injection of soft tissue lesions around the heel in chronic inflammatory arthritis. Clin Radiol 1995;50(2):120–2.
56. Frey C, Rosenberg Z, Shereff MJ, Kim H. The retrocalcaneal bursa: anatomy and bursography. Foot Ankle 1992;13(4):203–7.

57. Canoso JJ, Wohlgethan JR, Newberg AH, Goldsmith MR. Aspiration of the retrocalcaneal bursa. Ann Rheum Dis 1984;43(2):308–12.
58. Bennett GL, Graham CE, Mauldin DM. Morton's interdigital neuroma: a comprehensive treatment protocol. Foot Ankle Int 1995;16(12):760–3.
59. Rasmussen MR, Kitaoka HB, Patzer GL. Nonoperative treatment of plantar interdigital neuroma with a single corticosteroid injection. Clin Orthop Relat Res 1996;326:188–93.
60. Greenfield J, Rea J Jr, Ilfeld FW. Morton's interdigital neuroma. Indications for treatment by local injections versus surgery. Clin Orthop Relat Res 1984;185:142–4.
61. Thomson CE, Gibson JN, Martin D. Interventions for the treatment of Morton's neuroma. Cochrane Database Syst Rev 2004;(3):CD003118.
62. Reddy PD, Zelicof SB, Ruotolo C, Holder J. Interdigital neuroma. Local cutaneous changes after corticosteroid injection. Clin Orthop Relat Res 1995;317:185–7.
63. Hassouna H, Singh D, Taylor H, Johnson S. Ultrasound guided steroid injection in the treatment of interdigital neuralgia. Acta Orthop Belg 2007;73(2):224–9.
64. Hughes RJ, Ali K, Jones H, Kendall S, Connell DA. Treatment of Morton's neuroma with alcohol injection under sonographic guidance: follow-up of 101 cases. AJR Am J Roentgenol 2007;188(6):1535–9.
65. Fanucci E, Masala S, Fabiano S, Perugia D, Squillaci E, Varrucciu V et al. Treatment of intermetatarsal Morton's neuroma with alcohol injection under US guide: 10-month follow-up. Eur Radiol 2004;14(3):514–8.
66. Mozena JD, Clifford JT. Efficacy of chemical neurolysis for the treatment of interdigital nerve compression of the foot: a retrospective study. J Am Podiatr Med Assoc 2007; 97(3):203–6.
67. Magnan B, Marangon A, Frigo A, Bartolozzi P. Local phenol injection in the treatment of interdigital neuritis of the foot (Morton's neuroma). Chir Organi Mov 2005;90(4):371–7.
68. Younger AS, Claridge RJ. The role of diagnostic block in the management of Morton's neuroma. Can J Surg 1998;41(2):127–30.
69. Okafor B, Shergill G, Angel J. Treatment of Morton's neuroma by neurolysis. Foot Ankle Int 1997;18(5):284–7.
70. Kuwada GT. Long-term retrospective analysis of the treatment of sinus tarsi syndrome. J Foot Ankle Surg 1994;33:28–29.
71. HV Debrunner. Das Sinus Tarsi Syndrome. Schweiz Med Wochenschr 1963;93:1660–1664.
72. Zwipp H, Swoboda B, Holch M, Maschek HJ, Reichelt S. Sinus tarsi and canalis tarsi syndromes. A post-traumatic entity. Unfallchirurg 1991;94(12):608–13.
73. Tachibana S, Saegusa H, Suzuki S, Yamazaki Y, Iida H. Latent tarsal tunnel syndrome with the provocation of flexor spasms in a paraplegic person. Case report. Paraplegia 1995;33(8):482–4.
74. Waldman SD. Posterior Tarsal Tunnel Syndrome. Atlas of Pain Management Injection Techniques. Philadelphia, PA: WB Saunders company; 2007:524–8.
75. Tallia AF, Cardone DA. Diagnostic and therapeutic injection of the ankle and foot. Am Fam Physician 2003;68(7):1356–62.
76. Haddad SL, Sabbagh RC, Resch S, Myerson B, Myerson MS. Results of flexor-to-extensor and extensor brevis tendon transfer for correction of the crossover second toe deformity. Foot Ankle Int 2000;21(10):872.
77. Koenig MJ, Torp-Pedersen S, Qvistgaard E, Terslev L, Bliddal H. Preliminary results of colour Doppler-guided intratendinous glucocorticoid injection for Achilles tendonitis in five patients. Scand J Med Sci Sports 2004;14(2):100–6.
78. Boesen MI, Boesen M, Jensen KE, Bliddal H, Torp-Pedersen S. Imaging of intratendinous distribution of glucocorticosteroid in the treatment of Achilles tendinopathy. Pilot study of low-field magnetic resonance imaging correlated with ultrasound. Clin Exp Rheumatol 2006;24(6):664–9.
79. Gill SS, Gelbke MK, Mattson SL, Anderson MW, Hurwitz SR. Fluoroscopically guided low-volume peritendinous corticosteroid injection for Achilles tendinopathy. A safety study. J Bone Joint Surg Am 2004;86-A(4):802–6.
80. Waldman SD. Posterior Tibialis Tendinitis. Atlas of Pain Management Injection Techniques. Philadelphia, PA: WB Saunders company; 2007:560–562.

Procedure Instructions

Injection Procedure: Retrocalcaneal Bursa (Achilles Bursa) Injection

1. Indications:
   (a) Differentiation of retrocalcaneal bursitis (Achilles bursitis) from Achilles tendonitis
   (b) Achilles bursitis treatment

2. Contraindications especially pertinent to this procedure:
   (a) None documented

3. Possible side effects especially pertinent to this procedure:
   (a) Achilles tendon rupture [1]
   (b) Injury to sural nerve if lateral approach
   (c) Injury to tibial nerve or artery if medial approach

4. Technical details of note for this procedure (Fig. 12.1):
   (a) Preferred needle gauge; length; type:
       • Aspiration ±/- injection: 25 gauge; short
   (b) Need for image guidance: Both blind and ultrasound-guided injections have been described [2–5].

5. Step-by-step procedure:
   (a) Informed consent
   (b) Preprocedural testing: Identify and record the response to a physical examination preprocedural provocative maneuver if the procedure is a diagnostic injection.
   (c) Image guidance: Optional: Ultrasound-guided
   (d) Patient positioning:
       • Place the patient in a prone position with the affected foot hanging over the edge of the table in slight plantarflexion.
       • Passively dorsiflex and plantarflex the ankle so that you can firmly grasp the Achilles tendon between your thumb and index fingers. This will allow one to direct the needle under the Achilles tendon and into the bursa.
       • Palpate the skin entry site, identifying a spot 2–3 cm proximal to the calcaneal insertion site of the Achilles tendon and just above the posterior superior aspect of the calcaneus [3].
   (e) Identification and marking of injection site:
       • Mark the target using a marker or by depressing the skin with a plastic needle cap.
   (f) Skin preparation: Initial: Betadine® preparation using the no-touch technique.
   (g) Medication preparation:

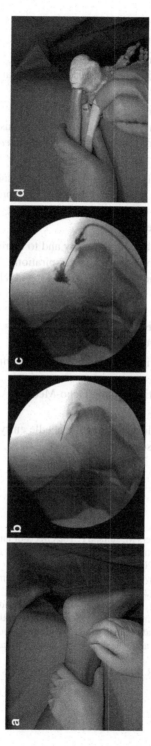

Fig. 12.1 Achilles bursa injection (fluoroscopic-guided). (**a**) Achilles bursa injection–human model. (**b**) Fluoroscopic image of needle entry into achilles bursa. (**c**) Fluoroscopic image of achilles bursogram. (**d**) Skeletal representation of achilles bursa injection

- Diagnostic injection:
  - 1 mL 1% preservative-free lidocaine
- Therapeutic injection:
  - 40 mg Depo-Medrol® and 1 mL 1% preservative-free lidocaine

(h) Skin preparation: Final: Alcohol prep
(i) Local anesthesia administration:
  - Anesthetize the overlying skin and soft tissue using a *small amount of 1% lidocaine* delivered via a *30-gauge-1-in. needle.*

(j) Needle Placement:
  - Pierce the previously anesthetized skin and subcutaneous tissue site with the appropriate needle and direct 2–3 cm proximal and deep to the calcaneal insertion of the Achilles tendon at the posterior superior aspect of the calcaneus.

(k) Aspiration: Rule out intravascular entry and to confirm entry into bursa (if enough bursal fluid is present to allow aspiration).
(l) Injection: Unclamp the aspiration syringe and clamp on the injection syringe.
(m) Postprocedural testing:
  - If applicable, reassess response to the aforementioned preprocedural provocative maneuver.

(n) If (+) response, repeat injection with therapeutic injectate:
  - Repeat steps (d)–(f).
  - Medication preparation: 40 mg Depo-Medrol®
  - Repeat steps (h)–(l).

(o) *Adhesive bandage* application over the needle entry site
(p) Postprocedural care discussion

References

1. Hugate R, Pennypacker J, Saunders M, Juliano P. The effects of intratendinous and retrocalcaneal intrabursal injections of corticosteroid on the biomechanical properties of rabbit achilles tendons. J Bone Joint Surg Am 2004;86:794–801.
2. Canoso JJ, Wohlgethan JR, Newberg AH, Goldsmith MR. Aspiration of the retrocalcaneal bursa. Ann Rheum Dis 1984;43(2):308–12.
3. Cunndne G, Brophy D, Gibney R, FitzGerald O. Diagnosis and treatment of heel pain in chronicinflammatory arthritis using ultrasound. Semin Arthritis Rheum 1996;25(6):383–89.
4. Brophy DP, Cunnane G, Fitzgerald O, Gibney RG. Technical report: ultrasound guidance for injection of soft tissue lesions around the heel in chronic inflammatory arthritis. Clinical Radiology 1995;50:120–2.
5. Sofka CM, Adler RS, Positano R. Haglund's syndrome: diagnosis and treatment using sonography. HSS J 2006;2(1):27–9.

Injection Procedure: Achilles Tendon Peritendinous Injection

1. Indications:
   (a) Differentiation of Achilles tendonitis from retrocalcaneal bursitis
   (b) Achilles tendonitis treatment

2. Contraindications especially pertinent to this procedure:
   (a) None documented

3. Possible side effects especially pertinent to this procedure:
   (a) Achilles tendon rupture[1, 2]

4. Technical details of note for this procedure (Fig. 12.2):
   (a) Preferred needle gauge; length; type:
       • Aspiration ±/– injection: 25 gauge; short; spinal
   (b) Need for image guidance: Recommended: Fluoroscopy or Ultrasound (if used for peritendinous injection)
       • The use of corticosteroid injections for Achilles tendonitis has received controversial reviews due to a reported associated risk of Achilles tendon rupture. The actual risk of Achilles tendon rupture with or without corticosteroid injection is not known with certainty. Although there are case reports of Achilles tendon rupture following corticosteroid injection, it is unclear if these occurred due to inadvertent intratendinous injection. Intratendinous injections are almost universally believed to significantly increase the risk of rupture. Animal studies have shown that intratendinous injections temporarily weaken the tendon [2]. In contrast, peritendinous injections have not been shown to do this [2]. In fact, injecting the peritendinous space reportedly decreases vascular proliferation and fibrosis, reducing the amount of inflammatory mediators that can migrate to the area. Corticosteroids also help to limit the adhesions between the tendon and the paratendon, which seem to be the primary cause of the tenderness and stiffness associated with Achilles tendonitis. Given the potential risk of tendon rupture with inadvertent tendon injection, image-guided injections are a logical alternative.
       • A retrospective study conducted by Gill and colleagues reported no incidence of tendon rupture in patients receiving peritendinous injections with the use of fluoroscopic guidance [3].
       • In contrast to the use of fluoroscopic guidance for peritendinous injections, ultrasound has been studied as a method for guiding injections into the tendon itself. As noted previously, while it is generally believed that intratendinous injections are potentially dangerous, Koenig and coworkers performed a study in which corticosteroids were directly injected into the Achilles tendon under ultrasound guidance [4]. With the use of ultrasound Doppler, they reported increased vascular activity within the tendon. They concluded that the presence of increased activity was indicative of an inflammatory reaction occurring inside the tendon, for which installation

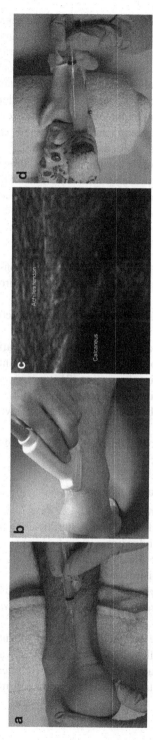

Fig. 12.2 Achilles tendon sheath injection (ultrasound-guided). (**a**) Achilles tendon sheath injection–human model. (**b**) Ultrasound transducer positioning for visualizing achilles tendon–human model. (**c**) Ultrasonogram corresponding to previous image. (**d**) Skeletal representation of achilles tendon sheath injection

of an anti-inflammatory agent directly into the region was desirable. This would theoretically decrease the vascularization and subsequently the pain in the area. They found that subjects had an average VAS score of 35 at rest and 56 during exercise prior to their injections. For up to 2 months following treatment, all of their patients were pain-free both at rest and during activity and were without any reported tendon ruptures [2]. Another ultrasound-guided intratendinous injection study on three patients found a total regression of hyperemia and intratendinous edema as seen on serial ultrasounds and MRIs, respectively [5].

- In summary, the authors at the time of this writing recommend the use of image guidance for peritendinous injections. The authors are not yet convinced that intratendinous injection has been proven to be safe enough to recommend it.

5. Step-by-step procedure:
   (a) Informed consent
   (b) Preprocedural testing: Identify and record the response to a physical examination preprocedural provocative maneuver if the procedure is a diagnostic injection.
   (c) Image guidance: Recommended: Fluoroscopic-guided or Ultrasound-guided
   (d) Patient positioning:
       - Place the patient in a prone position with the affected foot in a dorsiflexed position. Palpate the skin entry site, identifying a spot 2–3 cm proximal to the calcaneal insertion [3].
   (e) Identification and marking of injection site:
       - Mark the spot with a plastic needle cap with or without image guidance.
   (f) Skin preparation: Initial: Betadine® preparation using the no-touch technique
   (g) Medication preparation:
       - Diagnostic injection:
         – 3 mL 1% preservative-free lidocaine
       - Therapeutic Injection:
         – 20 mg Depo-Medrol®, 0.5 mL sterile saline solution and 2 mL 1% preservative-free lidocaine
   (h) Skin preparation: Final: Alcohol prep
   (i) Local anesthesia administration:
       - Anesthetize the overlying skin and soft tissue using a *small amount of 1% lidocaine* delivered via a 30-*gauge-1-in. needle.*
   (j) Needle Placement:
       - Pierce the previously anesthetized skin and subcutaneous tissue site with the appropriate needle, directing the needle towards a position 2–3 cm proximal to the calcaneal insertion of the Achilles tendon.
   (k) Aspiration: Rule out intravascular entry and confirmation of entry into target structure.
   (l) Contrast injection:

- Inject the region with enough contrast to confirm entry into the target structure. Connecting the contrast dye syringe to the needle using extension tubing is recommended to prevent a shift in needle position during attachment and detachment to and from the spinal needle. Adjust needle position, if necessary, in order to clearly define dye in the region of the pre-Achilles fat [3].

(m) Injection: Unclamp the aspiration syringe and clamp on the injection syringe.

(n) Postprocedural testing:
- If applicable, reassess response to the aforementioned preprocedural provocative maneuver.

(o) If (+) response, repeat injection with therapeutic injectate:
- Repeat steps (d)–(f).
- Medication preparation: 20 mg of triamcinolone, 0.5 mL of sterile saline solution, and 0.5 mL 1% lidocaine
- Repeat steps (h)–(m).

(p) Adhesive bandage application over the needle entry site

(q) Postprocedural care discussion

References

1. Hugate R, Pennypacker J, Saunders M, Juliano P. The effects of intratendinous and retrocalcaneal intrabursal injections of corticosteroid on the biomechanical properties of rabbit Achilles tendons. J Bone Joint Surg Am 2004;86:794–801.
2. Shrier I, Mathesoa G, Kohl H. Achilles tendonitis: Are corticosteroid injections useful or harmful? Clin J Sport Med 1996;6(4):245–250.
3. Gill S, Gelbke M, Mattson S, Anderson M, Hurwitz S. Fluoroscopically guided low-volume peritendinous corticosteroid injection for Achilles tendinopathy. J Bone Joint Surg 2004;86-A(4):802–806.
4. Koenig M, Torp-Pedersen S, Qvistgaard E, Terslev L, Bliddal H. Preliminary results of colour Doppler-guided intratendinous glucocorticoid injection for Achilles tendonitis in five patients. Scand J Med Sci Sports 2004;14:100–6.
5. Boesen MI, Boesen M, Jensen KE, Bliddal H, Torp-Pedersen S. Imaging of intratendinous distribution of glucocorticosteroid in the treatment of Achilles tendinopathy. Pilot study of low-field magnetic resonance imaging correlated with ultrasound. Clin Exp Rheumatol 2006;24(6):664–9.

Injection Procedure: Ankle Joint (Tibiotalar Joint) Injection

1. Indications:
   (a) Ankle osteoarthritis (OA) diagnosis as pain generator or treatment
   (b) Intra-articular ankle viscosupplementation:
      • To date, FDA approval has not been given for viscosupplementation of the tibiotalar joint. However, there have been several studies on its effectiveness for the use of treating ankle OA pain. Salk and colleagues performed a pilot study in which they compared the effectiveness of sodium hyaluronate with saline solution injected into the ankle. They concluded that while both solutions provided statistically significant relief in a 6-month period, 56% of the sodium hyaluronate group had a decrease >30 mm Ankle Osteoarthritis Scale (AOS) score from baseline compared with 13% of the saline solution group [1]. Similarly, Sun and coworkers found a decrease of total AOS from 5.1 ± 1.9 at baseline to 2.4 ± 1.9 at 6 months follow-up after a series of five hyaluronate injections. In this same study, they noted a significant decrease in acetaminophen use following viscosupplementation injections, with a use of 14.3 + 2.4 tablets/week at baseline compared to 3.3 + 2.2 tablets/week at 6 month follow-up [2]. More importantly, they documented positive patient satisfaction rates at different follow-up visits. Their results showed a 100% satisfaction rate 1 week and 1 month following injection, 90.7% satisfaction at 3 weeks follow-up, and 86.7% satisfaction 6 months after injection.
   (c) Ankle joint pathology treatment [3, 4]

2. Contraindications especially pertinent to this procedure:
   (a) None documented

3. Possible side effects especially pertinent to this procedure:
   (a) Infection in diabetic patients

4. Technical details of note for this procedure (Fig. 12.3):
   (a) Preferred needle gauge; length; type:
      • Aspiration ±/− injection: 22–25 gauge; short
   (b) Need for image-guidance: Recommended:
      • The use of image guidance is a highly recommended practice when injecting the foot and ankle regions, as the area is extremely compact with intricate articulations. The use of image guidance allows the physician to confirm the appropriate placement of the needle into the intra-articular space [4]. In contrast, when performed with the use of anatomic landmarks as a guide, these procedures can often miss their intended target [5]. Accuracy becomes particularly imperative when attempting to differentiate among pain generators within the foot and ankle regions. The use of standard radiography without conducting diagnostic injections is not necessarily helpful in determining the

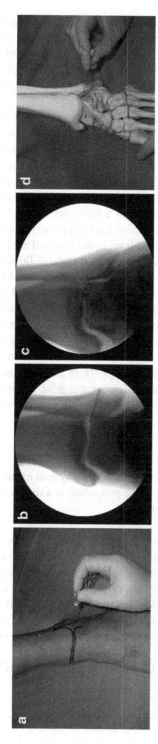

Fig. 12.3 Ankle joint injection (fluoroscopic-guided). (**a**) Ankle joint injection-human model. (**b**) Fluoroscopic image of needle entry into ankle joint. (**c**) Fluoroscopic image of ankle joint arthrogram. (**d**) Skeletal representation of ankle joint injection

primary pain generator. Structures that appear normal on radiographic findings can often be the primary source of pain, while joints appearing pathologic may not be the culprit [3]. Documenting the exact position of the needle within the desired joint allows the physician to determine if the suspected structure is the primary pain generator based on the response to local anesthetic.

- Lucas and coworkers demonstrated that the use of fluoroscopic guidance in foot and ankle injections led to a statistically significant difference in the confidence level of surgeons to identify a pain generator within the area. They showed that with the use of image-guided local anesthetic and steroid injections, the surgeon's level of confidence in regard to the cause of pain was altered in 82% of the cases [4]. This allowed them to structure a treatment plan more decisively. In a study performed by Remedios and colleagues, it was also shown that the use of fluoroscopic guidance enhanced the efficacy of steroid injections in the foot and ankle. They found that the average duration of pain relief with the use of fluoroscopy was 38 weeks, while the mean duration without fluoroscopy was 14 weeks [6].

- As per Sofka and coworkers, the use of ultrasound guidance for tibiotalar injections allows for detection of an effusion, which could subsequently be aspirated. Sonography also allows the physician to identify alternative etiologies for the pain, while localizing "active sites of inflammation" in cases of "nonspecific ankle swelling," while increasing the efficacy of local corticosteroid injections [5, 7]. In addition, this technique helps the physician avoid inadvertently contaminating a joint by "passing a needle though an infected periarticular bursa or septic tenosynovitis " [5].

5. Step-by-step procedure:
   (a) Informed consent
   (b) Preprocedural testing:
      - Identify and record the response to a physical examination preprocedural provocative maneuver if the procedure is a diagnostic injection.
   (c) Image guidance: Recommended
   (d) Patient positioning:
      - Place the patient in a supine position with the affected leg extended or in minimal external rotation, maintaining the ankle in a neutral position or in slight plantar flexion. Palpate the skin entry site, identifying the anterior tibial/dorsalis pedis artery [8]. Identify a spot to be injected between the anterior tibial tendon and the medial malleolus [9].
   (e) Identification and marking of injection site:
      - Mark the target using a marker or by depressing the skin with a plastic needle cap.
   (f) Skin preparation: Initial: Betadine® preparation using the no-touch technique
   (g) Medication preparation:
      - Diagnostic injection:
         - 5 ml 1% preservative-free lidocaine

- Therapeutic injection:
  - 40 mg Depo-Medrol® and 0.5 mL 1% preservative-free lidocaine
(h) Skin preparation- final: Alcohol prep
(i) Local anesthesia administration:
  - *Anesthetize* the overlying skin and soft tissue using a *small amount of 1% lidocaine* delivered via a *30-gauge-1-in. needle.*
(j) Needle placement:
  - *Pierce* the previously anesthetized skin and subcutaneous tissue site with the appropriate needle and direct "slightly cephalad angle to pass under the anterior lip of the tibia." [8]
(k) Aspiration: Rule out intravascular entry and confirm entry into bursa (if enough bursal fluid is present to allow aspiration).
(l) Contrast injection:
  - If fluoroscopic guidance: Inject the knee joint with *several cc of Omnipaque™ using a 5-cc syringe* connected to the straight needle via extension tubing. Adjust needle position, if necessary, in order to clearly define an arthrogram.
(m) Injection: Unclamp the aspiration syringe and clamp on the injection syringe.
  - If resistance is encountered early during the injection, rotate the needle to dislodge the bevel from the side of the joint.
(n) Postprocedural testing:
  - If applicable, reassess response to the aforementioned preprocedural provocative maneuver.
(o) If (+) response, repeat injection with therapeutic injectate:
  - Repeat steps (d)–(f).
  - Medication preparation: 40 mg Depo-Medrol®
  - Repeat steps (h)–(m).
(p) *Adhesive bandage* application over the needle entry site
(q) Postprocedural care discussion

References

1. Salk R, Chang T, D'Costa W, Soomekh, DJ, Grogan KA. Sodium hyaluronate in the treatment of osteoarthritis of the ankle: a controlled, randomized, double-blind pilot study. J Bone Joint Surg 2006;88-A(2):295–302.
2. Sun SF, Chou YJ, Hsu CW, Hwang C-W, Hsu P-T, Wang JL et al. Efficacy of intra-articular hyaluronic acid in patient with osteoarthritis of the ankle: a prospective study. Osteoarthritis Cartilage 2006;14:867–74.
3. Khoury NJ, El-Khoury GY, Saltzman C, Brandser E. Intraarticular foot and ankle injections to identify source of pain before arthrodesis. AJR Am J Roentgenol 1996;167:669–73.
4. Lucas PE, Hurwitz SR, Kaplan PA, Dussault RG, Maurer EJ. Fluoroscopically guided injections into the foot and ankle: Localization of the source of pain as a guide to treatment – prospective study. Radiology 1997;204:411–5.

5. Sofka CM, Adler RS. Ultrasound-guided interventions in the foot and ankle. Semin Musculoskelet Radiol 2002;6(2):163–8.
6. Remedios D, Martin K, Kaplan G, Mitchell R, Woo P, Rooney M. Juvenile chronic arthritis: diagnosis and management of tiobio-talar and sub-talar disease. Br J Rheumatol 1997; 36:1214–7.
7. D'Agostino MA, Ayral X, Baron G, Ravoud P, Breban M, Dougados M. Impact of ultrasound imaging on local corticosteroid injections of symptomatic ankle, hind-, and mid-foot in chronic inflammatory diseases. Arthritis Rheum 2005;53(2):284–92.
8. Newman J. Diagnostic and therapeutic injections of the foot and ankle. Semin Roentgenol 2004;39(1):85–94.
9. Trnka HJ, Ivanic G, Trattnig S. Arthrography of the foot and ankle. Foot Ankle Clin 2000; 5(1):49–62.

Injection Procedure: Metatarsophalangeal Joint Injection

1. Indications:
    (a) Gout
    (b) Osteoarthritis
    (c) Psoriatic arthritis
    (d) Rheumatoid arthritis
    (e) Traumatic injury
    (f) Turf toe (injury to capsuloligamentous structure of the first metatarsopha-
        langeal joint most commonly caused by hyperextension of the first metatar-
        sophalangeal joint, associated with artificial playing surfaces)

2. Contraindications especially pertinent to this procedure:
    (a) None documented

3. Possible side effects especially pertinent to this procedure:
    (a) Cutaneous foot depigmentation [1]
    (b) Metatarsophalangeal joint dislocation [2]

4. Technical details of note for this procedure (Fig. 12.4):
    (a) Preferred needle gauge; length; type:
        • Aspiration ±/- injection: 25 gauge, short
    (b) Need for image guidance: Optional
        • An extensive review of the literature revealed that there are no docu-
          mented studies evaluating the need for image guidance for injection of
          any of the metatarsophalangeal joints. However, according to Boxer,
          accurate needle placement "proximal to the joint in the intermetatarsal
          space" is imperative in order to obtain the desired therapeutic effect [3].
          Due to the variable size and shape of the metatarsophalangeal joints, it is
          difficult to palpate the joints adequately to perform the injections blindly.
          This becomes particularly true in patients with advanced degenerative
          arthritis [4]. For this reason, the authors recommend considering the use
          of image guidance when injecting the metatarsophalangeal joints. Either
          fluoroscopy or ultrasound can be used for image guidance.

5. Step-by-step procedure:
    (a) Informed consent.
    (b) Preprocedural testing:
        • Identify and record the response to a physical examination preprocedural
          provocative maneuver if the procedure is a diagnostic injection.
    (c) Image guidance: Recommended
    (d) Patient positioning:
        • Place the patient in a supine position with the knee of the affected foot
          in a flexed position with a pillow under the knee. Keep the foot firmly
          supported on the procedure table. Palpate the proposed entry site, and
          passively flex and extend the affected toe to locate the joint line [4].

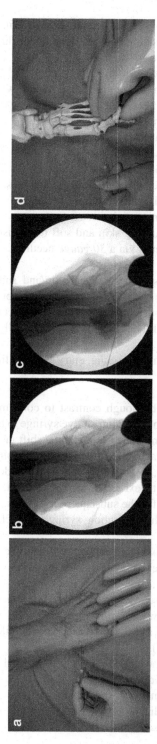

Fig. 12.4 Metatarsophalangeal (MTP) joint injection (fluoroscopic-guided). (**a**) MTP joint injection–human model. (**b**) Fluoroscopic image of needle entry into MTP joint. (**c**) Fluoroscopic image of MTP joint arthrogram. (**d**) Skeletal representation of MTP joint injection

- Have an assistant apply axial traction to the toe in order to help open up the joint. If the procedure is being done under fluoroscopic guidance, a lead glove can be worn.
(e) Identification and marking of injection site:
  - Mark the spot with a plastic needle cap with or without image guidance.
(f) Skin preparation: Initial: Betadine® preparation using the no-touch technique
(g) Medication preparation:
  - Diagnostic injection:
    - 1 mL of 2% preservative-free lidocaine
  - Therapeutic injection:
    - 20 mg Depo-Medrol® and 0.5 mL of 1% preservative-free lidocaine
(h) Skin preparation: Final: Alcohol prep
(i) Local anesthesia administration:
  - Anesthetize the overlying skin and soft tissue using a *small amount of 1% lidocaine* delivered via a *30 gauge* needle.
(j) Needle placement:
  - Pierce the previously anesthetized skin/and subcutaneous tissue site with the appropriate needle while continuing to provide distal traction to the toe, in order to open up the joint space. Direct the needle at a 60–70° angle to the plane of the foot and "pointed distally to match the slope of the joint"[4].
(k) Aspiration: Rule out intravascular entry and confirmation of entry into target structure
(l) Contrast injection:
  - Inject the joint with enough contrast to confirm entry into the target structure. Connecting the contrast dye syringe to the needle using extension tubing is recommended to prevent a shift in needle position during attachment and detachment to and from the spinal needle. Adjust the needle, if necessary, in order to obtain a clearly defined arthrogram. It is not recommended to exceed 1 mL of contrast, as this will limit the capacity necessary for the subsequent injections.
(m) Injection: Unclamp the aspiration syringe and clamp on the injection syringe.
  - If resistance is encountered early during the injection, rotate the needle to dislodge the bevel from the side of the joint.
(n) Postprocedural testing:
  - If applicable, reassess response to the aforementioned preprocedural provocative maneuver.
(o) If (+) response, repeat injection with therapeutic injectate:
  - Repeat steps (d)–(f).
  - Medication preparation: 20 mg Depo-Medrol® and 0.5 mL of 1% preservative-free lidocaine
  - Repeat steps (h)–(m).
(p) *Adhesive bandage* application over the needle entry site
(q) Postprocedural care discussion

References

1. Lemont H, Hetman J. Cutaneous foot depigmentation following intra-articular steroid injection. J Am Podiatr Med Assoc 1991;81(11):606–7.
2. Reis ND, Karkabi S, Zinman C. Metatarsophalangeal joint dislocation after local steroid injection. J Bone Joint Surg Br 1989;71-B:864.
3. Boxer M. Osteoarthritis involving the metatarsophalangeal joints and management of the metatarsophalangeal joint pain via injection therapy. Clin Podiatr Med Surg 1994;11(1):125–132.
4. Tallia A, Cardone D. Diagnostic and therapeutic injection of the ankle and foot. Am Fam Physician 2003;68(7):1356–1362.

Injection Procedure: Plantar Fascia Injection

1. Indications:
   (a) Differentiation of plantar fasciitis from other causes of heel pain of unclear etiology, especially including lumbar radiculopathy and tarsal tunnel syndrome involving the calcaneal branch of the tibial nerve
   (b) Plantar fasciitis treatment

2. Contraindications especially pertinent to this procedure:
   (a) None documented

3. Possible side effects especially pertinent to this procedure:
   (a) Biomechanical dysfunction of the foot including acquired hammertoe deformity [1]
   (b) Infection in diabetes patients
   (c) Lateral plantar nerve dysfunction [1]
   (d) Osteomyelitis [2]
   (e) Plantar fascia rupture [1]
   (f) Plantar fat pad atrophy

4. Technical details of note for this procedure (Fig. 12.5):
   (a) Preferred needle gauge; length; type:
      • If nonimage-guided: 25 gauge; short; straight
      • If image-guided: 25 gauge; short; spinal
   (b) Need for ultrasound guidance: Recommended
      • The use of ultrasound guidance is highly recommended for plantar fascia corticosteroid injections. Palpation-guided injections are estimated to have a 35% success rate presumably due to inaccurate injections with nonimage-guided injections [3]. It is often necessary to perform repeated procedures to attain the desired benefit. Due to the potential need for repeated injections, the patient can be put at increased risk of side effects such as fat pad atrophy and plantar fascia rupture. One study had documented that 10% of patients receiving steroid injections subsequently ruptured their plantar fascia at an average time of 10 weeks following corticosteroid injection [4]. These data reinforce the significance of accurately injecting the area during the first attempt, thus potentially avoiding subsequent injections as the efficacy of image-guided injections appears to be greater than that of nonimage guided injections.
      • A study by Tsai and colleagues compared the efficacy of injections using palpation versus ultrasound-guided injections. They determined that, while the pathologically thickened plantar fascia became thinner following corticosteroid injections with both methods, it regained its pathological thickness 1 year following injection using palpation, while remaining thin after the use of ultrasound guidance. They also noted that the recurrence rate of plantar fasciitis was much lower in the

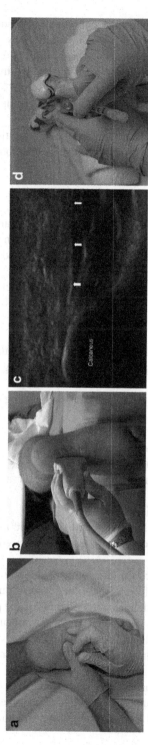

Fig. 12.5 Ankle plantar fascia injection (ultrasound-guided). (**a**) Ankle plantar fascia injection-human model. (**b**) Ultrasound transducer positioning for visualizing plantar fascia- human model. (**c**) Ultrasonogram corresponding to previous image. (**d**) Skeletal representation of ankle plantar fascia injection

ultrasound-guided group than the palpation-guided group (ultrasound: 1/12; palpation: 6/13). In the same study, they determined there was similar pain relief between the two groups at 2 weeks and 2 months postinjection. However, at 1-year follow-up, there was a significant decrease in visual analog-measured pain in the sonographically guided group compared with the palpation-guided group (palpation: 2.5 ± 2.6; ultrasound: 0.3 ± 0.98) [3].

- Kane and coworkers determined the mean duration of pain relief to be approximately 24 months with the use of ultrasound guidance [5].

5. Step-by-step procedure:
   (a) Informed consent
   (b) Preprocedural testing:
       - Identify and record the response to a physical examination preprocedural provocative maneuver if the procedure is a diagnostic injection.
   (c) Image guidance: Recommended: Ultrasound-guided
   (d) Patient positioning:
       - Place the patient in a prone position with the feet hanging over the edge of the examination table [3].
   (e) Identification and marking of injection site:
       - If ultrasound-guided:
         – Use the ultrasound transducer to image the underlying target structure.
       - Mark the target using a marker or by depressing the skin with a plastic needle cap
   (f) Skin preparation: Initial: Betadine® preparation using the no-touch technique.
   (g) Medication preparation:
       - Diagnostic injection:
         – 1 mL 2% preservative-free lidocaine
       - Therapeutic injection:
         – 40 mg Depo-Medrol® and 1 mL 1% preservative-free lidocaine
   (h) Skin preparation: Final: Alcohol prep pad wipe
   (i) Local anesthesia administration:
       - Anesthetize the overlying skin and soft tissue using a *small amount of 1% lidocaine* delivered via a *30-gauge-1-in. needle.*
   (j) Needle placement:
       - If ultrasound-guided: Use ultrasound to directly visualize needle placement into the plantar fascia. Real-time scanning during active dorsiflexion of the toes can help delineate the margins of the plantar fascia [3].
       - Pierce the previously anesthetized skin and subcutaneous tissue site with the appropriate needle and direct to the target.
   (k) Aspiration: Rule out intravascular entry and confirm entry into target structure.
   (l) Injection: Unclamp the aspiration syringe and clamp on the injection syringe.
       - If resistance is encountered early during the injection, rotate the needle to dislodge the bevel from the side of the structure.

(m) Postprocedural testing:
  • If applicable, reassess the response to the same aforementioned preprocedural provocative maneuver.
(n) If (+) response, repeat injection with therapeutic injectate:
  • Repeat steps (d)–(f)
  • Medication preparation: 40 mg Depo-Medrol®
  • Repeat steps (h)–(m)
(o) *Adhesive bandage* application over the needle entry site
(p) Postprocedural care discussion
  • Gentle stretching of the plantar fascia using exercise with or without the use of nighttime plantar fascia splints could be helpful. It is probably important to avoid excessive physical activity, as this potentially could place an accelerated stretch on the plantar fascia and perhaps lead to postprocedure pain exacerbation and/or plantar fascia rupture.

References

1. Acevedo J, Beskin J. Complications of plantar fascia rupture associated with corticosteroid injection. Foot Ankle Int 1998;19(2):91–7.
2. Ogden J, Alvarez R, Cross GL, Jaakkola JL. Plantar fasciopathy and orthotripsy: The effect of prior cortisone injection. Foot Ankle Int 2005;26(3):231–3.
3. Tsai WC, Hsu CC, Chen CP, Chen MJL, Yu T-Y, Chen Y-J. Plantar fasciitis treated with local steroid injection: Comparison between sonographic and palpation guidance. J Clin Ultrasound 2006;34(1):12–6.
4. Tsai WC, Wang CL, Tang FT, Tsu T-C, Hsu K-H, Wong M-K. Treatment of proximal plantar fasciitis with ultrasound-guided steroid injection. Arch Phys Med Rehabil 2000;81:1416–21.
5. Kane D, Greaney T, Bresnihan B, Gibney R, FitzGerald O. Ultrasound guided injection of recalcitrant plantar fasciitis. Ann Rheum Dis 1998;57:383–4.

Injection Procedure: Subtalar Joint Injection

1 *Indications*:
   (a) Differentiation of osteoarthritis from lower extremity neuropathy, confirming etiology of pain for site of os trigonum syndrome [1]
   (b) Chronic hindfoot pain and Juvenile idiopathic arthritis treatment
   (c) Diagnosis of foot pain to subtalar joint, rheumatoid arthritis, subtalar osteoarthritis, traumatic injury as pain generator [1]

2 Contraindications especially pertinent to this procedure:
   (a) None documented

3 Possible side effects especially pertinent to this procedure:
   (a) Anesthesia of medial/lateral plantar nerves [2]

4 Technical details of note for this procedure (Fig. 12.6):
   (a) Preferred needle gauge; length; type:
      • If nonimage-guided: 25 gauge; short; straight
      • If image-guided: 25 gauge; short; spinal
   (b) Need for image guidance: Recommended
      • The use of image guidance is a highly recommended practice when injecting the foot and ankle regions, as the area is extremely compact with intricate articulations. The use of image guidance allows the physician to confirm the appropriate placement of the needle into the intra-articular space [3]. In contrast, when performed with the use of anatomic landmarks as a guide, these procedures can often miss their intended target [4]. Accuracy becomes particularly imperative when attempting to differentiate among pain generators within the foot and ankle regions. The use of standard radiography without conducting diagnostic injections is not necessarily helpful in determining the primary pain generator. Structures that appear normal on radiographic findings can often be the primary source of pain, while joints appearing pathologic may not be the culprit [1]. Documenting the exact position of the needle within the desired joint allows the physician to determine if the suspected structure is the primary pain generator based on the response to local anesthetic.
      • The use of image guidance decreases the risk of damaging the neurovascular bundle during the procedure [2]. Imaging can also allow the physician to determine any communications that may exist between the joints in the foot. This provides information regarding the dispersal of the injectant, offering more accurate assessment of the pain generator in a diagnostic injection. In a number of cases, it has been determined that there is a communication between the subtalar and tibiotalar joints. In such a situation, the accuracy of localizing the subtalar joint as a pain generator with a diagnostic injection is markedly decreased.

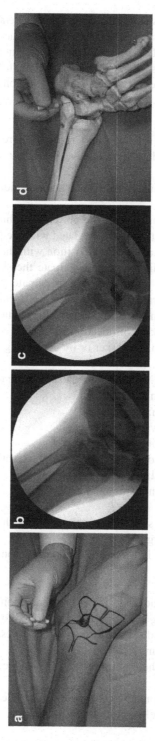

Fig. 12.6 Ankle subtalar joint injection (fluoroscopic-guided). (**a**) Ankle subtalar joint injection–human model. (**b**) Fluoroscopic image of needle entry into ankle subtalar joint. (**c**) Fluoroscopic image of ankle subtalar joint arthrogram. (**d**) Skeletal representation of ankle subtalar joint injection

(c) A study comparing posteromedial versus anterolateral approaches revealed that the latter was more specific for successful subtalar joint injection (38% vs. 84%, respectively) [2]. This approach did not result in cases of filling of additional structures (such as tendons) or in cases of digital anesthesia. Therefore, the recommended approach for subtalar joint injection is anterolateral.

5 Step-by-step procedure:
   (a) Informed consent
   (b) Preprocedural testing: Identify and record the response to a physical examination preprocedural provocative maneuver if the procedure is a diagnostic injection.
   (c) Image guidance: Recommended: Fluoroscopic-guided
   (d) Patient positioning:
       • The anterolateral approach is the preferred technique due to the fewer side effects and relative ease associated with the procedure.
       • Place the patient in a decubitus position with the affected side up with the knee and hip slightly flexed. Palpate the skin entry site over the anterior end of the joint. If unable to palpate the anterior end of the joint, palpate the crucial angle of Gissane, formed by the junction of the calcaneus and the anterior angle of the subtalar joint [2].
   (e) Identification and marking of injection site:
       • Mark the target using a marker or by depressing the skin with a plastic needle cap.
   (f) Skin preparation: Initial: Betadine® preparation using the no-touch technique
   (g) Medication preparation:
       • Diagnostic injection:
         – 2 mL 1% preservative-free lidocaine
       • Therapeutic injection:
         – 80 mg Depo-Medrol® and 2 mL 1% preservative-free lidocaine
   (h) Skin preparation: Final: Alcohol prep pad wipe
   (i) Local anesthesia administration: Not applicable
   (j) Needle placement:
       • Pierce the skin and subcutaneous tissue site with the appropriate needle and direct to the target.
   (k) Aspiration: Rule out intravascular entry and confirm entry into target structure.
   (l) Contrast injection:
       • If fluoroscopic guidance: Inject the knee joint with *several cc of Omnipaque™ using a 5-cc syringe* connected to the straight needle via extension tubing. Adjust needle position, if necessary, in order to clearly define an arthrogram.
   (m) Injection: Unclamp the aspiration syringe and clamp on the injection syringe.
       • If resistance is encountered early during the injection, rotate the needle to dislodge the bevel from the side of the joint.

(n) Postprocedural testing
  • If applicable, reassess response to the aforementioned preprocedural provocative maneuver.
(o) If (+) response, repeat injection with therapeutic injectate:
  • Repeat steps (d)–(f)
  • Medication preparation for therapeutic injection: 80 mg Depo-Medrol®
  • Repeat steps (h)–(m)
(p) Adhesive *bandage* application over the needle entry site
(q) Postprocedural care discussion:
  • Emphasis on the following considerations that are especially pertinent to this procedure: As mentioned previously, the anterolateral approach is the preferred technique due to the fewer side effects and relative ease associated with the procedure.

References

1. Khoury NJ, El-Khoury GY, Saltzman C, Brandser E. Intraarticular foot and ankle injections to identify source of pain before arthrodesis. AJR Am J Roentgenol 1996;167:669–73.
2. Ruhoy M, Newberg A, Yodlowski M, Mizel M, Trepman E. Subtalar joint arthrography. Semin Musculoskelet Radiol 1998;2(4):433–7.
3. Lucas PE, Hurwitz SR, Kaplan PA, Dussault RG, Maurer EJ. Fluoroscopically guided injections into the foot and ankle: Localization of the source of pain as a guide to treatment – prospective study. Radiology 1997;204:411–5.
4. Sofka CM, Adler RS. Ultrasound-guided interventions in the foot and ankle. Semin Musculoskelet Radiol 2002;6(2):163–8.

Injection Procedure Templates

Injection Procedure Template: Retrocalcaneal Bursa (Achilles Bursa) Injection

---

PROCEDURE: Retrocalcaneal Bursa (Achilles Bursa) Injection
Side: ☐-Right   ☐-Left   ☐-Bilateral
Procedure Type: Aspiration: ☐-Diagnostic aspiration
           Injection: ☐-Diagnostic   ☐-Therapeutic   ☐-Diagnostic then Therapeutic
Image guidance: None unless indicated as follows- ☐-Fluoroscopy ☐-Ultrasound
- The potential benefits and side effects of the procedure and alternative treatment options were explained to the patient, an opportunity for questions was provided, and the patient signed informed consent.
- ☐- If checked, the following physical examination pre-procedural provocative maneuver(s) was (were) performed: ☐-
  _____
- The patient was positioned for the procedure and the target structure was identified.
- The overlying skin was prepped with Betadine® followed by alcohol prep pad after the Betadine® dried.
- ☐- If checked, the overlying skin and soft tissue was anesthetized using a small amount of 1% lidocaine delivered via the following needle ☐-30G1"; ☐-25G1½ "; ☐-Other: _____
- The following needle was then used for the procedure:
      Type: Straight needle unless indicated as follows: ☐-Spinal needle; ☐-Other:_____
      Gauge: ☐-30; ☐-27; ☐-25; ☐-22; ☐-21; -18; Other:_____
      Length: ☐-5/8"; ☐- 1"; ☐- 1 ½"; ☐- 2"; ☐- 2 ½"; ☐- 3";☐- 3½"; ☐-Other:_____
- ○ Image guidance if indicated above was used to confirm needle entry into target structure.
- ○ ☐-If checked, contrast dye was then injected and the needle position was adjusted accordingly to confirm proper placement without inadvertent intravascular entry.
- Needle was adjusted accordingly to confirm proper placement without inadvertent vascular entry.
- An attempt was made to aspirate from the structure and then the following injectate was delivered into the target structure:
      ☐-Diagnostic injection: 1 mL 1% preservative-free lidocaine; ☐-Other injectate: _____
      ☐-Therapeutic injection: 40 mg Depo-Medrol® & ☐- 1 mL 1% preservative-free lidocaine
           ☐-Other injectate: _____
- The needle was removed and an adhesive bandage was placed over the needle entry site.

-If the above was a **diagnostic injection**, then proceed to section immediately below.
-If above was a **therapeutic injection procedure, aspiration only procedure,** or **aspiration and therapeutic injection,** then proceed to Procedure Summary Section.

For Diagnostic Injection Procedure:
- ☐-If checked, the above listed pre-procedural physical examination provocative maneuver was repeated and pain relief was: ☐-N/A; ☐-significant; ☐-some; ☐-equivocal; ☐-none; ☐-Other:_____
- Based on the amount of pain relief noted above:
      ☐-a therapeutic injection will be scheduled.
      ☐-a therapeutic injection will not be scheduled. See plan in corresponding office note.
      ☐-a therapeutic injection following the same procedure described above was done using
           ☐- 40 mg Depo-Medrol® & ☐- 1 mL 1% preservative-free lidocaine
           ☐- Other injectate: _____
- The needle was removed and an adhesive bandage was placed over the needle entry site.

Procedure Summary:
If fluid aspirated from the target structure during the procedure:
- Total volume of fluid aspirated: ____ mL; Fluid appearance: ☐- N/A; ☐-Clear yellow; ☐-Slightly cloudy;
      ☐-Cloudy; ☐-Purulent; ☐-Blood-tinged; ☐-Bloody; ☐-Other:_____
Patient tolerance for the procedure: ☐-Excellent; ☐-Good; ☐-Fair; ☐-Other:_____

Additional comments regarding the procedure: ☐-None; ☐-Other:_____
_____

Post-Procedural Treatment Advice:
Activity modification: Avoid non-essential use of the structure until seen for follow up. ☐-Other:_____

Orthotic instructions: N/A unless indicated as follows _____
Modalities: Apply ice over the injection site prn for 20-30 min. up to q2 hrs until seen for follow-up, unless instructed as follows:
☐-Heat; ☐-Other:_____

Injection Procedure Template: Achilles Tendon Peritendinous Injection

---

PROCEDURE: Achilles Tendon Peritendinous Injection
Side: ☐-Right   ☐-Left   ☐-Bilateral
Procedure Type: Aspiration: ☐-Diagnostic aspiration
      Injection: ☐-Diagnostic   ☐-Therapeutic   ☐-Diagnostic <u>then</u> Therapeutic
Image guidance: None unless indicated as follows- ☐-Fluoroscopy ☐-Ultrasound

- The potential benefits and side effects of the procedure and alternative treatment options were explained to the patient, an opportunity for questions was provided, and <u>the patient signed informed consent</u>.
- ☐ - If checked, the following physical examination <u>pre-procedural provocative maneuver(s)</u> was (were) performed: ☐-
_____
- The patient was positioned for the procedure and the target structure was identified.
- The overlying skin was prepped with <u>Betadine® followed by alcohol prep pad</u> after the Betadine® dried.
- ☐ - If checked, the overlying skin and soft tissue was anesthetized using a <u>small amount of 1% lidocaine</u> delivered via the following needle ☐-30G1"; ☐-25G1½ "; ☐-Other: _____
- The following needle was then used for the procedure:
  - <u>Type</u>: Straight needle unless indicated as follows: ☐-Spinal needle; ☐-Other:_____
  - <u>Gauge</u>: ☐-30; ☐-27; ☐-25; ☐-22; ☐-21; -18; Other:_____
  - <u>Length</u>: ☐-5/8"; ☐- 1"; ☐- 1 ½"; ☐- 2"; ☐- 2 ½"; ☐- 3";☐- 3½"; ☐-Other:_____
- ○ Image guidance if indicated above was used to confirm needle entry into target structure.
- ○ ☐-If checked, contrast dye was then injected and the needle position was adjusted accordingly to confirm proper placement without inadvertent intravascular entry.
- Needle was adjusted accordingly to confirm proper placement without inadvertent vascular entry.
- An attempt was made to aspirate from the structure and then the following injectate was delivered into the target structure:
  - ☐-Diagnostic injection: <mark>3 mL 1% preservative-free lidocaine</mark> ☐-Other injectate: _____
  - ☐-Therapeutic injection: <mark>20 mg Depo-Medrol®</mark> & ☐- <mark>2 mL 1% preservative-free lidocaine</mark>
  - ☐-Other injectate: _____
- The needle was removed and an <u>adhesive bandage</u> was placed over the needle entry site.

-If the above was a <u>diagnostic injection</u>, then proceed to section immediately below.
-If above was a <u>therapeutic injection procedure, aspiration only procedure,</u> or <u>aspiration and therapeutic injection,</u> then proceed to Procedure Summary Section.

For Diagnostic Injection Procedure:
- ☐-If checked, the above listed pre-procedural physical examination provocative maneuver was repeated and pain relief was: ☐-N/A; ☐-significant; ☐-some; ☐-equivocal; ☐-none; ☐-Other:_____
- Based on the amount of pain relief noted above:
  - ☐-a therapeutic injection will be scheduled.
  - ☐-a therapeutic injection will <u>not</u> be scheduled. See plan in corresponding office note.
  - ☐-a therapeutic injection following the same procedure described above was done using
    ☐- <mark>20 mg Depo-Medrol®</mark> & ☐- <mark>2 mL 1% preservative-free lidocaine</mark>
    ☐- Other injectate: _____
- The needle was removed and an <u>adhesive bandage</u> was placed over the needle entry site.

Procedure Summary:
If fluid aspirated from the target structure during the procedure:
- Total volume of fluid aspirated: ___ mL; Fluid appearance: ☐- N/A; ☐-Clear yellow; ☐-Slightly cloudy; ☐-Cloudy; ☐-Purulent; ☐-Blood-tinged; ☐-Bloody; ☐-Other:_____
Patient tolerance for the procedure: ☐-Excellent; ☐-Good; ☐-Fair; ☐-Other:_____

Additional comments regarding the procedure: ☐-None; ☐Other:_____
_____

Post-Procedural Treatment Advice:
Activity modification: Avoid non-essential use of the structure until seen for follow up. ☐-Other:_____
_____
Orthotic instructions: N/A unless indicated as follows _____
Modalities: Apply ice over the injection site prn for 20-30 min. up to q2 hrs until seen for follow-up, unless instructed as follows: ☐-Heat; ☐-Other:_____

Injection Procedure Template: Metatarsophalangeal Joint Injection

PROCEDURE: Metatarsophalangeal Joint Injection

Side: ☐-Right   ☐-Left   ☐-Bilateral
Procedure Type: Aspiration: ☐-Diagnostic aspiration
        Injection: ☐-Diagnostic   ☐-Therapeutic   ☐-Diagnostic then Therapeutic
Image guidance: None unless indicated as follows- ☐-Fluoroscopy ☐-Ultrasound

- The potential benefits and side effects of the procedure and alternative treatment options were explained to the patient, an opportunity for questions was provided, and the patient signed informed consent.
- ☐- If checked, the following physical examination pre-procedural provocative maneuver(s) was (were) performed: ☐-
_____
- The patient was positioned for the procedure and the target structure was identified.
- The overlying skin was prepped with Betadine® followed by alcohol prep pad after the Betadine® dried.
- ☐ If checked, the overlying skin and soft tissue was anesthetized using a small amount of 1% lidocaine delivered via the following needle ☐-30G1"; ☐-25G1½"; ☐-Other: _____
- The following needle was then used for the procedure:
  Type: Straight needle unless indicated as follows: ☐-Spinal needle; ☐-Other:_____
  Gauge: ☐-30; ☐-27; ☐-25; ☐-22; ☐-21; -18; Other: _____
  Length: ☐-5/8"; ☐- 1"; ☐- 1 ½"; ☐- 2"; ☐- 2 ½"; ☐- 3";☐- 3½"; ☐-Other:_____
- ○ Image guidance if indicated above was used to confirm needle entry into target structure.
- ○ ☐-If checked, contrast dye was then injected and the needle position was adjusted accordingly to confirm proper placement without inadvertent intravascular entry.
- Needle was adjusted accordingly to confirm proper placement without inadvertent vascular entry.
- An attempt was made to aspirate from the structure and then the following injectate was delivered into the target structure:
  ☐-Diagnostic injection: 1 mL 2% preservative-free lidocaine; ☐-Other injectate: _____
  ☐-Therapeutic injection: 20 mg Depo-Medrol® & ☐- 0.5 mL 1% preservative-free lidocaine
      ☐-Other injectate: _____
- The needle was removed and an adhesive bandage was placed over the needle entry site.

-If the above was a **diagnostic injection**, then proceed to section immediately below.
-If above was a **therapeutic injection procedure, aspiration only procedure,** or **aspiration and therapeutic injection,** then proceed to Procedure Summary Section.

For Diagnostic Injection Procedure:
- ☐-If checked, the above listed pre-procedural physical examination provocative maneuver was repeated and pain relief was: ☐-N/A; ☐-significant; ☐-some; ☐-equivocal; ☐-none; ☐-Other:_____
- Based on the amount of pain relief noted above:
  ☐-a therapeutic injection will be scheduled.
  ☐-a therapeutic injection will not be scheduled. See plan in corresponding office note.
  ☐-a therapeutic injection following the same procedure described above was done using
      ☐- 20 mg Depo-Medrol® & ☐- 0.5 mL 1% preservative-free lidocaine
      ☐- Other injectate:_____
- The needle was removed and an adhesive bandage was placed over the needle entry site.

Procedure Summary:
If fluid aspirated from the target structure during the procedure:
- Total volume of fluid aspirated: ___ mL; Fluid appearance: ☐- N/A; ☐-Clear yellow; ☐-Slightly cloudy; ☐-Cloudy; ☐-Purulent; ☐-Blood-tinged; ☐-Bloody; ☐-Other:_____
Patient tolerance for the procedure: ☐-Excellent; ☐-Good; ☐-Fair; ☐-Other:_____

Additional comments regarding the procedure: ☐-None; ☐Other:_____

Post-Procedural Treatment Advice:
Activity modification: Avoid non-essential use of the structure until seen for follow up. ☐-Other:_____

Orthotic instructions: N/A unless indicated as follows _____
Modalities: Apply ice over the injection site prn for 20-30 min. up to q2 hrs until seen for follow-up, unless instructed as follows:
☐-Heat; ☐-Other:_____

Injection Procedure Template: Plantar Fascia Injection

PROCEDURE: Plantar Fascia Injection

Side: ☐-Right   ☐-Left   ☐-Bilateral
Procedure Type: Aspiration: ☐-Diagnostic aspiration
         Injection: ☐-Diagnostic   ☐-Therapeutic   ☐-Diagnostic <u>then</u> Therapeutic
Image guidance: None unless indicated as follows- ☐-Fluoroscopy   ☐-Ultrasound
- The potential benefits and side effects of the procedure and alternative treatment options were explained to the patient, an opportunity for questions was provided, and <u>the patient signed informed consent</u>.
- ☐- If checked, the following physical examination <u>pre-procedural provocative maneuver(s)</u> was (were) performed: ☐-
  _____
- The patient was positioned for the procedure and the target structure was identified.
- The overlying skin was prepped with <u>Betadine® followed by alcohol prep pad</u> after the Betadine® dried.
- ☐- If checked, the overlying skin and soft tissue was anesthetized using a <u>small amount of 1% lidocaine</u> delivered via the following needle ☐-30G1"; ☐-25G1½"; ☐-Other:_____
- The following needle was then used for the procedure:
      <u>Type</u>: Straight needle unless indicated as follows: ☐-Spinal needle; ☐-Other:_____
      <u>Gauge</u>: ☐-30; ☐-27; ☐-25; ☐-22; ☐-21; -18; Other:_____
      <u>Length</u>: ☐-5/8"; ☐- 1"; ☐- 1 ½"; ☐- 2"; ☐- 2 ½"; ☐- 3";☐- 3½"; ☐-Other:_____
- ○ Image guidance if indicated above was used to confirm needle entry into target structure.
- ○ ☐-If checked, contrast dye was then injected and the needle position was adjusted accordingly to confirm proper placement without inadvertent intravascular entry.
- Needle was adjusted accordingly to confirm proper placement without inadvertent vascular entry.
- An attempt was made to aspirate from the structure and then the following injectate was delivered into the target structure:
  ☐-Diagnostic injection: 1 mL 2% preservative-free lidocaine; ☐-Other injectate:_____
  ☐-Therapeutic injection: 40 mg Depo-Medrol® & ☐- 1 mL 1% preservative-free lidocaine
          ☐-Other injectate:_____
- The needle was removed and an <u>adhesive bandage</u> was placed over the needle entry site.

-If the above was a <u>diagnostic injection</u>, then proceed to section immediately below.
-If above was a <u>therapeutic injection procedure</u>, <u>aspiration only procedure</u>, or <u>aspiration and therapeutic injection</u>, then proceed to Procedure Summary Section.

For Diagnostic Injection Procedure:
- ☐-If checked, the above listed pre-procedural physical examination provocative maneuver was repeated and pain relief was: ☐-N/A; ☐-significant; ☐-some; ☐-equivocal; ☐-none; ☐-Other:_____
- Based on the amount of pain relief noted above:
  ☐-a therapeutic injection will be scheduled.
  ☐-a therapeutic injection will <u>not</u> be scheduled. See plan in corresponding office note.
  ☐-a therapeutic injection following the same procedure described above was done using
      ☐- 40 mg Depo-Medrol® & ☐- 1 mL 1% preservative-free lidocaine
      ☐- Other injectate:_____
- The needle was removed and an <u>adhesive bandage</u> was placed over the needle entry site.

Procedure Summary:
If fluid aspirated from the target structure during the procedure:
- Total volume of fluid aspirated: ___ mL; Fluid appearance: ☐- N/A; ☐-Clear yellow; ☐-Slightly cloudy; ☐-Cloudy; ☐-Purulent; ☐-Blood-tinged; ☐-Bloody; ☐-Other:_____
Patient tolerance for the procedure: ☐-Excellent; ☐-Good; ☐-Fair; ☐-Other:_____

Additional comments regarding the procedure: ☐-None; ☐Other:_____
_____

Post-Procedural Treatment Advice:
Activity modification: Avoid non-essential use of the structure until seen for follow up. ☐-Other:_____

Orthotic instructions: N/A unless indicated as follows _____
Modalities: Apply ice over the injection site prn for 20-30 min. up to q2 hrs until seen for follow-up, unless instructed as follows: ☐-Heat; ☐-Other:_____

Injection Procedure Template: Subtalar Joint Injection

PROCEDURE: Subtalar Joint Injection

Side: ☐-Right ☐-Left ☐-Bilateral
Procedure Type: Aspiration: ☐-Diagnostic aspiration
     Injection: ☐-Diagnostic ☐-Therapeutic ☐-Diagnostic then Therapeutic
Image guidance: None unless indicated as follows- ☐-Fluoroscopy ☐-Ultrasound

- The potential benefits and side effects of the procedure and alternative treatment options were explained to the patient, an opportunity for questions was provided, and the patient signed informed consent.
- ☐- If checked, the following physical examination pre-procedural provocative maneuver(s) was (were) performed: ☐-
_____
- The patient was positioned for the procedure and the target structure was identified.
- The overlying skin was prepped with Betadine® followed by alcohol prep pad after the Betadine® dried.
- ☐- If checked, the overlying skin and soft tissue was anesthetized using a small amount of 1% lidocaine delivered via the following needle ☐-30G1"; ☐-25G1½"; ☐-Other: _____
- The following needle was then used for the procedure:
   Type: Straight needle unless indicated as follows: ☐-Spinal needle; ☐-Other: _____
   Gauge: ☐-30; ☐-27; ☐-25; ☐-22; ☐-21; -18; Other: _____
   Length: ☐-5/8"; ☐- 1"; ☐- 1 ½"; ☐- 2"; ☐- 2 ½"; ☐- 3";☐- 3½"; ☐-Other:_____
- o Image guidance if indicated above was used to confirm needle entry into target structure.
- o ☐-If checked, contrast dye was then injected and the needle position was adjusted accordingly to confirm proper placement without inadvertent intravascular entry.
- Needle was adjusted accordingly to confirm proper placement without inadvertent vascular entry.
- An attempt was made to aspirate from the structure and then the following injectate was delivered into the target structure:
   ☐-Diagnostic injection: 2 mL 1% preservative-free lidocaine; ☐-Other injectate: _____
   ☐-Therapeutic injection: 80 mg Depo-Medrol® & ☐- 2 mL 1% preservative-free lidocaine
      ☐-Other injectate: _____
- The needle was removed and an adhesive bandage was placed over the needle entry site.

-If the above was a diagnostic injection, then proceed to section immediately below.
-If above was a therapeutic injection procedure, aspiration only procedure, or aspiration and therapeutic injection, then proceed to Procedure Summary Section.

For Diagnostic Injection Procedure:
- ☐-If checked, the above listed pre-procedural physical examination provocative maneuver was repeated and pain relief was: ☐-N/A; ☐-significant; ☐-some; ☐-equivocal; ☐-none; ☐-Other:_____
- Based on the amount of pain relief noted above:
   ☐-a therapeutic injection will be scheduled.
   ☐-a therapeutic injection will not be scheduled. See plan in corresponding office note.
   ☐-a therapeutic injection following the same procedure described above was done using
     ☐- 80 mg Depo-Medrol® & ☐- 2 mL 1% preservative-free lidocaine
     ☐- Other injectate:_____
- The needle was removed and an adhesive bandage was placed over the needle entry site.

Procedure Summary:
If fluid aspirated from the target structure during the procedure:
- Total volume of fluid aspirated: ___ mL; Fluid appearance: ☐- N/A; ☐-Clear yellow; ☐-Slightly cloudy; ☐-Cloudy; ☐-Purulent; ☐-Blood-tinged; ☐-Bloody; ☐-Other:_____
Patient tolerance for the procedure: ☐-Excellent; ☐-Good; ☐-Fair; ☐-Other:_____

Additional comments regarding the procedure: ☐-None; ☐Other:_____
_____

Post-Procedural Treatment Advice:
Activity modification: Avoid non-essential use of the structure until seen for follow up. ☐-Other:_____
_____

Orthotic instructions: N/A unless indicated as follows _____
Modalities: Apply ice over the injection site prn for 20-30 min. up to q2 hrs until seen for follow-up, unless instructed as follows:
☐-Heat; ☐-Other:_____

Index